1992
YEAR BOOK OF
INFERTILITY

The 1992 Year Book® Series

Year Book of Anesthesia and Pain Management: Drs. Miller, Abram, Kirby, Ostheimer, Roizen, and Stoelting

Year Book of Cardiology®: Drs. Schlant, Collins, Engle, Frye, Kaplan, and O'Rourke

Year Book of Critical Care Medicine®: Drs. Rogers and Parrillo

Year Book of Dentistry®: Drs. Meskin, Currier, Kennedy, Leinfelder, Matukas, and Rovin

Year Book of Dermatologic Surgery: Drs. Swanson, Salasche, and Glogau

Year Book of Dermatology®: Drs. Sober and Fitzpatrick

Year Book of Diagnostic Radiology®: Drs. Federle, Clark, Gross, Madewell, Maynard, Sackett, and Young

Year Book of Digestive Diseases®: Drs. Greenberger and Moody

Year Book of Drug Therapy®: Drs. Lasagna and Weintraub

Year Book of Emergency Medicine®: Drs. Wagner, Burdick, Davidson, Roberts, and Spivey

Year Book of Endocrinology®: Drs. Bagdade, Braverman, Horton, Kannan, Landsberg, Molitch, Morley, Odell, Rogol, Ryan, and Sherwin

Year Book of Family Practice®: Drs. Berg, Bowman, Davidson, Dietrich, and Scherger

Year Book of Geriatrics and Gerontology®: Drs. Beck, Abrass, Burton, Cummings, Makinodan, and Small

Year Book of Hand Surgery®: Drs. Amadio and Hentz

Year Book of Health Care Management: Drs. Heyssel, Brock, King, and Steinberg, Ms. Avakian, and Messrs. Berman, Kues, and Rosenberg

Year Book of Hematology®: Drs. Spivak, Bell, Ness, Quesenberry, and Wiernik

Year Book of Infectious Diseases®: Drs. Wolff, Barza, Keusch, Klempner, and Snydman

Year Book of Infertility: Drs. Mishell, Paulsen, and Lobo

Year Book of Medicine®: Drs. Rogers, Bone, Cline, Braunwald, Greenberger, Utiger, Epstein, and Malawista

Year Book of Neonatal and Perinatal Medicine®: Drs. Klaus and Fanaroff

Year Book of Nephrology: Drs. Coe, Favus, Henderson, Kashgarian, Luke, Myers, and Strom

Year Book of Neurology and Neurosurgery®: Drs. Currier and Crowell

Year Book of Neuroradiology: Drs. Osborn, Harnsberger, Halbach, and Grossman

Year Book of Nuclear Medicine®: Drs. Hoffer, Gore, Gottschalk, Sostman, Zaret, and Zubal

Year Book of Obstetrics and Gynecology®: Drs. Mishell, Kirschbaum, and Morrow

Year Book of Occupational and Environmental Medicine: Drs. Emmett, Brooks, Harris, and Schenker

Year Book of Oncology®: Drs. Young, Longo, Ozols, Simone, Steele, and Weichselbaum

Year Book of Ophthalmology®: Drs. Laibson, Adams, Augsburger, Benson, Cohen, Eagle, Flanagan, Nelson, Reinecke, Sergott, and Wilson

Year Book of Orthopedics®: Drs. Sledge, Poss, Cofield, Frymoyer, Griffin, Hansen, Johnson, Simmons, and Springfield

Year Book of Otolaryngology–Head and Neck Surgery®: Drs. Bailey and Paparella

Year Book of Pathology and Clinical Pathology®: Drs. Gardner, Bennett, Cousar, Garvin, and Worsham

Year Book of Pediatrics®: Dr. Stockman

Year Book of Plastic, Reconstructive, and Aesthetic Surgery: Drs. Miller, Cohen, McKinney, Robson, Ruberg, and Whitaker

Year Book of Podiatric Medicine and Surgery®: Dr. Kominsky

Year Book of Psychiatry and Applied Mental Health®: Drs. Talbott, Frances, Freedman, Meltzer, Perry, Schowalter, and Yudofsky

Year Book of Pulmonary Disease®: Drs. Bone and Petty

Year Book of Sports Medicine®: Drs. Shephard, Eichner, Sutton, and Torg, Col. Anderson, and Mr. George

Year Book of Surgery®: Drs. Schwartz, Jonasson, Robson, Shires, Spencer, and Thompson

Year Book of Transplantation: Drs. Ascher, Hansen, and Strom

Year Book of Ultrasound: Drs. Merritt, Mittelstaedt, Carroll, and Nyberg

Year Book of Urology®: Drs. Gillenwater and Howards

Year Book of Vascular Surgery®: Dr. Bergan

Roundsmanship®: '92–'93: A Student's Survival Guide to Clinical Medicine Using Current Literature: Drs. Dan, Feigin, Quilligan, Schrock, Stein, and Talbott

1992

The Year Book of INFERTILITY

Editors

Daniel R. Mishell, Jr., M.D.

Lyle G. McNeile Professor and Chairman, Department of Obstetrics and Gynecology, University of Southern California School of Medicine, Los Angeles

C. Alvin Paulsen, M.D.

Professor of Medicine, University of Washington School of Medicine, NIH Population Center for Research in Reproduction; Chief of Endocrinology, Pacific Medical Center, Seattle

Rogerio A. Lobo, M.D.

Professor of Obstetrics and Gynecology, Department of Obstetrics and Gynecology; Chief, Division of Reproductive Endocrinology and Infertility, University of Southern California School of Medicine, Los Angeles

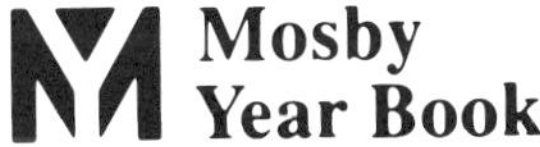

St. Louis Baltimore Boston Chicago London Philadelphia Sydney Toronto

Editor-in-Chief, Year Book Publishing: Kenneth H. Killion
Sponsoring Editor: Katherine Gill
Manager, Literature Services: Edith M. Podrazik
Senior Information Specialist: Terri Santo
Senior Medical Writer: David A. Cramer, M.D.
Assistant Director, Manuscript Services: Frances M. Perveiler
Associate Managing Editor, Year Book Editing Services: Connie Murray
Senior Production/Desktop Publishing Manager: Max F. Perez
Proofroom Manager: Barbara M. Kelly

A Year Book Medical Publishers imprint of Mosby–Year Book, Inc.

Mosby–Year Book, Inc.
11830 Westline Industrial Drive
St. Louis, MO 63146

Printed in the United States of America

Editorial Office:
Mosby–Year Book, Inc.
200 North LaSalle St.
Chicago, IL 60601

International Standard Serial Number: 0896-4475
International Standard Book Number: 0-8151-6023-2

Table of Contents

Journals Represented

Mosby–Year Book subscribes to and surveys nearly 900 U.S. and foreign medical and allied health journals. From these journals, the Editors select the articles to be abstracted. Journals represented in this YEAR BOOK are listed below.

Acta Endocrinologica
Acta Radiologica
American Journal of Industrial Medicine
American Journal of Obstetrics and Gynecology
American Journal of Physiology
Andrologia
Archives of Andrology
Australian and New Zealand Journal of Obstetrics & Gynecology
British Journal of Obstetrics and Gynaecology
British Medical Journal
European Journal of Cancer
European Urology
Fertility and Sterility
Gynecologic and Obstetric Investigation
Gynecological Endocrinology
Human Reproduction
International Journal of Andrology
International Journal of Fertility
Journal of Andrology
Journal of Clinical Endocrinology and Metabolism
Journal of Endocrinology
Journal of Health and Social Behavior
Journal of In Vitro Fertilization and Embryo Transfer
Journal of Reproductive Immunology
Journal of Reproductive Medicine
Journal of Urology
Lancet
New England Journal of Medicine
Obstetrics and Gynecology
Paraplegia
Radiology
Scandinavian Journal of Urology and Nephrology
Urologia Internationalis

STANDARD ABBREVIATIONS

The following terms are abbreviated in this edition: acquired immunodeficiency syndrome (AIDS), central nervous system (CNS), cerebrospinal fluid (CSF), computed tomography (CT), electrocardiography (ECG), human immunodeficiency virus (HIV), and magnetic resonance (MR) imaging (MRI).

Publisher's Preface

As Publishers, we feel challenged to seek ways of presenting complex information in a clear and readable manner. To this end the 1992 YEAR-BOOK OF INFERTILITY now provides structured abstracts in which the various components of a study can easily be identified through headings. These headings are not the same in all abstracts, but rather are those which most accurately designate the content of each particular journal article. We are confident that our readers will find the information contained in our abstracts to be more accessible than ever before. We welcome your comments.

Introduction

In addition to the large number of couples with primary infertility there are an even greater number of couples with secondary infertility. A recent survey from two studies in Great Britain estimated that 13% of couples have difficulty conceiving their first child, and 17% of couples with children have difficulty conceiving an additional time. They report that 25% of all couples have difficulty attempting to conceive during some part of their reproductive life. Many of those couples seek medical attention and request that practitioners provide them with the most recently developed diagnostic and therapeutic procedures to help them achieve pregnancy. It is impossible for busy clinicians to survey the entire medical literature related to infertility. It is also difficult for them to critically analyze the data presented in these scientific articles, as most of the studies are not prospective, not randomized, and not placebo controlled, making interpretation of the data very difficult. The annual volumes of the YEAR BOOK OF INFERTILITY are integrated to provide busy clinicians an opportunity to rapidly survey the entire world's most relevant literature dealing with infertility and to read a critical analysis of the articles by one of the three editors.

Each editor has reviewed the entire scientific literature published in his area and selected the most important relevant articles for abstracting and has then written a descriptive comment. Dr. Paulsen has selected the articles dealing with male infertility, Dr. Lobo has selected the articles relating to reproductive endocrinology, and I have selected the articles concerned with female infertility. In this volume we are also fortunate to have an excellent article summarizing current opinion regarding the puzzling relationship between endometrium and infertility written by a leading expert on the subject, Dr. Arthur Haney.

The editors believe that the information contained in this volume will be of great aid to practitioners when couples who have problems conceiving children seek their assistance. Readers are invited to send suggestions to the publisher for improvement of the material presented in this YEAR BOOK as well as subjects for future reviews.

Daniel R. Mishell, Jr., M.D.

The Correlation of Endometriosis and Infertility

A.F. Haney, M.D.
Professor and Director, Division of Reproductive Endocrinology & Infertility, Department of Obstetrics and Gynecology, Duke University Medical Center, Durham, North Carolina

Introduction

In most infertility centers today, the most frequently made diagnosis in infertile couples is endometriosis, with the majority of women having very modest amounts of disease (1). Before the advent of ambulatory endoscopy, endometriosis was almost always associated with severe pelvic pain, dysmenorrhea, dysparcunia, and nodular masses in the pelvis. This shift to a milder disease spectrum likely represents the fact that virtually all women have a laparoscopy in the course of their evaluation for infertility.

The technical ease with which we now can directly visualize the pelvis has preceded a thorough understanding of the pathophysiology of the infertility associated with endometriosis when there is no mechanical distortion of the pelvic viscera. The assumption was made that the observed gynecologic pathology (i.e., the endometriotic implant) was responsible for the patient's inability to conceive. As a result, a variety of medical and surgical therapies have evolved to treat the infertility, focusing on reducing or eradicating the ectopic endometrial implants. Unfortunately, the vast majority of the reports describing these therapies are anecdotal and do not include the appropriate control groups. Those clinical trials using adequate study designs have failed to confirm the earlier impression of efficacy (2-5). No treatment, sometimes referred to as "expectant management," has the same cycle fecundity as medical and surgical treatments designed to eliminate or reduce implants (Table 1). Based on the available data, it is just as plausible a hypothesis that infertility causes endometriosis as it is that endometriosis causes infertility.

Endometriosis-associated infertility remains one of the most frustrating

TABLE 1.—Cycle Fecundity With Expectant Management in Patients With Mild Endometriosis

Studies	N	Overall % Pregnant	Monthly Fecundity
Garcia, et al. (100)	17	64.7%	.050*
Shenken, et al. (101)	18	72.2%	.102*
Seibel, et al. (2)	28	50.0%	.111*
Portuondo, et al. (102)	31	61.2%	.083
Olive, et al. (103)	34	52.9%	.057
TOTALS	183	50.3%†	.080

*Estimated 6-month interval averages.
†Estimated 12-month interval averages.

clinical problems encountered in gynecologic practice. This unique disease has traditionally been defined by the presence of endometrial glands and stroma outside the uterus, but it undoubtedly represents a complex pathologic process, and a voluminous literature attests to the interest of gynecologists. Until we have better insight into the nature of the disease, it is unlikely that significant progress will be made in improving the outlook for fertility in patients with endometriosis. This article will be directed toward an exploration of the issues regarding the association of infertility and the presence of endometriosis, including pathogenesis, the relationship with infertility, and potential mechanisms by which endometriosis could prevent pregnancy.

Pathogenesis

The pathogenetic mechanisms leading to the presence of ectopic endometriotic implants have stimulated a contentious debate focused on 3 major possibilities including transplantation, celomic metaplasia, and congenital rests of ectopic endometrium. Only the transplantation of endometrial cells, primarily through retrograde menstruation, has any credible scientific supporting evidence (6, 7). The concept of celomic metaplasia evolved at the turn of the century, but there is still no scientifically critical supporting data. Similarly, the congenital rest theory has no embryologic basis because there has been no demonstration of "inactive" ectopic endometrial tissue associated with the peritoneum of the pelvis in an anatomical distribution consistent with that observed in women with endometriosis. As a consequence of these considerations, interest has focused on the regurgitation of viable endometrial cells into the peritoneal cavity, not only for the possibility of implantation, but also because of consequences on the immune system.

In the last half of the luteal phase of nonconceptive ovulatory cycles, the endometrium synthesizes prostaglandins that cause spiral arteriolar vasospasm culminating in autolysis and sloughing of the superficial layer of the endometrium (8). Simultaneously, the prostaglandins induce myometrial contractions that increase the pressure within the uterine cavity, expelling the menstrual effluent through the vagina (9). Although the majority of menstrual blood is most certainly expelled through the cervical canal, a portion is refluxed into the peritoneal cavity through the fallopian tubes. Some degree of retrograde menstruation into the peritoneal cavity apparently occurs during every menses in virtually all women because bloody peritoneal fluid is encountered in a high proportion (>90%) of all cycling women (10, 11). The likely explanation is that the human uterotubal junction has no functional or anatomical valve preventing passage of menstrual debris from the endometrial cavity into the fallopian tube. This lack of resistance to retrograde flow forms the basis for tests of tubal patency such as hysterosalpingography.

The factors leading to retrograde menstruation are only partially understood. The absence of a drainage route from the uterus (i.e., congenital absence of the cervix and/or vagina) is invariably associated with menstrual regurgitation through the fallopian tubes and a high probability of developing endometriosis. More subtle degrees of uterine outflow obstruction are less well-characterized, but the relative pressures and dimensions of the uterotubal junctions and the cervical canal should be the critical features in determining the volume of menstrual regurgitation (12). These are technically difficult measurements and, as a result, we know very little about intratubal and intracervical pressures in vivo.

Viable endometrial cells can be cultured from the follicular phase peritoneal fluid of virtually all cycling women (13). With a prolonged interval of cyclic menses, it is not surprising that some cells may attach to the peritoneal surfaces and form islands of transplanted endometrium, deriving blood supply from the underlying tissue. Similarly, eliciting a localized fibroproliferative reaction if the implant responds to the cycle of gonadal hormones would be expected. In humans, both iatrogenic (14) and experimental (15) endometriosis have been demonstrated, confirming the nature of the process.

The anatomical distribution of endometrial implants is accurately predicted by the simple tenants of transplantation biology. These include gravity, the receptivity of the donor site epithelium (or mesothelium), the mobility of the donor site, and the proximity of the portal of entry of the cells (i.e., the fimbrial ostia). When the uterus is anteflexed, a gravity-dependent pouch is created between the uterus and the bladder (the uterovesicle fold), and endometriosis is common at that site. By contrast, when the uterus is retroflexed, there is no dependent anterior pocket, and endometriosis is rarely encountered on the peritoneum overlying the bladder (1). Similarly, the natural location of the fimbrial ostia is adjacent to the uterosacral ligaments and the ovaries, the most common sites of implantation.

Factors that influence the likelihood of endometriosis are only now being systematically investigated. A prominent early study suggested a racial influence, with a higher frequency noted in white private patients (16). When corrected for different reproductive patterns and contraceptive use, however, these racial influences disappeared (17). These data suggest that the length and total number of menstrual periods likely are the major determinants for developing endometriosis. There is a positive correlation with a long interval of uninterrupted menstrual cycles. Typically, these are nulliparous women delaying childbearing (18, 19). A change in the character or an increase in the amount of the regurgitated menses could similarly be a factor. Although the name endometriosis implies that the primary pathology is the ectopic endometrium, the pathophysiologic process of retrograde menstruation may have its own reproductive consequences, of which implantation of endometrium is just one manifestation.

Are Women With Endometriosis Infertile?

Despite the high incidence of finding endometriosis in infertile couples, the relationship between infertility and endometriosis remains controversial. When significant mechanical distortion of the pelvic viscera is present, there seems little doubt that the infertility is, at least in part, attributable to these anatomic changes. However, in the absence of mechanical distortion of the pelvic viscera, there remains a great deal of controversy about whether women with less significant endometriosis are infertile. Presently, only clinical "intuition" suggests that women with endometriosis complain of infertility more often than women without the disease.

One strategy to examine the relationship of endometriosis and infertility would be to evaluate the prevalence of the disease in fertile and infertile women. Obviously, the true prevalence cannot be determined because it would be unethical to perform laparoscopies on asymptomatic fertile women. The incidence of endometriosis in the female partner of infertile couples undergoing laparoscopy is currently estimated to range from 20%–50%, and the incidence of endometriosis in the general population of women of reproductive age is between 2% and 10% (20). This has led many physicians to conclude that endometriotic implants are responsible for the concurrent infertility. Unfortunately, these data reinforce the notion of an association but cannot support a causal argument.

Another approach to determining whether a causal relationship exists would be to correlate the amount of endometriosis and the clinical outcome of interest, infertility. If a greater amount of disease is inversely correlated with some measure of therapeutic success, then a more reasonable case for causality could be made. Gynecologists have long attempted to stage endometriosis to develop a tool for comparing the effect of various treatments (21, 22). The staging systems have not been based on the presenting symptom of infertility, but rather are based on the premise that endometriosis is analogous to a gynecologic cancer and that the disease will inevitably be progressive and the prognosis will worsen in the presence of more extensive disease. In contrast to cancer, however, where the volume of the disease clearly correlates with survival, the situation with regard to fertility is far more complex. Clinical staging has not been prospectively validated and no data support a relationship between the amount of endometriosis and infertility. Additionally, the staging systems have mixed true peritoneal endometriotic implant volume with pelvic adhesions, intraovarian endometriomas, and extragenital disease. As a consequence, the relevance of the currently available staging systems for endometriosis to the symptom of infertility will remain controversial.

One line of evidence supports an association between endometriosis and infertility. Women preparing to undergo therapeutic donor insemination because of severe male factor were evaluated prospectively by laparoscopy. When endometriosis without mechanical distortion was encountered, no attempt was made to destroy the ectopic implants. Those women without endometriosis subsequently achieved a higher cycle fecundity with therapeutic donor insemination than when endometriosis was present (23). These data more strongly imply an association of endometriosis with a decrease in cycle fecundity but are also insufficient to confirm the often espoused causal link with infertility.

Any consideration of whether women with endometriosis are infertile must take into account the nature of endometriosis-associated infertility.

TABLE 2.—Cycle Fecundity of Various Treatments in Women With Mild Endometriosis

Treatment	N	No. of Pregnancies	% Pregnant	Monthly Fecundity
Conservative Surgery				
Rock, et al. (104)	45	28	62.2%	.022
Olive, et al. (105)	11	5	45.4%	.039
Laser Vaporization				
Olive, et al. (106)	45	18	40.0%	.035
Nezhat, et al. (107)	39	28	71.8%	.067
Danazol				
Seibel, et al. (2)	20	6	30.0%	.059
Buttram, et al. (108)	12	4	33.3%	.048
GnRH-Agonist				
Fedele, et al. (5)	35	17	61.0%	.036

These couples are not sterile, but, rather, have a lower monthly probability of pregnancy and are properly termed subfertile. Additionally, many of these women are in their latter reproductive years and have to contend with the normal age-related decline in cycle fecundity. In view of these issues, any therapeutic trials involving destruction or suppression of the endometrial implants and claiming an improvement in fertility must include untreated controls and must be age-matched for the female partner as well. Unfortunately, these features are missing from the vast majority of the reports. More importantly, when the proper untreated controls are included in a randomized fashion, no therapeutic efficacy has been demonstrated by medically suppressing the endometrial implants (2-5). Although no adequately designed studies have been reported for surgical treatments such as laser vaporization or cauterization, the cycle fecundities reported after surgical destruction/removal or medical suppression do not exceed those of expectant management (Table 2).

What Will Be Required to Demonstrate Causality?

The "rules" regarding causality are well defined for infectious diseases (i.e., Henle-Koch's postulates) (24). By contrast, they remain somewhat nebulous when dealing with noninfectious diseases. Previously, it was widely accepted that the endometrial implants, by virtue of their very presence, were responsible for the failure to conceive without a specific mechanism being sought. Whereas adnexal adhesions may certainly coexist with endometriosis, the majority of infertile women with endometriosis identified today have a relatively small amount of disease without mechanical compromise of the pelvic viscera (1). In the absence of a confirmed mechanism about how the peritoneal implants could alter the reproductive process, endometriosis may simply be a co-migrating factor. A plausible explanation for this situation is that some other, as yet unappreciated, pathologic phenomenon associated with the development of endometriosis may simultaneously have an adverse impact on fertility. Examples might include the retrograde menstruation responsible for the presence of inflammatory cells in the peritoneal cavity (25) or the altered cell-mediated immune response reported in women with endometriosis (26). Until more data suggest that the endometrial implants directly alter reproduction, this issue will remain controversial.

In treating clinical symptoms, it is not unusual to have no definite mechanism at which to direct therapy. Realistically, a substantial number of therapeutic schemes are undertaken that focus on a mechanism of disease, despite the absence of adequate data upon which to base causation. This is precisely the situation that exists currently with endometriosis-associated infertility. There is, however, value in identifying which current therapies have no evidence of efficacy. This will allow couples to make rational decisions regarding ostensibly useful but, in truth, unproven treatments. This is precisely the situation that occurred with the drug danazol. Whereas there is no doubt that danazol shrinks the volume of endometrial implants and reduces pain, there is now ample evidence it has no significant fertility-enhancing effect (2, 3). Furthermore, the couple cannot conceive while ovulation is suppressed with danazol, so, in effect, it allows the natural age-related fertility decline to occur without any opportunity for pregnancy during therapy and no benefit after ovulation returns. Unfortunately, this drug was used to treat infertility associated with endometriosis for many years based solely on anecdotal "experience." As a consequence of this experience, it is important that any therapy that claims efficacy, medical or surgical, be based on adequately designed clinical trials.

There are some guidelines that may be helpful in considering the issue of causality. These features include the consistency, strength, specificity, temporal relationship, and coherence (biologic plausibility) of infertility and endometriosis, the so-called "causal catechism" (27) (Table 3):

Consistency.—As noted earlier, it has been consistently observed that when endometriosis is noted at laparoscopy for infertility, women conceive at the same rate as infertile women without endometriosis. This is expectant management.

Strength.—The association of endometriosis and infertility could not be considered strong based on the rather small sample size available in the literature (28). A rather large experimental or prospective cohort study would be required to detect a difference in the reproductive performance of women with endometriosis from controls because there is a substantial spontaneous conception rate in these women. Furthermore, as noted earlier, there is no proven correlation of infertility with the amount of disease present, so a dose-response relationship has yet to be proven.

Specificity.—Unfortunately, the factors that lower the cycle fecundity below that of the general age-matched population of couples attempting to conceive remain largely unknown.

Many causes of infertility have been identified, independent from endometriosis, and undoubtedly more will become apparent. Other symptoms of endometriosis such as severe dysmenorrhea, dyspareunia, and pelvic pain are also frequently present, indicating infertility is clearly not a specific symptom for endometriosis and vice versa.

TABLE 3.—The Causal Catechism

- The consistency of the association: This refers to any evidence of reproducible results when the proposed association is studied by different methods.
- The strength of the association: This refers to the strength of the quantitative index of association (i.e., a relative risk) or a distinct dose-responsive relationship.
- The specificity of the association: This refers to the uniqueness of a specific association with one proposed causative agent.
- The temporal relationship of associated variables: This requires proof that the proposed causative agent temporally preceded the development of the disease of interest.
- The coherence of the association: This refers to the biologic plausibility that the proposed association would be predicted by established principles of biology.

The temporal relationship of the associated variables.—The precise time when endometriosis is present cannot be known for certain. It is impossible to determine because the symptom of ascertainment and infertility, will, by the nature of medical practice, precede the diagnostic test for the other variable. Because fertile women may also have endometriosis, it cannot be stated with authority whether they will ever become infertile in the evolution of the disease.

The coherence of the association.—Despite the lack of an established mechanism by which endometriosis, in the absence of mechanical distortion, causes infertility, this clearly makes biologic sense. Many potential mechanisms have been proposed, and, regardless of the outcome of the investigations into these individual mechanisms, a causal relationship is definitely plausible and continues to stimulate a great deal of clinical and laboratory interest. From an epidemiologic point of view, endometriosis and infertility tend to occur simultaneously in many women in their reproductive years, and the possibility of a causal relationship makes epidemiologic sense.

Thus, despite insufficient data to conclude that endometriosis causes endometriosis, this possibility is very attractive and will continue to attract clinical investigators. It is unlikely that further insight will be gained from retrospectively evaluating the occurrence of endometriosis and infertility. Given the nature and clinical presentation of infertility, the epidemiologic assessment of the possible role of endometriosis will likely continue to mislead and frustrate the clinician. However, progress in clarifying this relationship may be forthcoming with exploration of mechanisms by which minimal disease lowers cycle fecundity. This question can be approached from another perspective only if a clear mechanism can be established and specific therapeutic interventions evolve.

Potential Mechanisms of Endometriosis-Associated Infertility

A wide variety of mechanisms concerning how endometriosis might lower cycle fecundity have been proposed (Table 4), but none have sufficient data to unequivocally support an adverse impact on reproduction in humans. In evaluating each theoretical possibility, it is important to consider the clinical context in which this diagnosis is made and the nature of the infertility (subfertility) experienced by these couples.

Tubal Dysfunction

It has been proposed that peritoneal fluid prostaglandins produced by ectopic endometrium may have an adverse impact on fertility. This idea was based on the fact that luteal phase endometrium secretes prostaglandins, and elevated levels of prostaglandins have been found in the peritoneal fluid of infertile women with endometriosis (29-35). This has led to the hypothesis that the potent smooth muscle effects of prostaglandins cause tubal dysfunction and alter oocyte or embryo transport.

Not only is there no direct experimental evidence to support this idea, but several facts are at odds with it. First, oocytes and pre-implantation embryos are transported through the distal tube by ciliary action, which is not known to be prostaglandin-dependent. Second, a luteal phase secretory product of endometrium, prolactin, is not elevated in the luteal phase peritoneal fluid of women with endometriosis (36), questioning the secretory capability of ectopic implants of endometrium and the origin of the peritoneal fluid prostaglandins. Furthermore, controversy continues about whether prostaglandins are elevated in women with endometriosis (37-39). Other cells in the peritoneal cavity, such as macrophages, can produce prostaglandins and may represent the source of the peritoneal fluid prostaglandins. Lastly, and most importantly, prostaglandins have not been successful contraceptives, and the intravenous administration of extremely potent prostaglandin analogues does not alter oviductal transport of human oocytes (40).

TABLE 4.—Proposed Mechanisms for Infertility Associated With Endometriosis

Tubal dysfunction
Ovulatory dysfunction
The luteinized unruptured follicle syndrome
Habitual abortion
Altered immunity

T cells	(tolerance to endometrial cell autograft and NK cell deficiency)
B cells	(adaptive and nonspecific polyclonal activation)

Intraperitoneal inflammation

A single group of investigators has reported the preliminary identification of a soluble product in the peritoneal fluid of women with endometriosis that prevents the attachment of a cumulus-intact oocyte to the oviductal epithelium in the hamster (41, 42). Although these experimental observations are intriguing, there remains significant concern regarding the relevance of interspecies experiments to human reproduction.

Ovulatory Dysfunction

It has frequently been suggested that subtle ovulatory defects are associated with endometriosis despite the absence of convincing evidence that infertile women with endometriosis are anovulatory or have luteal phase dysfunction (43). Most observers have noted the disease exclusively in women who undergo long intervals of ovulatory menstrual cycles without conception. Delaying childbearing for socioeconomic, educational, and professional reasons is the basis for the frequently applied but misleading moniker, the "career woman's disease."

The elevated peritoneal fluid prostaglandin levels have been invoked to explain altered luteal function. There is little evidence to suggest that prostaglandins are luteolytic in primates, and prostaglandins failed to act as contraceptives. The data to support this contention are anecdotal, with some authors finding a higher rate of luteal phase deficiency in women with endometriosis (44, 45) and others unable to do so (46). Furthermore, treatment of luteal phase deficiency with clomiphene citrate or progesterone suppositories has failed to improve the cycle fecundity of women with endometriosis. The best available data suggest that the luteal phase in women with endometriosis is normal, based on the correlation between the histologic dating of the endometrium and the midcycle luteinizing hormone surge (47).

The Luteinized Unruptured Follicle Syndrome

It has been suggested that endometriosis is associated with luteinization of the mature dominant follicle in the absence of actual rupture of the ovarian capsule and release of the oocyte, the so-called "LUF" syndrome (48-50). The data supporting this hypothesis are based on several lines of investigation, including altered peritoneal fluid levels of gonadal steroids in the luteal phase, the lack of sonographic disappearance of the follicle at midcycle, and the absence of visualizing an ovulatory stigma during laparoscopy early in the luteal phase. Although seemingly compelling, these are all indirect markers of the mechanical event of ovulation, and the only unequivocal evidence of ovulation is pregnancy. To illustrate the difficulty in establishing this entity, pregnancies have been reported in cycles where laparoscopy was performed after ovulation and an ovulatory stigma was not present (51).

Several investigators have found no association between apparently unruptured luteinized follicles and infertile women with endometriosis (52-53). Furthermore, virtually no data are available regarding the frequency of unruptured luteinized follicles in women of normal fertility. Definitive confirmation of the existence of the LUF phenomenon will await the histologic demonstration of oocytes within a morphologic corpus luteum.

Habitual Abortion

The frequency of clinical spontaneous abortion has been suggested to be greater in infertile women after treatment for endometriosis compared with before establishing that diagnosis (18, 19, 54-61). The data suggesting an association are purely observational and retrospective in nature and are based on the rate of first trimester loss before the diagnosis. Because endometriosis is probably an acquired disease, it is unclear whether patients had endometriosis at the time of earlier pregnancy losses. Additionally, the patients were collected in referral infertility clinics, which, by definition, represent an alteration in reproductive status and the potential for significant selection bias. Using this referral population is obviously very concerning and may result in erroneous conclusions. Issues such as the age of the control population, the thoroughness with which early pregnancy events were detected, which typically is greater in infertile couples, and whether endometriosis was present at the time of the abortion complicate the data analysis.

No specific mechanism has been proposed to explain how the presence of extrauterine endometrium would affect an established intrauterine pregnancy. Furthermore, most infertile women with endometriosis have previously not had clinically apparent conceptions. A prospective study has now demonstrated a similar rate of spontaneous abortion in infertile women with endometriosis compared to infertile women without endometriosis (62). Similarly, using a sensitive assay for serum human chorionic gonadotropin late in the luteal phase, no preclinical abortions were noted in women with endometriosis (63). Thus, it seems unlikely that repetitive spontaneous abortions can account for the infertility experienced by these couples.

An Altered Immune Response: T Cells

Pelvic endometriosis is caused by the transplantation of autologous endometrium to ectopic sites. For this reason, the T cell-mediated immune system, involved in rejection of homologous transplants, has long been suspected of being altered in women with endometriosis. If alterations in the cell-mediated immune system are present in women with endometriosis, the pattern of circulating white cells might be changed. The data are confusing because some investigators have reported lower numbers of lymphocytes (64), while others have not found alterations in the number or distribution of subsets of leukocytes (65-66). To make the picture even more confusing, higher numbers of T cells, B cells, and CD4/CD8 ratios in blood and peritoneal fluid of women with endometriosis have also been reported (67). The reason(s) for these discrepancies may well be methodologic, but there is no clear and consistent change in the number or pattern of circulating leukocytes.

Several groups of investigators have explored the possibility of an alteration of T lymphocyte function in women with endometriosis. An abnormality was reported in monkeys manifested by a reduction in leukocyte infiltration around autologous endometrial antigens injected under the skin of monkeys with spontaneous pelvic endometriosis. Similarly, when lymphocytes were collected from the peripheral blood of these monkeys and incubated with endometrial antigens, a lower rate of lymphocyte proliferation was observed (68). This suggested a deficiency in cell-mediated immunity in animals with endometriosis and uncharacteristic tolerance to their autograft. The same investigators noted suppression of peripheral lymphocyte-mediated lysis of autologous endometrial cells in women with endometriosis, and the degree of the cytotoxicity was inversely proportional to the extent of the disease (26). Interestingly, no alteration in lymphocyte proliferation in response to endometrial antigens was noted in vitro in infertile women with endometriosis. The discrepancy between women and monkeys with regard to lymphocyte proliferation in vitro remains unexplained.

Recently, this deficiency in lymphocyte-mediated cytotoxicity toward autologous endometrial cells was confirmed (66). This effect was apparently specific for endometrium because it was not observed when using K562 cells, the specific targets for natural killer (NK) lymphocytes, as targets. The degree of cytotoxicity was slightly greater for endometrial stromal cells compared with endometrial epithelial cells. Similar experiments by another group have confirmed the reduced cell-mediated cytotoxic effect directed toward endometrial cells, even when heterologous lymphocytes were used, although to a lesser extent (69). However, a lowering of the lymphocyte cytotoxicity for K562 cells was noted, suggesting NK cell dysfunction was responsible for the reduced cytotoxicity directed toward autologous endometrial cells. When the NK cells were depleted in the assay system with pretreatment with an antibody directed toward NK cells, anti-leu-11b, the cytotoxicity was reversed. The reason for the discrepancy with regard to the lymphocyte-mediated cytotoxicity toward the K562 cell line and, thus, whether the NK lymphocytes are the lymphocytes involved in endometrial cell cytotoxicity remains unresolved.

A mechanistic role for altered T cell function in the associated infertility has not been demonstrated. Because endometrial cells are regularly sloughed and regenerated at an immunologically competent site, the endometrium, it is unclear why T cells would have specific cytotoxicity toward autologous endometrial cells to which they are regularly exposed during menstruation. Accordingly, further progress in this area awaits additional and more consistent data as well as a comprehensive hypothesis regarding how the observed alterations in T cell function would influence reproduction. No consistent clinical immune dysfunction is apparent in these women. This raises the possibility that any unusual immune phenomena observed may be a consequence of endometriosis or the associated retrograde menstruation rather than an intrinsic immunological defect in these women.

An Altered Immune Response: B Cell Activation

The occurrence of anti-endometrial antibodies in the serum of women with endometriosis has been reported (70-76), but this remains controversial. Some investigators have found antibodies directed toward endometrial glands, stroma, and other genital tract tissues (70) while others have found antibodies directed only against the endometrial glands (75). Additionally, some investigators have been unable to identify antibodies by indirect immunofluorescence and could only identify them by radial immunodiffusion (73). The existence of anti-endometrial antibodies remains controversial because others have not been able to identify anti-endometrial antibodies with virtually the same methodology (77). The specificity of these observations is also of concern. Another group reported finding antibodies to endometrium in women with diverse pelvic pathology (74). A mechanism by which these circulating antibodies impede the establishment of pregnancy has not been demonstrated.

A distinct autoimmune syndrome characterized by a nonspecific polyclonal B cell activation has been suggested to be the cause of infertility in women with endometriosis, as it has in women with repetitive pregnancy loss (78). Antiphospholipid antibodies and low levels of antibodies directed against a wide variety of unrelated antigens were reported to be present in women with endometriosis. Whether this is a unique syndrome comparable to that observed in women with active connective tissue diseases remains controversial. An alternative explanation is that these findings may simply represent an artifact secondary to the sophisticated antibody testing used that identifies a high rate of clinically inconsequential autoimmune responses in women of reproductive age compared to the general male and female population. A clear mechanism of how these low level nonspecific antibodies could adversely impact the establishment of a pregnancy is lacking. Virtually all identifiable autoimmune diseases are more common in young women, and it may be that a very reactive B cell immune response may confer some evolutionary advantage to the gestational sex. Until more clinical data are available regarding this possibility, an antibody-dependent mechanism for the infertility associated with endometriosis will remain tenuous.

Peritoneal Fluid Inflammation

Primates ovulate within the peritoneal cavity, and the peritoneal environment is in continuity with the ovary and the distal fallopian tube. Factor(s) in the peritoneal environment that are toxic to gametes or embryos have the potential to impede reproduction. Fertilization in humans occurs within the ampullary portion of the fallopian tube. Human peritoneal fluid has been reported to have an adverse influence on the survival of human sperm (79-81), the rate of human sperm penetration of zona-free Hamster oocytes (82, 83), and the fertilization and embryo growth rates of nonprimate mammalian embryos (84, 85).

Normally, there is a small resident population of leukocytes in the peritoneal cavity (86) of all women. The function of these leukocytes is likely to be to remove sperm and any bacteria or particulate material ascending through the genital tract. The number of these leukocytes varies with the stage of the menstrual cycle, being greater immediately after menses (87). The largest subgroup of cells is mononuclear phagocytes (i.e., macrophages) with a smaller number of lymphocytes and rare desquamated mesothelial cells (86, 87).

Infertile women with endometriosis have evidence of a mononuclear cell exudate in the peritoneal cavity manifested by increased peritoneal fluid volume (86) and macrophage number (N = 101–106) (86-91), as well as an elevated degree of macrophage activation (88, 92) and increased concentrations of macrophage secretory products (i.e., proteolytic enzymes, monokines, and growth factors) (93-96). This peritoneal fluid exudate is present not only in those women with visible endometriosis, but also in those with unexplained infertility (97). The stimulus responsible for eliciting the peritoneal fluid exudate appears to be retrograde menstruation (10, 11, 98). Paradoxically, the extent of endometrial implantation has recently been inversely correlated with quantitative markers of intraperitoneal inflammation, suggesting that a highly reactive intraperitoneal monocytic response may actually remove viable endometrial cells and protect against their implantation (25).

The finding of intraperitoneal inflammation with the potential to injure gametes/embryos raises the intriguing possibility that the visual identification of endometrial implants is unrelated to the mechanism of reduced fecundity in women with endometriosis-associated infertility. This concept is consistent with the well-documented observation that removal or destruction of the endometrial implants, either medically or surgically, does not alter the likelihood of pregnancy (99).

Summary

Despite the intense clinical interest in endometriosis and the increasingly sophisticated diagnostic techniques available, we know surprisingly little about the relationship of endometriosis and infertility. Most of the available data are derived from retrospective studies of infertile women in whom endometriosis was identified at laparoscopy. It is unlikely that definitive epidemiologic information will be forthcoming under the clinical circumstances in which this diagnosis is made. A causal relationship between endometriosis and infertility has yet to be established. This is consistent with the observation that, in the absence of mechanical distortion of the pelvic viscera, no therapy, medical or surgical, directed toward the endometriotic implants improves the likelihood of pregnancy for these couples. At present, it would be most accurate to consider these couples to have unexplained infertility. Only with further effort directed toward determining the possible mechanisms by which lowered fecundity might result will a more effective therapy be found.

References

1. Jenkins S, Olive DL, Haney, AF: Endometriosis: Pathogenetic implications of the anatomic distribution. *Obstet Gynecol* 67:335, 1986.
2. Seibel MM, Berger MJ, Weinstein FG, et al: The effectiveness of danazol on subsequent fertility in minimal endometriosis. *Fertil Steril* 38:435, 1982.
3. Hull ME, Moghissi KS, Magyar DF, et al: Comparison of different treatment modalities of endometriosis in infertile women. *Fertil Steril* 47:40, 1987.

4. Thomas EJ, Cooke ID: Impact of gestrinone on the course of asymptomatic endometriosis. *BMJ* 294:272, 1987.
5. Fedele L, Parazzini F, Radici E, et al: Buserelin acetate versus expectant management in the treatment of infertility associated with minimal or mild endometriosis: A randomized clinical trial. *Am J Obstet Gynecol* 166:1345, 1992.
6. Olive DL, Haney AF: Endometriosis, in DeCherney AH (ed): *Reproductive Failure*. New York, Churchill Livingstone, 1986, p 153.
7. Haney AF: Pelvic endometriosis: Etiology and pathology, in Gondos B, Riddick DH (eds): *Pathology of Infertility*. New York, Thieme Medical Publishers, 1987, p 85.
8. Markee JE: Morphological basis for menstrual bleeding. *Bull NY Acad Med* 24:253, 1948.
9. Vijaykumar R, Walters WAW: Myometrial prostaglandins during the human menstrual cycle. *Am J Obstet Gynecol* 141:313, 1981.
10. Blumenkrantz MJ, Gallager N, Bashore RA, et al: Retrograde menstruation in women undergoing chronic peritoneal dialysis. *Obstet Gynecol* 57:677, 1981.
11. Halme J, Hammond MG, Hulka JF, et al: Retrograde menstruation in healthy women and in patients with endometriosis. *Obstet Gynecol* 64:151, 1984.
12. Barbieri RL, Callery M, Perez SE: Directionality of menstrual flow: Cervical os diameter as a determinant of retrograde menstruation. *Fertil Steril* 57:727, 1992.
13. Kruitwagen RFPM, Poels LG, Willemsen WNP, et al: Endometrial epithelial cells in peritoneal fluid during the early follicular phase. *Fertil Steril* 55:297, 1991.
14. Sampson JA: Pathogenesis of postsalpingectomy endometriosis in laparotomy scars. *Am J Obstet Gynecol* 50:597, 1945.
15. Ridley JH, Edwards IK: Experimental endometriosis in the human. *Am J Obstet Gynecol* 76:783, 1958.
16. Scott RB, TeLinde RB: External endometriosis—scourge of the private patient. *Ann Surg* 131:697, 1950.
17. Lloyd FP: Endometriosis in the Negro woman. *Am J Obstet Gynecol* 89:468, 1964.
18. Norwood GE: Sterility and fertility in women with pelvic endometriosis. *Clin Obstet Gynecol* 3:456, 1960.
19. Olive DL, Franklin RR, Gratkins LV: Association between endometriosis and spontaneous abortions: A retrospective clinical study. *J Reprod Med* 27:333, 1982.
20. Candiani GB, Vercellini P, Fedele L, et al: Mild endometriosis and infertility: A critical review of epidemiologic data, diagnostic pitfalls, and classification limits. *Obstet Gynecol Surv* 46:374, 1991.
21. The American Fertility Society: Classification of endometriosis. *Fertil Steril* 32:633, 1979.
22. The American Fertility Society: Classification of endometriosis: 1985. *Fertil Steril* 43:351, 1985.
23. Jansen RPS: Minimal endometriosis and reduced fecundability: Prospective evidence from an artificial insemination by donor program. *Fertil Steril* 46:141, 1986.
24. Henle J: *On Miasmata and Contagie*. Baltimore, Johns Hopkins University Press, 1978.
25. Haney AF, Jenkins SJ, Weinberg JB: The stimulus responsible for the peritoneal fluid inflammation observed in infertile women with endometriosis. *Fertil Steril* 56:408, 1991.
26. Steele RW, Dmowski WP, Marmer DJ: Immunologic aspects of human endometriosis. *Am J Reprod Immunol* 6:33, 1984.
27. Feinstein AR: Theoretical perspectives in causality assessment. *Drug Inform J* 18:219, 1984.
28. Wheeler JM, Malinak, LR: Does mild endometriosis cause infertility? *Semin Reprod Endocrinol* 6:239, 1988.
29. Drake TS, O'Brien WF, Ramwell PW, et al: Peritoneal fluid thromboxane B_2 and 6-keto-prostaglandin E_{2a} in endometriosis. *Am J Obstet Gynecol* 140:401, 1981.

30. Soundheimer SJ, Flickinger G: Prostaglandin E_{2a} in the peritoneal fluid of patients with endometriosis. *Int J Fertil* 27:73, 1982.
31. Badawy SZA, Marshall L, Gabal AA, et al: The concentration of 13,14-dihydro-15-keto-prostaglandin F_{2a} and prostaglandin E_2 in peritoneal fluid of infertile patients with and without endometriosis. *Fertil Steril* 38:166, 1982.
32. Yikorkala O, Koskinies A, Laatikainen T, et al: Peritoneal fluid prostaglandins in endometriosis, tubal disorders and unexplained infertility. *Obstet Gynecol* 63:616, 1984.
33. Koskinies AL, Tenhunen A, Yikorkala O: Peritoneal 6-keto-prostaglandin F_{1a}, thromboxane B_2 in endometriosis and unexplained infertility. *Acta Obstet Gynecol Scand Suppl* 123:19, 1984.
34. DeLeon FD, Vijayakumar R, Brown M, et al: Peritoneal fluid volume, estrogen, progesterone, prostaglandin, and epidermal growth factor concentrations in patients with and without endometriosis. *Obstet Gynecol* 68:189, 1986.
35. Chacho KJ, Strankowski-Chacho MS, Andresen PJ, et al: Peritoneal fluid in patients with and without endometriosis: Prostanoids and macrophages and their effect on the spermatozoa penetration assay. *Am J Obstet Gynecol* 154:1290, 1986.
36. Haney AF, Handwerger S, Weinberg JB: Peritoneal fluid prolactin in infertile women with endometriosis: Lack of evidence of secretory activity by endometrial implants. *Fertil Steril* 42:935, 1984.
37. Rock JA, Dubin NH, Ghodganokar RB, et al: Cul-de-sac fluid in women with endometriosis: Fluid volume and prostanoid concentration during the proliferative phase of the cycle-days 8 to 12. *Fertil Steril* 37:747, 1982.
38. Sqarlata CS, Hetelendy F, Mikhail G: The prostanoic content in peritoneal fluid and plasma of women with endometriosis. *Am J Obstet Gynecol* 147:563, 1983.
39. Dawood MY, Khan-Dawood FS, Wilson L Jr: Peritoneal fluid prostaglandins and prostanoids in women with endometriosis, chronic pelvic inflammatory disease and pelvic pain. *Am J Obstet Gynecol* 148:391, 1984.
40. Croxatto HB, Ortiz M-E, Guiloff E, et al: Effect of 15(S)-15-methylprostaglandin F_{2a} on human oviductal motility and ovum transport. *Fertil Steril* 30:408, 1978.
41. Suginami H, Yano K, Watanabe K, et al: A factor inhibiting ovum capture by the oviductal fimbriae present in endometriosis peritoneal fluid. *Fertil Steril* 46:1140, 1986.
42. Suginami H, Yano K: An ovum capture inhibitor (OCI) in endometriosis peritoneal fluid: An OCI-related membrane responsible for fimbrial failure of ovum capture. *Fertil Steril* 50:648, 1988.
43. Pittaway DE, Maxson W, Daniell J, et al: Luteal phase defects in infertility patients with endometriosis. *Fertil Steril* 39:712, 1983.
44. Grant A: Additional sterility factors in endometriosis. *Fertil Steril* 17:514, 1966.
45. Hargrove JT, Abraham GE: Abnormal luteal function in endometriosis. *Fertil Steril* 34:302, 1980.
46. Pittaway DE, Maxson W, Daniell J, et al: Luteal phase defects in infertility patients with endometriosis. *Fertil Steril* 39:712, 1983.
47. Koninckx PR, Goddeeris PG, Lauweryns JM, et al: Accuracy of endometrial biopsy dating in relation to the midcycle luteinizing hormone peak. *Fertil Steril* 28:443, 1977.
48. Koninckx PR, Brosens IA, Corvelyn, PA: A study of plasma progesterone, oestradiol-17B, prolactin and LH levels and of the luteal phase appearance of the ovaries in patients with endometriosis and infertility. *Br J Obstet Gynaecol* 85:246, 1978.
49. Marik J, Hulka J: Luteinized unruptured follicle syndrome: A subtle cause of infertility. *Fertil Steril* 29:270, 1978.
50. Dmowski WP, Rao R, Scommegna A: The luteinized unruptured follicle syndrome and endometriosis. *Fertil Steril* 33:30, 1980.
51. Portuondo JA, Peña J, Otaloa C, et al: Absence of ovulation stigma in the conception cycle. *Int J Fertil* 28:51, 1983.
52. Koninckx PR, Ide P, Vandenbrouche W, et al: New aspects of the pathophysiology of endometriosis and associated infertility. *J Reprod Med* 24:257, 1980.

53. Dhont M, Serreyn R, Duvivier P, et al: Ovulation stigma and concentration of progesterone and estradiol in peritoneal fluid: Relation with fertility and endometriosis. *Fertil Steril* 41:872, 1984.
54. Devereux WP: Endometriosis: Long-term observations, with particular reference to incidence of pregnancy. *Obstet Gynecol* 22:444, 1963.
55. Petershon L: Fertility in patients with ovarian endometriosis before and after treatment. *Acta Obstet Gynecol Scand* 49:331, 1970.
56. Spangler DB, Jones GS, Jones HW: Infertility due to endometriosis: Conservative surgical therapy. *Am J Obstet Gynecol* 109:850, 1971.
57. Naples JD, Batt RE, Sadigh A: Spontaneous abortion rate in patients with endometriosis. *Obstet Gynecol* 57:509, 1981.
58. Rock JA, Guzick DA, Sengos C, et al: The conservative surgical treatment of endometriosis: Evaluation of pregnancy success with respect to the extent of the disease as categorized using contemporary classification systems. *Fertil Steril* 35:131, 1981.
59. Wheeler JM, Johnston BM, Malinak LR: The relationship of endometriosis to spontaneous abortion. *Fertil Steril* 39:656, 1983.
60. Metzger DA, Olive DL, Stohs GF, et al: Association of endometriosis and spontaneous abortion: Effect of control group selection. *Fertil Steril* 45:18, 1986.
61. FitzSimmons J, Stahl R, Gocial B, et al: Spontaneous abortion in women with endometriosis. *Fertil Steril* 47:696, 1987.
62. Pittaway DE, Vernon C, Fayez JA: Spontaneous abortions in women with endometriosis. *Fertil Steril* 50:711, 1988.
63. Pittaway DE, Ellington CP, Klimek M: Preclinical abortions and endometriosis. *Fertil Steril* 49:221, 1988.
64. Startseva NV: Clinico-immunological aspects in genital endometriosis. *Akush Ginekol (Sofiia)* 3:23, 1980.
65. Gleicher N, Dmowski WP, Seigel I, et al: Lymphocyte subsets in endometriosis. *Obstet Gynecol* 63:463, 1984.
66. Vigano P, Vercelini P, Di Blasio AM, et al: Deficient antiendometrium lymphocyte-mediated cytotoxicity in women with endometriosis. *Fertil Steril* 56:894, 1991.
67. Badawy SZA, Cuenca V, Kaufman L, et al: The regulation of immunologic production by B cells in patients with endometriosis. *Fertil Steril* 51:770, 1989.
68. Dmowski WP, Steele RW, Baker GF: Deficient cellular immunity in endometriosis. *Am J Obstet Gynecol* 141:377, 1981.
69. Oosterlynck DJ, Cornillie FJ, Waer M, et al: Women with endometriosis show a defect in natural killer activity resulting in a decreased cytotoxicity to autologous endometrium. *Fertil Steril* 56:45, 1991.
70. Mathur S, Peress MR, Williamson HO, et al: Autoimmunity to endometrium and ovary in endometriosis. *Clin Exp Immunol* 50:259, 1982.
71. Wild RA, Shivers CA: Antiendometrial antibodies in patients with endometriosis. *Am J Reprod Immunol Microbiol* 8:84, 1985.
72. Chihal HJ, Mathur S, Holtz GL, et al: An endometrial antibody assay in the clinical diagnosis and management of endometriosis. *Fertil Steril* 46:408, 1986.
73. Meek SC, Hodge DD, Musich JR: Autoimmunity in infertile patients with endometriosis. *Am J Obstet Gynecol* 158:1365, 1988.
74. Kreiner D, Gromowitz FB, Richardson DA, et al: Endometrial immunofluorescence associated with endometriosis and pelvic inflammatory disease. *Fertil Steril* 46:243, 1986.
75. Wild RA, Stayaswarop PG, Shivers AC: Epithelial localization of antiendometrial antibodies associated with endometriosis. *Am J Reprod Immunol Microbiol* 13:62, 1987.
76. Mathur S, Chihal HJ, Homm RJ, et al: Endometrial antigens involved in the autoimmunity of endometriosis. *Fertil Steril* 50:860, 1988.
77. Switchenko AC, Kauffman RS, Becker M: Are there antiendometrial antibodies in sera of women with endometriosis? *Fertil Steril* 56:235, 1991.
78. Gleicher N, El-Roeiy A, Cofino E, et al: Is endometriosis an autoimmune disease? *Obstet Gynecol* 70:115, 1987.

79. Burke RK: Effect of peritoneal washings from women with endometriosis on sperm velocity. *J Reprod Med* 32:743, 1987.
80. Oak MK, Chantler EN, Vaughan-Williams CA, et al: Sperm survival studies in peritoneal fluid from infertile women with endometriosis and unexplained infertility. *Clin Reprod Fertil* 3:297, 1985.
81. Soldati G, Piffaretti-Yanez A, Campana A, et al: Effect of peritoneal fluid on sperm motility and velocity distribution using objective measurements. *Fertil Steril* 52:113, 1989.
82. Chacho KJ, Stronkowski-Chacho M, Andressen PJ, et al: Peritoneal fluid in patients with and without endometriosis: Prostanoids and macrophages and their effect on the spermatozoa penetration assay. *Am J Obstet Gynecol* 154:1290, 1986.
83. Sueldo CE, Lambert H, Steinleitner A, et al: The effect of peritoneal fluid from patients with endometriosis on murine sperm-oocyte interaction. *Fertil Steril* 48:697, 1987.
84. Morcos RN, Gibbons WE, Findley, WE: Effect of peritoneal fluid on in vitro cleavage of 2-cell mouse embryos: A possible role in infertility associated with endometriosis. *Fertil Steril* 44:678, 1985.
85. Prough SG, Aksel S, Gilmore SM, et al: Peritoneal fluid fractions from patients with endometriosis do not promote two-cell mouse embryo growth. *Fertil Steril* 54:927, 1990.
86. Haney AF, Muscato JJ, Weinberg, JB: Peritoneal fluid cell populations in infertility patients. *Fertil Steril* 35:696, 1981.
87. Syrop CH, Halme J: Cyclic changes of peritoneal fluid parameters in normal and infertile patients. *Obstet Gynecol* 69:419, 1987.
88. Halme J, Becker S, Hammond MG, et al: Increased activation of pelvic macrophages in infertile women with endometriosis. *Am J Obstet Gynecol* 145:333, 1983.
89. Haney AF, Misukonis MA, Weinberg JB: Macrophages and infertility: Oviductal macrophages as potential mediators of infertility. *Fertil Steril* 39:310, 1983.
90. Badawy SZA, Cuenca V, Marshall L, et al: Cellular components in peritoneal fluid in infertile women with and without endometriosis. *Fertil Steril* 42:704, 1984.
91. Olive DL, Weinberg JB, Haney AF: Peritoneal macrophages and infertility: The association between cell number and pelvic pathology. *Fertil Steril* 44:772, 1985.
92. Muscato JJ, Haney AF, Weinberg, JB: Sperm phagocytosis by human peritoneal macrophages: A possible cause of infertility in endometriosis. *Am J Obstet Gynecol* 144:503, 1982.
93. Fakih H, Baggett B, Holtz G, et al: Interleukin-1: A possible role in the infertility associated with endometriosis. *Fertil Steril* 47:212, 1987.
94. Eisermann J, Gast MJ, Pineda J, et al: Tumor necrosis factor in peritoneal fluid of women undergoing laparoscopic surgery. *Fertil Steril* 50:573, 1988.
95. Weinberg JB, Haney AF, Xu FJ, et al: Peritoneal fluid and plasma levels of human macrophage colony-stimulating factor in relation to peritoneal fluid macrophage content. *Blood* 78:513, 1991.
96. Halme J: Release of tumor necrosis factor-alpha by human peritoneal macrophages in vivo and in vitro. *Am J Obstet Gynecol* 161:1718, 1989.
97. Olive DL, Haney AF, Weinberg, JB: The nature of the intraperitoneal exudate associated with infertility: Peritoneal fluid and serum lysozyme activity. *Fertil Steril* 48:802, 1987.
98. Haney AF, Weinberg, JB: Reduction of the intraperitoneal inflammation associated with endometriosis by treatment with medroxyprogesterone acetate. *Am J Obstet Gynecol* 159:450, 1988.
99. Olive DC, Haney AF: Endometriosis-associated infertility: A critical review of therapeutic approaches. *Obstet Gynecol Surv* 41:538, 1986.
100. Garcia CR, David SS: Pelvic endometriosis: Infertility and pelvic pain. *Am J Obstet Gynecol* 129:740, 1877.
101. Shenken RS, Malinak LR: Conservative surgery vs. expectant management for the infertile patient with mild endometriosis. *Fertil Steril* 37:183, 1982.

102. Portuondo JA, Echanojauregui AD, Herran C, et al: Early conception in patients with untreated mild endometriosis. *Fertil Steril* 39:22, 1983.
103. Olive DL, Stohs GF, Metzger DA, et al: Expectant management and hydrotubations in the treatment of endometriosis associated infertility. *Fertil Steril* 44:35, 1985.
104. Rock JA, Guzick DS, Sengol C, et al: The conservative surgical treatment of endometriosis: Evaluation of pregnancy success with respect to the extent of disease as categorized using contemporary classification system. *Fertil Steril* 35:31, 1981.
105. Olive DL, Lee KL: Analysis of sequential treatment protocols for endometriosis associated infertility. *Am J Obstet Gynecol* 154:613, 1986.
106. Olive DL, Martin DC: Treatment of endometriosis-associated infertility with CO_2 laser laparoscopy: The use of one- and two-parameter exponential models. *Fertil Steril* 48:18, 1987.
107. Nezhat C, Crowgey R, Nezhat F: Videolaseroscopy for the treatment of endometriosis associated with infertility. *Fertil Steril* 51:237, 1989.
108. Buttram VC Jr, Beleu JB, Reiter R: Interim report of a study of danazol for the treatment of endometriosis. *Fertil Steril* 37:478, 1982.

1 Reproductive Endocrinology

Suppression of the Pituitary-Gonadal Axis in Children With Central Precocious Puberty: Effects on Growth, Growth Hormone, Insulin-Like Growth Factor-I, and Prolactin Secretion

Sklar CA, Rothenberg S, Blumberg D, Oberfield SE, Levine LS, David R (New York Univ; Columbia Univ)

J Clin Endocrinol Metab 73:734–738, 1991 1–1

Background.—The relationship between the changes in sex steroids, growth hormone (GH), and insulin-like growth factor-I (IGF-I) occurring at puberty and the accelerated growth velocity in both normal and precocious children is unclear. The impact of gonadal suppression on growth and GH, prolactin, and IGF-I levels in children with precocious puberty was studied.

Methods.—Ten girls and 1 boy with central precocious puberty were examined before and during gonadal suppression with the gonadotropin-releasing hormone agonist leuprolide acetate. Before and 3–6 months after pituitary-gonadal suppression, nocturnal sampling for plasma levels of GH and prolactin was done, and the GH response to GH-releasing factor-(1-44) and plasma IGF-I levels were determined.

Findings.—Treatment significantly reduced the luteinizing hormone and follicle-stimulating hormone responses to gonadotropin-releasing hormone and the plasma level of estradiol. The mean height velocity standard deviation score for chronological age dropped significantly from 3.8 to .9. Nocturnal GH secretion and the mean IGF-I levels were not changed significantly, but the mean peak GH response to GH-relesing factor-(1-44) declined significantly after gonadal suppression. Prolactin secretion before and after suppression was similar.

Conclusions.—Pituitary-gonadal suppression produced no change in IGF-I levels or nocturnal GH and prolactin secretion. It partly inhibited the GH release stimulated by growth hormone releasing factor. The decrease in height velocity occurred independently of changes in GH and IGF-I secretion, but it paralleled the declining levels of gonadal sex steroids, suggesting a direct and GH-independent effect of sex steroids on bone growth.

▶ What is it that is responsible for the abnormal accelerated growth in precocious puberty? This paper suggests that it is primarily estrogen and is not related to activation of the GH-IGF axis. The problem in idiopathic precocious puberty is that unexpected activation of the hypothalamic-pituitary axis occurs;

this results in estrogen production, which in turn mediates the accelerated bone growth along with sexual maturation. The activation of bone growth has been thought to be related to activation of IGF and other factors. In this study, however, the gonadotropin-releasing hormone agonist was used to cause estrogen suppression, and a reduction in peak bone growth was noted. But, although there was no correlation with GH or IGF, there was a direct correlation with declining levels of estrogen. Estrogen receptors have been found on bone, and it is perhaps through this direct interaction that bone growth can be inhibited by the use of the agonist. Nevertheless, the effect of GH-releasing hormone that normally stimulates GH was blunted by the action of the agonist. Indeed, GH secretion can be modulated by the estrogen status. Whereas we cannot absolutely discount a GH/IGF effect, these data suggest strongly a direct effect of estrogen on bone.—R.A. Lobo, M.D.

Inhibition of Endogenous Catecholamine Synthesis Augments Early Follicular Phase Luteinizing Hormone Secretion

Plosker SM, Rabinovici J, Jaffe RB (Univ of California, San Francisco)

J Clin Endocrinol Metab 73:549–554, 1991 1–2

Background.—The physiologic role of catecholamines, especially dopamine and norepinephrine, in regulating gonadotropin secretion in humans has not been defined. An experimental paradigm using tyrosine hydroxylase inhibitor α-methyl-*p*-tyrosine was developed to compare total and pulsatile luteinizing hormone (LH) secretion under catecholamine synthesis inhibition conditions in 1 group of women to LH secretion in women not receiving α-methyl-*p*-tyrosine.

Methods.—α-Methyl-*p*-tyrosine, 500 mg at 8:00 AM and 10:00 AM, was administered to 5 women in the early follicular phase of their menstrual cycle. Secretion patterns of LH were compared with those in 5 untreated women. Blood was drawn every 15 minutes to determine LH and prolactin levels beginning at 8:00 AM until 4:00 PM.

Findings.—α-Methyl-*p*-tyrosine increased prolactin levels from a baseline of 14.72 μg/L to a peak of 102.2 μg/L. The group with inhibition of catecholamine synthesis had higher LH levels as well as greater LH area under the curve and LH pulse amplitude. There were no between-group differences in pulse frequency.

Conclusions.—Inhibition of endogenous catecholamine synthesis augments LH levels in the early follicular phase. Elevated LH secretion during catecholamine synthesis inhibition is caused, at least in part, by increased LH pulse amplitude but not increased LH pulse frequency.

▶ The whole area of the interaction of catecholamines and LH secretion is controversial. Data that made it fairly clear in the past have recently been challenged. It is because of this controversy that this paper was abstracted for review. Very nicely demonstrated here is that, by inhibition of tyrosine hydroxylase (which is important for the production of both dopamine and norepinephrine), an increase in LH occurs. Therefore, it is suggested that catecholamines, either dopamine or norepinephrine, or both, are important for the inhibitory effects of LH secretion. Whereas dopamine has been considered for years to be inhibitory to LH, these data have been controversial, and it has been suggested that, under some circumstances, dopamine may actually do the opposite. Even more difficult to ferret out is the fact that there is an interaction between opioid peptides and dopamine and that opioid peptides are inhibitory to LH secretion; perhaps this, in turn, is also mediated by dopamine.

Nevertheless, in clinical terms, when dopamine is used to try to inhibit LH, this has not really panned out. Bromocriptine has been used in attempts to inhibit LH secretion in patients with polycystic ovary syndrome, but this has not been successful. It is not clear whether these catecholamine effects are purely hypothalamic, or whether there are pituitary effects as well. Nicely demonstrated in this paper is that inhibition of catecholamines synthesis did not affect pulse frequency, which is thought to represent hypothalamic gonadotropin-releasing hormone (GnRH) secretion. It was stimulating to pulse amplitude, although GnRH pulsations largely reflect the pituitary translation of GnRH boluses.

Another difficulty in interpretation of studies such as this is that these are acute effects similar to dopamine infusions, which have inhibitory effects on gonadotropin secretion. How this would translate into changes were adaptive responses likely to ensue is not clear. Difficulties in interpreting studies such as these include whether these are hypothalamic and/or pituitary effects, or acute or chronic changes, and whether it is dopamine or norepinephrine that is working in light of the rapid interconversion between the 2. The measurement of dopamine and norepinephrine peripherally is also difficult because this primarily reflects adrenal catecholamine activity. Although it seems that our basic concept, i.e., that dopamine decreases LH and norepinephrine stimulates LH, may still hold, we are still a far cry from having pharmacologic means to deal with suppression and stimulation because of the multiple variables discussed here.—R.A. Lobo, M.D.

The Source of Inhibin Secretion During the Human Menstrual Cycle

Illingworth PJ, Reddi K, Smith KB, Baird DT (Univ of Edinburgh; Ctr for Reproductive Biology, Edinburgh)

J Clin Endocrinol Metab 73:667–673, 1991 1–3

Objective.—The corpus luteum may be an important source of inhibin. A study was conducted to determine the source of inhibin secretion during the human menstrual cycle.

Methods.—Inhibin concentrations were measured in the peripheral and ovarian veins of 41 women aged 29–45 years who were undergoing hysterectomy at different stages of the menstrual cycle. In addition, the peripheral concentration of inhibin was measured before and for 24 hours after enucleation of the corpus luteum in 13 women. Inhibin was assayed by a heterologous radioimmunoassay with an antiserum raised against 31-kilodalton bovine inhibin.

Results.—During the early follicular phase, the mean inhibin concen-

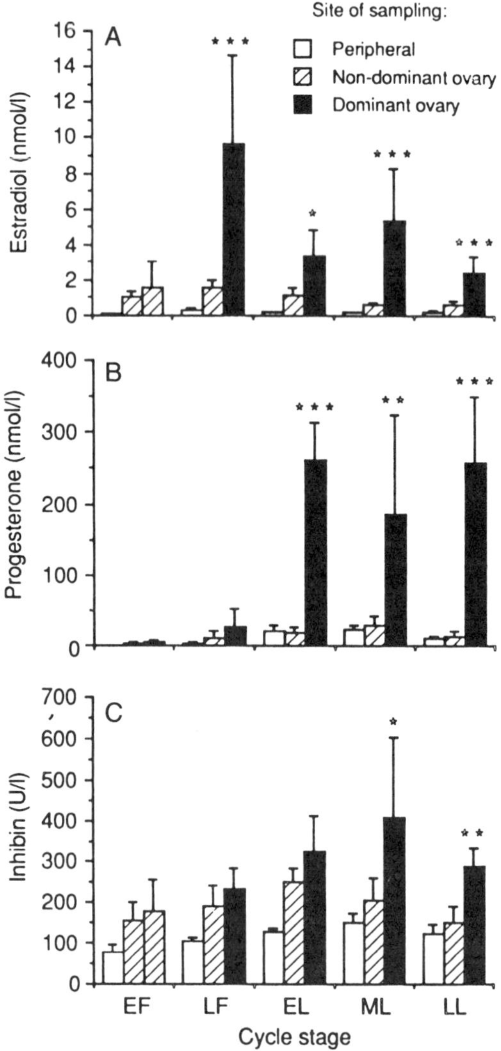

Fig 1–1.—Geometric mean (with 67% confidence intervals shown) concentrations of *(A)* estradiol, *(B)* progestrone, and *(C)* inhibin in the peripheral, nondominant, and dominant ovarian veins during the LF, EL, ML, and LL stages of the menstrual cycle. In the EF, where dominance is not yet apparent, the data shown refer to the right and left ovaries. Nondominant ovarian vein vs. dominant ovarian vein:*, $P < .02$; **, $P < .01$; ***, $P < .001$. (Courtesy of Illingworth PJ, Reddi K, Smith KB, et al: *J Clin Endocrinol Metab* 73:667–673, 1991.)

trations in the right and left ovarian veins were significantly higher than those in the peripheral vein (Fig 1–1). During the late follicular phase, the mean inhibin concentrations did not differ significantly between the dominant ovarian vein (the vein of the ovary bearing a follicle larger than 10 mm) and the nondominant ovarian vein. During the mid and late luteal phases, the mean inhibin concentration in the vein draining the ovary bearing the corpus luteum was significantly higher than that in the contralateral ovarian vein. After enucleation of the corpus luteum, the peripheral concentrations of inhibin fell significantly from 134.4 units per liter before lutectomy to 80 units per liter 24 hours afterward. A crude estimate of the half-life of the initial decline in peripheral inhibin concentration was 86 minutes.

Conclusion.—There is conclusive evidence for the secretion of inhibin into the circulation by the human corpus luteum. The lack of a significant increase in inhibin secretion from the dominant follicle in the late follicular phase suggests that inhibin may not be the factor responsible for the fall in plasma follicle-stimulating hormone concentrations during the follicular phase.

▶ Several interesting concepts emerge from this paper on the effect of inhibin during the menstrual cycle. The controversy is that the dominant follicle during the late follicular phase is not the major source of inhibin and therefore is not inhibitory to follicle-stimulating hormone (FSH) which decreases as the follicle grows. From this and other papers, we know that the corpus luteum is the predominant source of inhibin. The authors suggest here that the dominant follicle does not secrete sufficient inhibin to be responsible for the decline in FSH (see Fig 1–1). There is a potential problem in the assays for inhibin, and considerable controversy is currently raging as to the specificity of different antibodies used in the inhibin assay. Nevertheless, it is entirely possible that inhibin increases in the follicular phase, not because of secretion from the dominant follicle, but because of secretion from the total mass of small follicles.

It could be that the estrogen produced by the dominant follicle as it grows is primarily responsible for the decline in FSH, as suggested by these investigators. However, these data are somewhat at odds with previous papers showing a direct correlation between granulosa cell production of inhibin by the dominant follicle and that of estradiol. A piece is missing from these data; inhibin is only one of many products of the granulosa cell of the dominant follicle. Others include activin and follistatin, which also may be important in feedback interactions with FSH.—R.A. Lobo, M.D.

Elevation of Follicular Phase Inhibin and Luteinizing Hormone Levels in Mothers of Dizygotic Twins Suggests Nonovarian Control of Human Multiple Ovulation

Martin NG, de Kretser DM, Robertson DM, Osborne J, Chenevix-Trench G, Burger HG (Queensland Inst of Med Research and Royal Women's Hosp, Brisbane, Australia; Monash Univ, Melbourne)

Fertil Steril 56:469–474, 1991 1–4

Background.—The increased rate of multiple pregnancies after ovulation induction in anovulatory women suggests a physiologic cause such as alteration of maternal hormone levels. An earlier report found nonsignificant midcycle elevations of follicle-stimulating hormone (FSH) and luteinizing hormone (LH) in mothers of twins. In a previous study, FSH

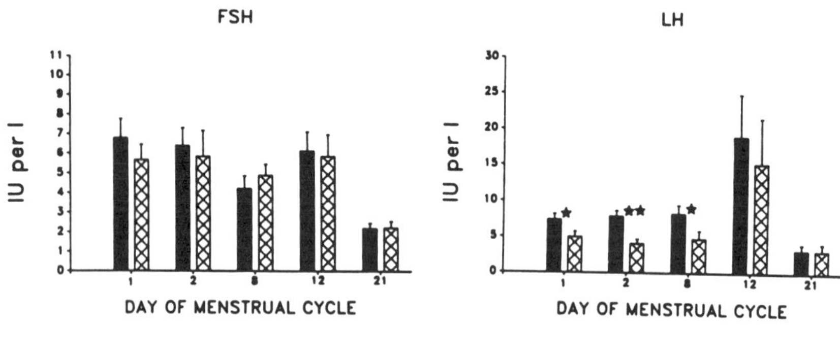

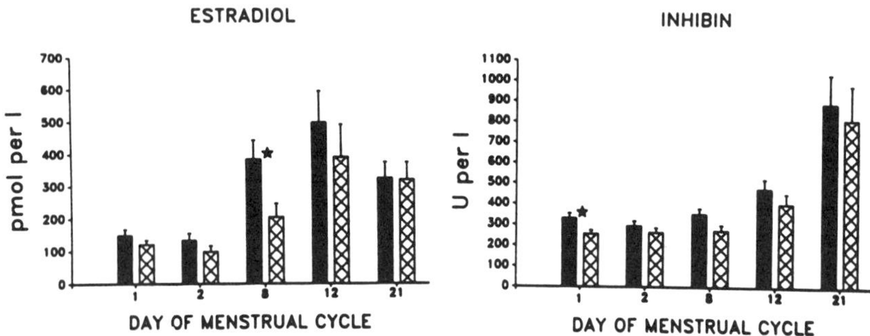

Fig 1–2.—Mean ±SE hormone levels for mothers of DZ twins (filled area) and controls (stippled area). *, Means differ at $P < .05$ level; **, means differ at $P < .01$ level. (Courtesy of Martin NG, de Kretser, DM, Robertson DM, et al: *Fertil Steril* 56:469–474, 1991.)

and LH levels were elevated in the early follicular phase of mothers of 2 natural sets of dizygotic (DZ) twins compared with matched controls. The question of whether the elevation of FSH levels is the result of greater hypothalamic stimulation or is in response to lower serum levels of ovarian inhibin was addressed.

Methods.—Eight volunteers with at least 1 set of spontaneous DZ twins were paired with matched controls. Serum hormone levels were measured 5 times throughout the menstrual cycle and ovarian ultrasonography was performed on day 12. Serum inhibin, FSH, LH, and estradiol (E_2) levels were measured on approximate cycle days 1, 2, 8, 12, and 21.

Findings.—As in the previous study, the mothers of twins had much higher levels of LH throughout the follicular phase, significantly so on days 1, 2, and 8, and higher levels of E_2 in the early to midfollicular phase (Fig 1–2). In the mothers of twins, serum inhibin levels were elevated throughout the cycle, and FSH levels were elevated in the early follicular phase. The overall elevated levels were indicative of greater follicular activity.

Conclusions.—The decrease in inhibin secretion from the ovary does not appear to be the primary cause of multiple ovulation in humans. The increased secretion of FSH and LH may be caused by elevated secretion of, or sensitivity to, gonadotropin-releasing hormone; the elevated levels of inhibin and E_2 are a response to the increased release.

▶ What is the cause of dizygotic twinning in women? This study tries to determine whether it is a hypothalamic-pituitary response or an ovarian response. Whereas previous studies suggested that gonadotropins are elevated in women with a history of twinning, the ability to measure inhibin afforded the opportunity to determine whether it is in reality an ovarian aberration, i.e., a reduction in inhibin that signals the gonadotropin elevations in these patients. Inhibin, in point of fact, was slightly elevated in these individuals, as were gonadotropins in the early follicular phase (see Fig 1–2). These data suggest that the gonadotropins are produced in increased amounts either because of pituitary sensitivity or because of an exaggerated gonadotropin-releasing hormone stimulus that results in higher levels of both estradiol and inhibin in the early follicular phase and therefore stimulates increased follicular development. It would be interesting to test the sensitivity of the pituitary and to study pulse frequency in these individuals to determine the hypothalamic-pituitary interactions that cause this interesting phenomenon.—R.A. Lobo, M.D.

Amplification of Pulsatile LH Secretion by Exogenous Melatonin in Women

Cagnacci A, Elliott JA, Yen SSC (Univ of California, San Diego, La Jolla)

J Clin Endocrinol Metab 73:210–212, 1991 1–5

Purpose.—There is increasing interest in the role of melatonin during reproductive quiescence in humans. The effect of exogenous melatonin on the pulsatile secretion of luteinizing hormone (LH) was investigated in 11 women during the early follicular phase of the menstrual cycle.

Methods.—The women received placebo or melatonin orally for 2 consecutive days in a random, double-blind fashion. Two dosages of melatonin were used: 6 patients received 100 mg of melatonin once and 5 received 2.5 mg of melatonin in 3 divided doses at 2-hour intervals. Blood samples were collected every 10 minutes between 9:00 AM and 5:00 PM.

Findings.—Compared with placebo, the administration of melatonin significantly augmented LH pulse amplitude without changing LH pulse frequency. Consequently, the integrated LH secretion was significantly greater after melatonin administration. There was a 38-fold increase in circulating melatonin levels after the 100-mg dose was given, but there were no significant differences in LH pulsatile characteristics between the 2 dosages. Nor were there significant changes in serum follicle-stimulating hormone and ovarian steroid levels after melatonin administration.

Discussion.—This is the first study to clearly demonstrate the stimulatory effect of exogenous melatonin on pulsatile LH secretion in the early follicular phase. Previous studies have described putative melatonin receptors in the hypothalamus and median eminence as well as the modifying effects of melatonin on the hypothalamic release of neurotransmitters and prostaglandins, which are involved in the regulation of gonadotropin-releasing hormone (GnRH). Thus the stimulatory effect of exogenous melatonin on LH pulse amplitude may be mediated by an action at the level of the hypothalamus and median eminence by increasing the amplitude of GnRH pulses.

▶ This paper was selected for review because we will be hearing more and more about the effects of melatonin in reproduction. These nicely demonstrated data are of interest but suggest the opposite of what would be anticipted. Melatonin up to now has been thought to have an inhibitory effect on the gonadotropin axis. Could it be that there is a bimodal effect, and that there is augmentation in the early phase of the cycle and a decrease in subsequent phases? More data are needed to clarify these differences. Well established here is that pulse amplitude, but not pulse frequency, can be increased in the early phases of the menstrual cycle with doses as low as 2.5 mg. This is a pharmacologic dose but obviously quite different from the 100-mg dose used in this study. Melatonin was shown to augment gonadotropin responses. Putting this observation together with previous reports of a decrease in gonadotropin pulse dynamics with melatonin administration clearly demonstrates the potential for melatonin to exert a role in reproductive function. In terms of its pharmacologic mode of action, it is being considered as a contraceptive agent together with progestins.—R.A. Lobo, M.D.

Follicular Arrest During the Midfollicular Phase of the Menstrual Cycle: A Gonadotropin-Releasing Hormone Antagonist Imposed Follicular-Follicular Transition

Kettel LM, Roseff SJ, Chiu TC, Bangah ML, Vale W, Rivier J, Burger HG, Yen SSC (Univ of California, San Diego; Salk Inst, La Jolla; Prince Henry's Inst of Med Research, South Melbourne, Vic, Australia)

J Clin Endocrinol Metab 73:644–649, 1991 1–6

Background.—Hypothalamic gonadotropin-releasing hormone (GnRH)-mediated pulsatile gonadotropin release is essential for folliculogenesis and maturation. The availability of rapidly acting GnRH antagonists has provided an important probe to assess the functional dependency of the dominant follicle on pulsatile gonadotropin inputs.

Methods.—Twelve normal cycling women were studied during 2 consecutive menstrual cycles; the first cycle served as a control and the second as a treatment cycle. During the latter, each woman received daily injections of Nal-Glu GnRH antagonist, 50 μg/kg, for 3 days in the midfollicular phase (days 7–9). Daily blood samples were obtained for luteinizing hormone (LH), follicle-stimulating hormone (FSH), estradiol (E_2), progesterone, and immunoreactive inhibin (i-INH) measurements by radioimmunoassay during and after administration of Nal-Glu. In 5 women, LH pulsatility was assessed by 10-minute blood sampling for 12 hours before, during, and after Nal-Glu treatment.

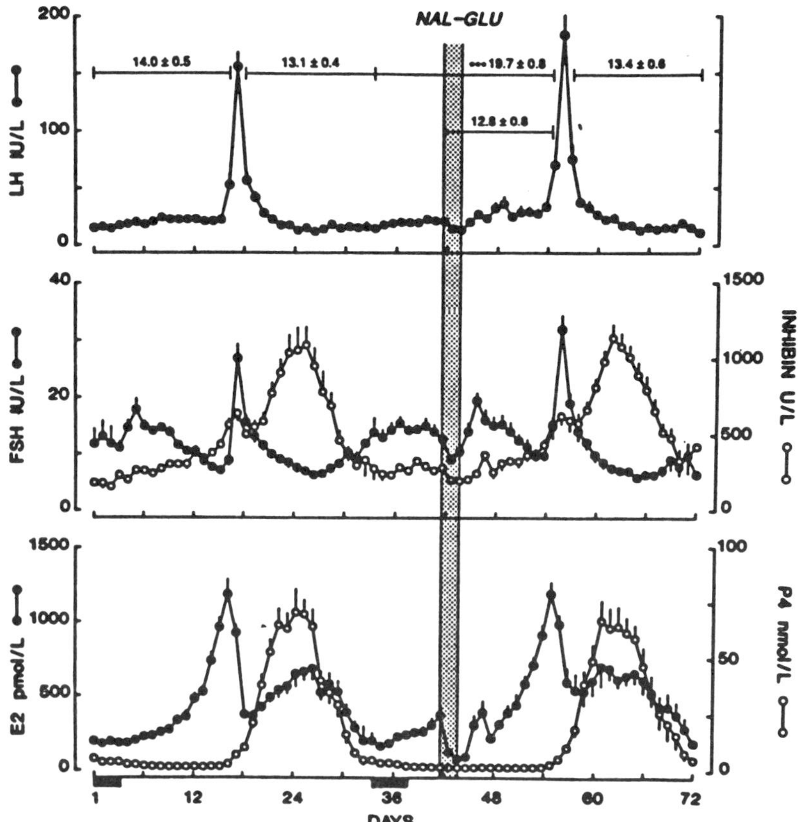

Fig 1–3.—Mean (±SE) daily serum LH, FSH, E_2, P_4, and i-INH concentrations during control and treatment cycles in 12 women. Data are centered around the LH peak. Nal-Glu GnRH antagonist (50 μg/kg, intramuscularly) was administered for 3 days in the midfollicular phase of the second cycle. ***, $P < .0001$. (Courtesy of Kettel LM, Roseff SJ, Chiu TC, et al: *J Clin Endocrinol Metab* 73:644–649, 1991.)

Results.—Administration of Nal-Glu significantly prolonged both the follicular phase and total cycle length compared with control cycles. Furthermore, Nal-Glu maximally reduced the mean serum levels of LH by 62.2% and those of FSH by 45.3% and significantly reduced LH pulse amplitude by 56% (Fig 1–3). The number of LH pulses was reduced by 36%, but pulse remained discernible. There were concomitant significant reductions in E_2 and i-INH levels. The degree of gonadotropin suppression was maintained throughout the 3-day treatment period. Within 24–48 hours after Nal-Glu was discontinued, all hormones returned to pretreatment levels. There was prompt reinitiation of follicular growth and maturation, as reflected by a rapid increase in E_2 and i-INH levels, timely ovulation, and normal luteal function.

Conclusion.—In this study administration of Nal-Glu antagonist at midfollicular phase for 3 days resulted in an approximately 50% decrease in gonadotropin support to the dominant follicle, leading to functional arrest. The follicular apparatus retains its ability to reinitiate its original functionality once appropriate gonadotropin inputs return.

Prevention of Premature Luteinizing Hormone and Progesterone Rise With a Gonadotropin-Releasing Hormone Antagonist, Nal-Glu, in Controlled Ovarian Hyperstimulation

Frydman R, Taieb J, Cornel C, Spitz IM, de Ziegler D, Bouchard P (Hôpital Antoine Béclère, Clamart, France; Hôpital Bicêtre, Bicêtre; Population Council, New York)

Fertil Steril 56:923–927, 1991 1–7

Background.—Administration of the gonadotropin-releasing hormone (GnRH) antagonist, Nal-Glu, during the follicular phase of the menstrual cycle delays the luteinizing hormone (LH) surge by 8–10 days. Administration of GnRH may also interrupt growth of the dominant ovarian follicle. Timely administration of Nal-Glu was investigated to determine whether it can prevent the premature LH and progesterone (P) rise in controlled ovarian hyperstimulation using clomiphene citrate and human menopausal gonadotropin (hMG).

Treatment.—Eleven women aged 25–34 years with normal menstrual cycles and using barrier methods of contraception received 100 mg of clomiphene citrate daily on days 2–6. In addition, 150 IU of hMG was given intramuscularly on days 4, 6, and 8. When serum estradiol (E_2) levels exceeded 600 pg/mL, 5 mg of Nal-Glu was given subcutaneously on the same day and repeated 48 hours later. Five women received 5000 IU of human chorionic gonadotropin (hCG) 48 hours after the second Nal-Glu injection to study the effects of Nal-Glu on the luteal phase.

Results.—After the first Nal-Glu administration on day 11.2 (mean), the plasma E_2 level continued to increase to 1159 pg/mL at 24 hours and 1,610 pg/mL 48 hours later. The mean number of follicles ±15 mm in diameter increased from 2.3 to 57. The plasma levels of LH and P remained low for at least 96 hours after the first Nal-Glu administration in 10 women. The plasma level of LH was already slightly elevated in 1 woman before the first Nal-Glu administration. In the 5 women who received hCG, the length of the luteal phase was similar to that in normal or hyperstimulated cycles, and plasma P levels were not different from those in other controlled ovarian hyperstimulation cycles. Plasma E_2 and P levels reached a maximum of 1258 pg/mL and 50.3 ng/mL 6 day after hCG administration.

Conclusion.—Timely administration of Nal-Glu during the late follicular phase of controlled ovarian hyperstimulation induced with clomiphene citrate and hMG prevents premature elevation of LH and P levels for at least 96 hours despite increasing plasma E_2 levels. In addition, Nal-Glu does not interfere with a rise in E_2 or disrupt follicular growth and the post-hCG hormonal profile.

▶ The article reviewed in Abstract 1–6 furthers our understanding of the LH requirements of midcycle and the potential clinical use of the antagonist, Nal-Glu. This GnRH antagonist was used to probe the dynamics of the menstrual cycle. Its administration in the midfollicular phase showed that a 50% reduction in gonadotropin arrests follicle development, but the follicle survives and within 3 days is able to reinitiate its original function and development (Fig 1–3). Parallel reductions in estrogen and inhibin production also were observed. These data suggest the significant dependence of the dominant follicle on gonadotropin support; this follicle is relatively hardy, however, and demise does not occur unless it is deprived of support for about 3 days.

The group from Paris (Abstract 1–7) showed that if Nal-Glu is given at midcycle in clomiphene-hMG-induced cycles, estradiol levels are not disturbed yet premature luteinization and the LH surge are avoided (see Fig 1–4). Clearly, this dose is also sufficient to continue to block the LH surge and allow timely folliculogenesis and prevent premature ovulation, an event that plagued us when timing in vitro fertilization before this GnRH agonist became available. A similar approach is described in Abstract 1–8. Of interest, however, is that estradiol levels did not plummet with the acute onset of Nal-Glu use. This is at variance of some of our own findings and suggests that the timing of Nal-Glu administration is extremely critical. If given late in folliculogenesis when the oocyte is competent and sensitive to circulating gonadotropins, no decrement in E_2 would be anticipated. At earlier stages of folliculogenesis, however, before this competence is achieved, even small doses of Nal-Glu disrupt follicular growth and E_2 levels need to be maintained by exogenous gonadotropins. Again, this is a beautiful illustration of how Nal-Glu can be used to achieve greater understanding of menstrual cycle dynamics and to determine practical ways to better handle the induction of ovulation.—R.A. Lobo, M.D.

Comparison of Intermittent and Continuous Use of a Gonadotropin-Releasing Hormone Antagonist (Nal-Glu) in In Vitro Fertilization Cycles: A Preliminary Report

Cassidenti DL, Sauer MV, Paulson RJ, Ditkoff EC, Rivier J, Yen SSC, Lobo RA
(Univ of Southern California; Univ of California, San Diego; Salk Inst, La Jolla)
Am J Obstet Gynecol 165:1806–1810, 1991 1–8

Background.—The use of gonadotropin-releasing hormone (GnRH) agonist in in vitro fertilization (IVF) cycles requires an extended treatment period to achieve down-regulation, resulting in longer treatment cycles and increased costs. The GnRH antagonist Nal-Glu lacks an agonistic effect and directly blocks the pituitary, preventing hypothalamic GnRH-induced gonadotropin release. When used as an adjunct for stimulation with gonadotropins, down-regulation is achieved more readily with Nal-Glu, and total cycle length is reduced as a result of elimination of the agonistic phase.

Treatment.—A simplified new protocol involving the intermittent use of Nal-Glu was applied in 7 women undergoing ovarian hyperstimulation for IVF or gamete donation. All women had previously undergone treatment with leuprolide and human menopausal gonadotropins (hMG). In these control cycles the patients received leuprolide acetate, 1 mg/day subcutaneously, in the midluteal phase until down-regulation was achieved (estradiol <30 pg/mL). Thereafter, leuprolide, 500 μg, was given in conjunction with hMG, 3–4 ampules per day intramuscularly. In the treatment cycles, the women received 50 μg of Nal-Glu per kg daily intramuscularly on cycle day 1 or 2 for 3 days or until down-regulation was achieved. Thereafter, Nal-Glu was discontinued and hMG, 3–4 ampules per day was given intramuscularly. When the follicles reached 14–16 mm, Nal-Glu was resumed and administered daily in conjunction with hMG.

Outcome.—The time required to achieve down-regulation was significantly reduced with the use of Nal-Glu (mean, 1.6 days) compared with the leuprolide acetate-hMG cycles (mean, 20 days). Similarly, the mean cycle length was significantly shorter in the Nal-Glu cycles (11 vs 31 days). Furthermore, serum luteinizing hormone (LH) levels in the group given Nal-Glu and hMG were significantly lower after down-regulation and on the day of human chorionic gonadotropin administration, compared with the levels in the group given leuprolide acetate and hMG. There were no significant differences between groups in the mean number of days of treatment with hMG, the mean number of ampules of hMG, peak estradiol levels, number of oocytes, and percentage of oocytes fertilized. The use of Nal-Glu was well tolerated, and 5 pregnancies resulted.

Conclusion.—The intermittent administration of Nal-Glu provides a convenient and effective regimen for use in IVF, achieving rapid pituitary down-regulation and preventing premature luteinization and LH surges. The use of Nal-Glu may allow as high oocyte and embryo yield as the leuprolide acetate-hMG regimen does.

▶ This is a companion report on preliminary data using Nal-Glu for IVF. The hypothesis has been that if the GnRH agonist is used to cause down-regulation before gonadotropin stimulation, the recruitment phase would be more synchronous and the ovary more sensitive to gonadotropins. When continued with gonadotropin stimulation, the agonist blocks the premature LH surge. In the previous paper (Abstract 1–7) it was shown that Nal-Glu can prevent spontaneous luteinization and increases in progesterone levels. Here, Cassidenti et al. attempted to develop a practical means of administering Nal-Glu instead of the agonist by giving it at 2 separate times—once in the early follicular phase to induce acute ovarian down-regulation and again late in the follicular phase to block the spontaneous LH surge. That this was accomplished without difficulty shows the feasibility of this intermittent approach of Nal-Glu administration without the GnRH agonist, which often prolongs the treatment cycle and increases the requirement for gonadotropins. In this study, although the requirement for gonadotropins was comparable to the requirements of these same patients given an agonist and hMG, the data suggest that this approach is practical and more beneficial in that the treatment time was decreased dramatically.—R.A. Lobo, M.D.

Suppression of Corpus Luteum Function by the Gonadotropin-Releasing Hormone Antagonist Nal-Glu: Effect of the Dose and Timing of Human Chorionic Gonadotropin Administration

Dubourdieu S, Marraoui J, Charbonnel B, Spitz I, Massai MR, Bouchard P (Hôtel-Dieu, Nantes, France; Service d'Endocrinologie Hôpital Bicêtre, Le Kremlin Bicêtre; Ctr for Biomedical Research, New York)

Fertil Steril 56:440–445, 1991 1–9

Background.—In primates it appears that endogenous luteinizing hormone (LH) is required to sustain corpus luteum function. Interruption of pulsatile gonadotropin-releasing hormone (GnRH) administration in the luteal phase results in a decline of serum progesterone levels. The viability of the corpus luteum appears to be preserved without LH support for at least 72 hours and can be rescued if pulsatile GnRH therapy is reinitiated. A contraceptive strategy based on GnRH antagonist treatment in the luteal phase may be successful, but the presence of human chorionic gonadotropin (hCG) may rescue the corpus luteum function. The effect of the GnRH antagonist Nal-Glu administered in the luteal phase and the potential rescue of the corpus luteum by exogenous hCG after antagonist treatment were assessed.

Methods.—An Nal-Glu dose required for luteolysis was administered to 29 women for 3 consecutive days. A low dose of hCG was administered either simultaneously or 48 or 72 hours after the Nal-Glu administration. Six additional women received pharmacologic doses of hCG 48 hours after the luteolytic dose of Nal-Glu. Radioimmunoassay measurements of follicle-stimulating hormone, LH, estradiol, and progesterone levels were performed before, during, and after the regimens.

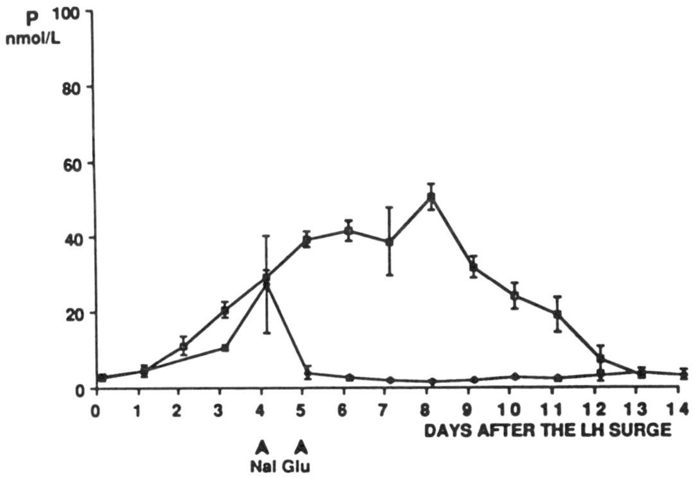

Fig 1–4.—Mean (±SE) serum P during the luteal phase, in women treated with Nal-Glu (10 mg, subcutaneously) on days 4 and 5 after the LH surge (day 0) (filled squares) and during the control cycles (open squares). (Courtesy of Dubourdieu S, Marraoui J, Charbonnel B, et al: *Fertil Steril* 56:440–445, 1991.)

Results.—Complete luteolysis occurred in women who received 10 mg of Nal-Glu daily 4–5 days after the LH surge. The coadministration of Nal-Glu and hCG overrode the effect of the antagonist compared to treatment with hCG alone. Treatment with hCG started 48 hours after Nal-Glu resulted in partial luteolysis, when hCG was administered 72 hours after Nal-Glu, complete luteolysis occurred, and higher doses of hCG resulted in a significant rescue of corpus luteum function. Serum progesterone levels in the luteal phase are shown in Figure 1–4.

Conclusions.—As observed previously in primates and women, suppression of LH support of the corpus luteum for at least 3 days induces luteolysis. After 3-day suppression, compromise of the corpus luteum cannot be reversed by administration of low doses of hCG, which mimics early pregnancy, but the corpeus luteum can be at least partially restored by pharmacologic doses of hCG.

▶ The use of Nal-Glu, the GnRH antagonist, has given us a beautiful way to investigate follicular dynamics and trophic requirements during the menstrual cycle. This potent third-generation antagonist is highly effective in inhibiting LH and follicle-stimulating hormone throughout the menstrual cycle. Doses of anywhere from 50 to 150 μg/kg on a daily basis are highly effective in this regard. This study shows how dependent the corpus luteum is on LH during the luteal phase. The results are fairly clear that beyond 3 days of LH decrement the corpus luteum can no longer be rescued and is irrevocably compromised (see Fig 1–4). There is a possibility of rescue within this period of time and, clearly, a pharmacologic dose of hCG may be the rescuer. This is analogous to other studies of follicular rescue during the menstrual cycle before ovulation. Even in the presence of a decline in estradiol levels to baseline follicular levels, the dominant follicle can be rescued and ultimately result in ovulation. It is suggested therefore that the dominant follicle and the corpus luteum are fairly hardy and can withstand 2 to 3 days of trophic deprivation before demise.—R.A. Lobo, M.D.

Recognition of Gonadotroph Adenomas in Women

Daneshdoost L, Gennarelli TA, Bashey HM, Savino PJ, Sergott RC, Bosley TM, Snyder PJ (Univ of Pennsylvania; Wills Eye Hosp, Philadelphia)

N Engl J Med 324:589–594, 1991 1–10

Introduction.—Gonadotroph adenomas are rarely reported, possibly because they are more difficult to recognize in women than in men. These tumors are usually found in men older than 50 years; increased serum gonadotropin levels in women of this age could come from normal gonadotroph cells.

Methods.—Thyrotropin-releasing hormone (TRH) was given to 16 women who apparently had nonsecreting pituitary macroadenomas. Serum gonadotropins and the glycoprotein hormone α subunit levels were monitored for 90 minutes after TRH injection. In addition, 16 age-matched healthy women and 10 with macroadenomas secreting prolactin, growth hormone, or corticotropin were studied.

Results.—Eleven women in the study group had a significant increase in the β subunit of luteinizing hormone (LH) in the serum after TRH. Three had a follicle-stimulating hormone (FSH) response and 4 had an LH response. None of the healthy women and none of those with secreting adenomas had an LHβ, FSH, or LH response to TRH. Of the 12 nonsecreting adenomas that were cultured, 10 secreted readily detected amounts of FSH, LH, and LHβ. The in vitro findings correlated with the patients' responses to TRH.

Conclusions.—Most women presumed to have nonsecreting pituitary macroadenomas probably have adenomas of gonadotroph origin. Many of these patients have a serum LHβ response to TRH.

▶ This is an interesting report about gonadotropin-secreting tumors. This entity has not been well described in women, although there have been several reports in men. A high percentage of nonfunctioning macroadenomas have been found to be functional and to produce gonadotropins. Also, at least in men, these tumors appear to be very common, and up to 25% of macroadenomas in men secrete gonadotropins. In women these adenomas have largely been called nonfunctional, primarily because it is difficult to determine whether the levels of gonadotropins at baseline are in any way elevated, particularly in postmenopausal women. Therefore, it is not possible to diagnose these largely nonfunctional macroadenomas, which are actually gonadotropin-secreting, by baseline measurements of gonadotropins.

This study found that TRH induces an increase in LHβ as well as in LH and FSH in women as well as in men. What is the value of this finding? In women with nonfunctioning adenomas, a gonadotropin-secreting adenoma may be diagnosed by administering TRH to differentiate these "nonfunctional" tumors from other intersellar lesions. As the authors also point out, it might be feasible to use the TRH test as a mechanism of following up patients with these adenomas post treatment. It is intriguing that, if these tumors are truly secrete gonadotropins, gonadotropin-releasing hormone agonist therapy may prove to be a new nonsurgical treatment for these nonsecreting macroadenomas, or least shrink them to the point at which a transsphenoidal approach may be contemplated. Also intriguing is why these gonadotropin-secreting adenomas are so common. Clearly, they have a benign course and probably are largely asymptomatic. Why they occur with this frequency is not as yet known.—R.A. Lobo, M.D.

Exercise Induces Two Types of Human Luteal Dysfunction: Confirmation by Urinary Free Progesterone

Beitins IZ, McArthur JW, Turnbull BA, Skrinar GS, Bullen BA (Univ of Michigan; Boston Univ; CSI/PAREXEL Internatl Corp, Wellesley, Mass)

J Clin Endocrinol Metab 72:1350–1358, 1991 1–11

Background.—Previous reports indicate that strenuous exercise in untrained young women with documented ovulatory menstrual cycles results in secondary oligomenorrhea and luteal phase defects. These abnormalities may be caused by altered neuroendocrine regulation of menstrual hormone secretion, and weight loss may potentiate such effects.

Methods.—In a prospective study, 28 untrained women with documented ovulatory menstrual cycles participated in a 2-month program of strenuous exercise. Overnight urine samples were collected daily during a control ovulatory menstrual cycle and during the 2 exercise months, covering a total of 53 menstrual cycles. Changes in urinary levels of luteinizing hormone (LH), follicle-stimulating hormone (FSH), estriol (E_3), and free progesterone (P) during the menstrual cycles with abnormal corpus luteum function were compared to those during the control ovulatory cycles. The area under the curve (AUC) for each hormone was calculated for the follicular and luteal phases of each cycle.

Results.—Eighteen women (64%) had a total of 20 cycles (38%) with luteal phase defects. Six cycles were classified as inadequate, characterized by a luteal phase of 9 days or longer and a reduced mean integrated P value during the period between the urinary LH peak and the onset of menses, compared with corresponding control cycles. Fourteen other cycles were classified as short, with luteal phases of less than 9 days in duration and a decreased mean integrated P level compared with corresponding control cycles. Other abnormalities (e.g., an increase in the length and AUC for E_3 of the follicular phase and a decrease in the AUC for LH during the luteal phase) occurred only in the short luteal phase cycles. There was a relatively minor but statistically significant weight loss in women with both short and inadequate luteal phase cycles.

Discussion.—The initiation of strenuous exercise in previously ovulating untrained women frequently leads to corpus luteum dysfunction associated with insufficient P secretion and decreased luteal phase lengths. The delay in the ovulatory LH peak despite increased E_3 excretion and decreased LH excretion during the luteal phase suggest that exercise may alter the neuroendocrine system. The lack of positive feedback to estrogens and the decreased LH secretion during the luteal phase could compromise corpus luteum function. In contrast, decreased P excretion is the sole abnormality noted in menstrual cycles with an inadequate luteal phase.

▶ Exercise-induced menstrual dysregulation has been a focus of attention for many years now. The luteal defect, as suggested in this paper, was also determined some time ago; indeed, luteal deficiency is thought to be just part of the spectrum of defective folliculogenesis. Nevertheless, this study, although not necessarily novel, was nice to see because it was well controlled and very well carried out in a prospective manner. Urinary determinations showed the integrated daily production of the hormones in question. Of some interest, as was confirmed here, both short and inadequate luteal phases were hormonally incompetent. The bottom line in the evolution of this abnormality is that there is some dysregulation of the signaling, and some studies have suggested that LH pulsations are aberrant in this kind of situation.

Interestingly an increase in LH pulse frequency in the early follicular phase was suggested by Soules to result in an inadequate luteal phase (1). Studies of amenorrhea induced by exercise have suggested the opposite, namely, a decrease in LH pulse frequency. Also of interest is the authors' observation that despite a higher estrogen excretory pattern there was an inadequate LH response, suggesting that there may be a disassociation in the feedback system between estrogen and the hypothalamic-pituitary axis. Nevertheless, it is important to note that these urinary measurements of estrogen were of E_3, which, although reflective of estrogen status, is not the major metabolite of estradiol. Further refinements in assay techniques may allow other findings.— R.A. Lobo, M.D.

Reference

1. Soules MR: *Obstet Gynecol Clin North Am* 14:865, 1987.

High-Resolution Endovaginal Ultrasonography of the Endometrium: A Noninvasive Test for Endometrial Adequacy

Grunfeld L, Walker B, Bergh PA, Sandler B, Hofmann G, Navot D (Mount Sinai Med Ctr, New York)

Obstet Gynecol 78:200–204, 1991 1–12

Purpose.—The ability of endometrial texture, as depicted on endovaginal ultrasonography, to predict endometrial development was studied. Ultrasonographic features of the endometrium were correlated with morphological assessment of endometrial biopsy specimens.

Methods.—Nineteen cycles were studied in 18 women with ovarian failure undergoing sequential transdermal 17β-estradiol (E_2) and intramuscular progesterone replacement for oocyte transfer. Endovaginal sonography was performed before progesterone initiation (luteal day +1) and continued throughout the midsecretory phase. Endometrial echogenicity was classified by using a modification of the criteria of Sakamoto et al. Endometrial biopsy was performed 6–8 days after initiation of progesterone replacement, the criteria of Noyes et al. being used for endometrial dating.

Findings.—On luteal day +1, ultrasonography showed a multilayered endometrium consisting of a hyperechoic perimeter (endometrial-myometrial interface), a hypoechoic functionalis, and a hyperechoic basalis in all but 2 cycles (pattern I). On luteal day +7, 8 cycles showed increased echogenicity of the basalis and functionalis, but not encompassing the entire endometrium (pattern II). Eleven cycles showed a homogeneous hyperechoic functionalis (pattern III) on luteal day +7, and endometrial biopsy specimens showed normal stromal development. The appearances of the 3 patterns on ultrasonography are shown in Figure 1–5. Three patients had endometrial specimens consistent with chronological development but did not have a hyperechoic endometrium by luteal day +7. Ultrasonography detected all 5 biopsy specimens that were histologically

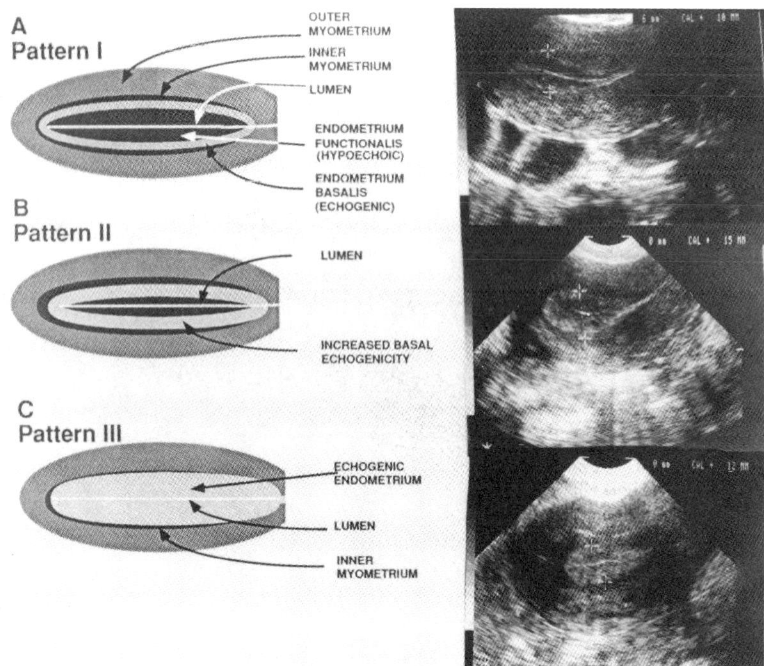

Fig 1–5.—Ultrasonography of the endometrium throughout the late follicular and early- and mid-luteal phases. **A,** Pattern I is characteristic of the late follicular phase. The midline echo represents the endometrial lumen. This is surrounded by a hypoechoic area and an echogenic basalis. **B,** Pattern II is a transitional phase. There is increased echogenicity of the basalis, but still a hypoechoic functionalis. C, Pattern III demonstrates echogenicity of the entire functionalis. (Courtesy of Grunfeld L, Walker B, Bergh PA, et al: *Obstet Gynecol* 78:200–204, 1991.)

out of phase. Thus ultrasonography had a sensitivity of 100% and a specificity of 62% for the detection of histologically normal endometrial development. Endometrial histology demonstrated inadequate glandular development but advanced stroma in 9 patients, but in 7 of these ultrasonography showed pattern III, suggesting that increased echogenicity may reflect stromal edema. Endometrial thickness failed to distinguish between biopsy samples that were normal and those out of phase, and there was poor correlation between serum steroid values and sonographic patterns.

Conclusion.—The presence of a homogeneous hyperechoic endometrium on endovaginal sonography on luteal day +7 is reassuring. Its absence should raise suspicion of a luteal phase deficiency.

▶ The purpose of this paper is to show the orderly transition of the endometrium through the follicular phase and into the luteal phase. The endometrium of the luteal phase is very well organized; the thickness is extremely characteristic and not at all reminiscent of the thick endometrium of endometrial hyperplasia. The thickness in pattern III (see Fig 1–5) consists of a homogeneous hyperechoic functional zone and correlates best with the stromal maturation of the endometrium. Whereas the authors suggest that dating the endometrium is possible by ultrasound, stromal maturational events correlate but glandular morphological changes, which are also important, do not seem to do so as well. Hormonal data concerning estrogen and progesterone did correlate well; the estrogen level has been shown in other study to correlate well with endometrial thickness and total uterine volume. If the normalcy of endometrial organization, but not its thickness per se, can be used as a prognostic indicator in cycles of induction of ovulation and in vitro fertilization, a pattern III would be reassuring. However, I do not believe that these data can be used prospectively, as yet, to substitute for the use of biopsies in endometrial dating.— R.A. Lobo, M.D.

Effect of Recombinant Activin on Androgen Synthesis in Cultured Human Thecal Cells

Hillier SG, Yong EL, Illingworth PJ, Baird DT, Schwall RH, Mason AJ (Univ of Edinburgh; Genentech Inc, South San Francisco)

J Clin Endocrinol Metab 72:1206–1211, 1991 1–13

Background.—In vitro studies show that activin-A inhibits luteinizing hormone (LH)-stimulated androgen production by rat ovarian thecal/interstitial tissues, suggesting an intraovarian function for this protein. The effect of recombinant activin-A on androgen production was studied in vitro in human thecal cells.

Methods.—Thecal cell monolayers were incubated for 4 days in serum-free culture medium containing LH (10 mg/mL) and insulin-like growth factor-1 (IGF-1) (±30 ng/mL) with and without activin-A (1–100 ng/mL). Both LH and IGF-1 were added to induce maximal androgen (androstenedione and dehydroepiandrosterone) production.

Results.—The addition of activin-A in culture medium resulted in dose-dependent inhibition of thecal cell androgen production in response to LH and IGF-1. A 50% maximal inhibition was observed with an activin-A dose of 10 mg/mL. However, suppression of progesterone production occurred only at high doses (100 ng/mL) of activin-A. Inhibition of steroid production occurred without inhibition of DNA synthesis, as measured by tritiated thymidine uptake.

Discussion.—Activin-A has a potent and selective inhibitory action on androgen production by human thecal cells in vitro. This is consistent with a paracrine function for activin in modulating follicular androgen biosynthesis in human ovaries.

▶ This is a nice paper suggesting ovarian paracrine interaction, giving credence to the 2-cell theory of estrogen production. Human thecal cells were used in these in vitro cultures and recombinant activin was used to study androgen production. The 2-cell theory suggests that androgen is produced by thecal cells; then, when diffusing to granulosa cells, it is aromatized to estrogen. If this theory is correct, activin, which is produced along with inhibin by the granulosa cells, inhibits androgen production by thecal cells. Therefore, in early follicular development, when inhibin and activin levels are low, this lack of inhibition of activin allows androgen substrate to be produced from the theca and to be transported for aromatization in granulosa cells. As the follicle grows and more activin is produced, presumably there is inhibition of further androgen production; because there is a reduction in the requirement, excessive or uncontrolled androgen production may somehow be detrimental to the process of follicular development. Again, it is important to note that although this model seems relatively straightforward, it is not quite that simple because there are multiple additional factors involved, including follistatin, which appears to be a binding protein.—R.A. Lobo, M.D.

Polycystic Ovarian Disease: Contribution of Vaginal Endosonography and Reassessment of Ultrasonic Diagnosis

Ardaens Y, Fossati P, Robert Y, Dewailly D, Lemaitre L (Ctr Hospitalier Regional de Lille, Lille, France

Fertil Steril 55:1062–1068, 1991 1–14

Objective.—Vaginal ultrasonography allows more precise analysis of internal ovarian morphology. The effectiveness of vaginal and abdominal ultrasound in the diagnosis of polycystic ovarian disease (PCOD) was compared and previously reported ultrasonic signs of PCOD on abdominal ultrasonography were assessed.

Methods.—The ultrasonic findings in 144 patients aged 15–44 years in whom PCOD was diagnosed on the basis of endocrine parameters were compared with those in 62 patients with primary hyperprolactinemia or hypothalamic anovulation.

Findings.—In the 64 patients with PCOD who underwent both abdominal and vaginal ultrasonography, the external ovarian features of PCOD (e.g., increased ovarian area, uterine width/ovarian length ±1, and excessive roundness index) were observed with similar frequency on both examinations. The internal ovarian features (e.g., abnormal ovarian stroma and polycystic appearance) were significantly more apparent on vaginal than on abdominal ultrasound. The frequencies of polycystic appearance and uterine width/ovarian area ±1 on abdominal and vaginal ultrasound did not differ significantly between patients with PCOD and those with primary hyperprolactinemia or hypothalamic anovulation. In contrast, an increased ovarian area, excessive roundness index, and abnormal ovarian stroma were noted almost exclusively in patients with PCOD. The most striking difference between patients with and without PCOD was the abnormal ovarian stroma only when investigated by the vaginal route.

Conclusion.—An increased ovarian stroma appears to be the most sensitive and specific ultrasonic sign of PCOD, provided that it is evaluated by vaginal ultrasonography. Other criteria of PCOD used previously with abdominal ultrasonography are much less informative.

▶ I, for one, am a firm believer that polycystic ovaries should not be called a disease, as suggested by these authors; also, I do not believe that the diagnosis is made by ultrasound findings. Anyway, this report is of interest because it characterizes some of the ultrasonographic findings in this entity and compares them with findings in other patients with anovulation. Here is where the study falls down a little: The authors studied patients who had hyperprolactinemia or hypothalamic dysfunction; normal patients, who can also have "polycystic"-looking ovaries were not included. Of no surprise, these authors found that vaginal ultrasound was superior to abdominal ultrasound. Nevertheless, an important finding here of a confirmatory nature is that it is really the stromal thickness of the ovaries that distinguishes the so-called polycystic ovary from other morphological changes. Not all of the patients with polycystic ovaries, defined hormonally in this study, had evidence of abnormalities on ultrasound. On vaginal ultrasound only 31% had increased ovarian areas and only 68% had a polycystic pattern. The converse is true as well; the polycystic pattern as described here also appears in some "normal" women, as we have found. Nevertheless, abnormal ovarian stroma was present in 64% of the patients compared to only 8% of those with other anovulatory disorders.

All of this discussion does not mean that ultrasound of polycystic ovaries is not valuable. I think it is. However, I do not rely on this technique to make the diagnosis of polycystic ovaries, but, rather, to suggest the type of ovaries that one will encounter and consider for purposes of induction of ovulation.— R.A. Lobo, M.D.

Serum Bioactive and Immunoreactive Luteinizing Hormone and Follicle-Stimulating Hormone Levels in Women With Cycle Abnormalities, With or Without Polycystic Ovarian Disease

Fauser BCJM, Pache TD, Lamberts SWJ, Hop WCJ, de Jong FH, Dahl KD (Dijkzigt Univ Hosp, Rotterdam; Erasmus Univ, Rotterdam; VA Med Ctr, Seattle)
J Clin Endocrinol Metab 73:811–817, 1991 1–15

Objective.—Apart from high serum androgen levels in most women with polycystic ovarian disease (PCOD), inappropriate gonadotropin secretion, with selectively elevated luteinizing hormone (LH), has been emphasized. Circulating gonadotropin levels were determined using both immunologic methods and in vitro bioassays in 35 women with oligomenorrhea or amenorrhea and infertility. Eight healthy, regularly cycling women also were studied. Eleven of the former women had a diagnosis of PCOD.

Findings.—Women with PCOD had significant elevations of α-subunit, free androgen index, androstenedione, estrone, and estradiol. Levels of LH, determined by both immunoradiometric assay and radioimmunoassay, were distinctly increased compared with control values but were comparable with values in patients without PCOD. The median LH level on bioassay was nearly sixfold higher in patients with PCOD than in the other patients, and fourfold higher than control values in the early follicular phase of the cycle.

Implications.—Immunoradiometric values of LH may not help to identify women with PCOD. The ratio of bioassay to immunoradiometric LH values is more helpful in distinguishing between PCOD and other cyclic abnormalities. Polycystic ovarian disease may be viewed as a clinical model in which to study the steroidal regulation of LH biopotency.

▶ Renewed interest in measurements of gonadotropins in patients with polycystic ovaries (PCO) is the subject of this report. It was noted here that measurements of LH by immunoradiometric assay (IRMA) are not useful for the biochemical diagnosis of PCO. But this paper confirms that the biological activity of PCO is enhanced. Luteinizing hormone is extremely heterogeneous and, depending on the assay system chosen, there will be differences in the results that are obtained. Conventional radioimmunoassay often demonstrates an increased level of LH in patients with PCO, but the bioactivity of LH is more significantly increased. As noted above, however, the IRMA assay is not particularly useful in making a biochemical diagnosis of PCO. Recent data, however, have found fluorometric assays to be helpful in that they better reflect biological activity. Of interest in this paper was that for the first time to my knowledge, bio-follicle-stimulating hormone levels were reported in PCO, and they were noted to be normal. Further, although LH levels are helpful for the biochemical characterization of patients with PCO, particularly in acknowledging the increase in biological activity, we do not necessarily rely on these measurements for the clinical diagnosis or management of this syndrome.—R.A. Lobo, M.D.

3α-Androstanediol Glucuronide in Virilizing Congenital Adrenal Hyperplasia: A Useful Serum Metabolic Marker of Integrated Adrenal Androgen Secretion

Pang S, MacGillivrary M, Wang M, Jeffries S, Clark A, Rosenthal I, Wiegensberg M, Riddick L (Univ of Illinois, Chicago; Children's Hosp of Buffalo)
J Clin Endocrinol Metab 73:166–174, 1991 1–16

Background.—The goal of long-term treatment of congenital virilizing adrenal hyperplasia is to achieve genetic potential for stature, normal maturation of secondary sex characteristics, reproductive function, electrolyte and water homeostasis maintenance, and normal blood pressure. Whether serum 3α-androstanediol glucuronide (3AG) reflects the overall effect of integrated adrenal androgen secretion in congenital virilizing adrenal hyperplasia was determined.

Methods.—Seven patients with classic 21-hydroxylase deficiency and 1 with classic 11β-hydroxylase deficiency were studied. Circadian levels of serum 3AG and 17-hydroxyprogesterone or 11-deoxycortisol, androstenedione, testosterone, and 24-hour urinary 17-ketosteroids (17KS) were assessed.

Findings.—In 5 poorly controlled patients, highly increased baseline morning serum levels of 17-hydroxyprogesterone or 11-deoxycortisol and androstenedione, and in 3 patients elevated morning testosterone levels, dropped markedly in the evening. The elevated serum level of 3AG did not change significantly; 17-ketosteroid levels were markedly high for age. During dexamethasone administration, moderately or slightly increased morning 17-hydroxyprogesterone androstenedione, or testosterone in 2–4 patients with 21-hydroxylase deficiency dropped to normal in the evening; 11-deoxycortisol, androstenedione, and testosterone levels were suppressed in the patient with 11β-hydroxylase deficiency. Serum 3α-androstanediol glucuronide levels were increased modestly or normal in these patients, without circadian changes; 17-ketosteroid levels were high or normal. In 2 other patients with 21-hydroxylase deficiency, modestly raised morning baseline 17-hydroxyprogesterone and androstenedione levels dropped in the evening. Increased morning testosterone dropped in 1 patient in the evening. Modestly increased 3AG levels demonstrated no circadian changes, and 17-ketosteroid levels were increased modestly. During dexamethasone treatment, normal or slightly high serum steroids and 17-ketosteroid levels were associated with normal or high normal 3AG levels, with no circadian changes. Overall, excellent correlation was observed between either 8:00 AM (mean) or 8:00 PM serum 3AG levels and 17-ketosteroids. Morning and evening serum 3AG levels in 5 normal women were comparable.

Conclusions.—The high correlation between serum 3AG and urinary 17-ketosteroids, and the absence of a significant circadian variation in 3AG, indicate that serum 3AG is a useful metabolic index of integrated adrenal androgen secretion in congenital virilizing adrenal hyperplasia. This is true regardless of the time of sampling.

▶ The purpose of this report is not so much to discuss the management of patients with virilizing congenital adrenal hyperplasia but to discuss in general the clinical utility of serum 3AG. These authors suggest that the measurement of serum 3AG largely reflects total adrenal androgen production. Nevertheless, it is important to realize that this marker of peripheral androgen metabolism is dependent on the level of 5α-reductase activity in tissue, specifically in skin. In this instance, patients with congenital adrenal hyperplasia (CAH) often have normal or slightly increased levels of 5α-reductase activity. Therefore, as androgen from the adrenal goes up and down, levels of 3AG will be commensurate and reflect total adrenal androgen activity. Nevertheless, there are situations when 5α-reductase activity is not increased (even in CAH) and may, in fact, be decreased, resulting in a dissociation between and androgen secretion by adrenal or ovary and the lives of 3AG levels in blood. This has led to much confusion about the clinical use of 3AG, as well as the use of this marker in patients receiving various types of treatment. The part of the equation that needs to be considered is how substrate (androstenedione testosterone) is secreted by adrenal or ovary, and how much 5α-reductase activity is really present endogenously or is affected by the treatment modality.—R.A. Lobo, M.D.

Ovarian Hyperandrogenism: The Role of and Sensitivity to Gonadotropins

McClamrock HD, Bass KM, Adashi EY (Univ of Maryland)

Fertil Steril 55:73–79, 1991

1–17

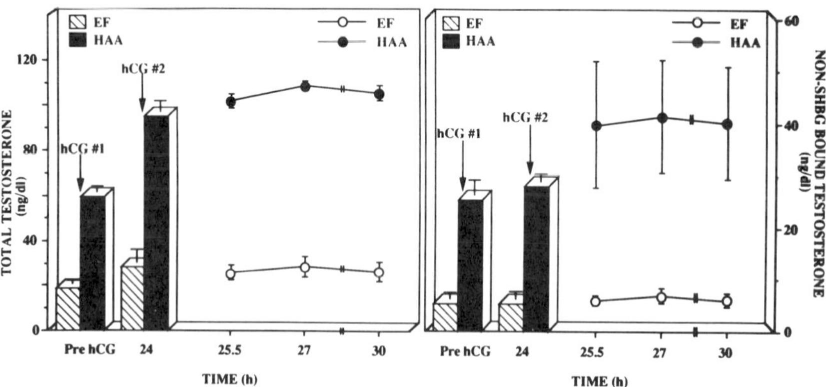

Fig 1–6.—Ovarian androgenic responsiveness to exogenous hCG administration: total T and non-SHBG–bound T-hyperandrogenic anovulatory subjects (n = 4) and early follicular controls (n = 4) were given 2 intramuscular injections of 10,000 IU of HCG at 24-hour intervals. Immediately before the second hCCG injection, a single blood sample was obtained for the determination of the circulating levels of total T and non-SHBG–bound T. Immediately after the second hCG injection, blood samples were intermittently obtained at the indicated time points over a 6-hour period, during which time the circulating levels of total T and non-SHBG–bound T were determined by RIA. (Courtesy of McClamrock HD, Bass KM, Adashi EY: *Fertil Steril* 55:73–79, 1991.)

Background.—Patients with chronic normogonadotropic anovulation commonly have ovarian hyperandrogenism as well; however, the cause-and-effect relationship behind this association remains unknown. To determine whether the hyperandrogenism results from enhanced availability of gonadotropins, hyperandrogenic anovulatory patients were compared with normal controls as to ovarian exposure and sensitivity to endogenous or exogenous gonadotropins.

Methods.—The patients were 4 symptomatic women aged 25–39 years with hyperandrogenic anovulation. Their mean circulating total testosterone level was 59.5 ng/dL. Controls were 4 normally ovulating women aged 22–35 years who were studied in the early follicular phase. The 2 groups were comparable in height. The 24-hour integrated concentrations of serum total testosterone and luteinizing hormone (LH) were measured by means of a portable Cormed pump. In addition, the ovarian testosterone response to 2 intramuscular injections of human chorionic gonadotropin, given 24 hours apart, was measured between injections and up to 6 hours after the second injection.

Results.—The mean 24-hour concentration of LH was 20.1 mIU/mL in subjects with hyperandrogenism, 2.4 times higher than in controls. The total testosterone level was 3.2 times higher. The integrated concentrations of bioactive LH were 1.9 times higher, but this difference did not attain significance. On exogenous stimulation, circulating levels of total T reached 94.8 ng/dL in the subjects with hyperandrogenism before the second injection vs. 28.6 ng/dL in controls (Fig 1–6). Additional increments were seen after the second injection in women with hyperandrogenism—up to 81.3% over baseline—but not in controls.

Conclusions.—Ovarian hyperandrogenism appears to reflect an overall increase in gonadotropic support as well as augmented ovarian sensitivity to gonadotropic stimulation. The contributions of these 2 factors may vary among individuals.

▶ Although there are no major surprises in this report, it is a nice demonstration of the ovarian androgen problems of patients with hyperandrogenic chronic anovulation also known as polycystic ovary (PCO) syndrome. This study suffers a little from being small, including only 4 patients and because these disorders are extremely heterogeneous, it is difficult to generalize from the data. Yet, as stated above, the demonstration is clear and of importance (see Fig 1–6). In this study, human chorionic gonadotropin (hCG) was used to stimulate ovarian androgen production. Commercial preparations of hCG also can stimulate adrenal androgens to some extent, although the differentiation here is somewhat difficult and this issue cannot be specifically addressed. Because hCG is a much more potent stimulus than LH, it therefore produced perhaps a pharmacologic response in this series. The LH that circulates in PCO syndrome, however, has greater biological activity and thus has a greater propensity for ovarian androgen stimulation.

So, we see at least 2 things operative in PCO syndrome to result in the hyperandrogenism of ovarian origin: increased biological activity of LH, and increased ovarian sensitivity. Why is the ovary more sensitive in PCO syndrome? Well, there is evidence in the rat that there is an up-regulation of LH receptors. Data reviewed previously suggest that there is a dysregulation of the enzymes 17-hydroxylase/17-20 desmolase, resulting in accentuation of the androgenic response to gonadotropin stimulation.

How all this fits together is not as yet clear. Nevertheless, the aim in treating hyperandrogenism would ideally be to try the inhibition of gonadotropins as well as androgen, perhaps by making the ovary less sensitive to gonadotropic stimulation. Whereas it is easy at this point to turn off or suppress gonadotropic stimulation, to alter the inherent sensitivity of the ovary at this point remains a challenge.—R.A. Lobo, M.D.

Adrenal Androgen Secretion in Postadolescent Acne: Increased Adrenocortical Function Without Hypersensitivity to Adrenocorticotropin

Laue L, Peck GL, Loriaux DL, Gallucci W, Chrousos GP (Natl Inst of Child Health and Human Development; Natl Cancer Inst, Bethesda, Md; Georgetown Univ)

J Clin Endocrinol Metab 73:380–384, 1991 1–18

Background.—As many as 50% of women with acne have elevated levels of plasma androgens and androgen precursors. These include free testosterone, Δ^4-androstenedione, dehydroepiandrosterone (DHEA), and DHEA sulfate; it is unknown whether this excess comes from the ovary and/or the adrenal gland. Levels of these androgens and precursors were compared in patients with acne and in controls.

Methods.—The patients were 11 women (mean age, 30.5 years) with therapeutically resistant acne. Ten normal controls (mean age, 33.3

years) also were studied. All of the women underwent five 1-hour adrenocorticotropic hormone (ACTH) stimulation tests, performed at least 3 days apart. A different dose of ACTH (1–24) was used for each test in random order—0, .003, .01, and 1 μg/kg by intravenous bolus. Blood samples were taken for measurement of plasma cortisol, Δ^4-androstenedione, and DHEA by radioimmunoassay at 0, 10, 30, and 60 minutes.

Results.—At baseline, the women with acne had a mean cortisol level of 237 nmol/L, a mean Δ^4-androstenedione level of 4.6 nmol/L, and a mean DHEA level of 16 nmol/L, all slightly higher than in the normal controls. In response to ACTH, this group had higher peak and time-integrated DHEA concentrations. There was no significant difference between the groups in either the mean effective dose or slope of the dose-response curve, however, suggesting that there were no differences in the sensitivity of the adrenal cortex to ACTH. The patients with acne had a significantly higher ratio of DHEA to cortisol response; this suggested some preponderance of the Δ^5 pathway of steroidogenesis in acne.

Conclusions.—Women with postadolescent acne appear to have basal and ACTH-stimulated hypersecretion of Δ^5 androgens. This finding is consistent with the hypothesis of an increased volume of androgen-secreting tissue rather than hypersensitivity of the adrenal zona reticularis to ACTH. Thus the role of ACTH in acne continues to be unknown; it may play a permissive role only.

▶ This paper, which discusses acne, is brought to your attention because this is truly an androgen-related problem that is often forgotten. There is evidence for both ovarian as well adrenal androgen excess. Recent data also suggest that there is a peripheral or sebaceous tissue abnormality in androgen metabolism in patients with acne. This paper focuses primarily on the adrenal gland, and graded responses to ACTH were assessed. These authors suggest that there is no inherent adrenal hypersensitivity. However, there is a larger volume of tissue for production of adrenal androgens. This distinction is relatively arbitrary because, in essence, the adrenal is most likely more sensitive, or at least was more sensitive initially, resulting in a greater volume of tissue.

Of clinical importance, if there is evidence of adrenal androgen excess, or at other times ovarian androgen excess, success might be achieved only be adequate suppression of the offending increased glandular secretion. Data have emerged recently suggesting that the increased peripheral androgen response in patients with acne is related primarily to sebaceous tissue overproducing metabolites of androstenedione, specifically androsterone. Indeed, an increase in these metabolites has been found even in patients with normal circulating levels of testosterone and androstenedione, suggesting that in difficult-to-manage patients with acne who don't clearly have elevated levels of ovarian and adrenal androgens, a trial course of antiandrogen therapy may be initiated.—R.A. Lobo, M.D.

Peripheral Androgen Blockade Versus Glandular Androgen Suppression in the Treatment of Hirsutism

Carmina E, Lobo RA (Università di Palermo, Italy; Univ of Southern California)

Obstet Gynecol 78:845–849, 1991 1–19

Objective.—Hirsutism in women has been attributed to increased peripheral androgen metabolism. The clinical efficacy of dexamethasone and spironolactone was compared in the treatment of hirsutism in women. Also, whether serum markers of ovarian, adrenal, or peripheral androgen production may be helpful determinants of treatment was evaluated.

Treatment.—Twenty hyperandrogenic women with hirsutism were treated for up to 2 years. Based on their sensitivity to dexamethasone, as assessed by a short-term dexamethasone suppression test, 11 women were treated with that drug, 0.37 mg/day, and 9 received spironolactone, 100 mg daily, for at least 1 year. Thereafter, the 11 patients treated with dexamethasone were treated with dexamethasone and spironolactone combined for an additional year. Hirsutism was quantified with a modified Ferriman-Gallwey score.

Outcome.—In the patients treated with dexamethasone, androgen levels were suppressed into the normal range, but the Ferriman-Gallwey scores decreased by only 20%, although this decrease was significant. In contrast, in the patients treated with spironolactone, serum androgen levels did not change significantly, but the Ferriman-Gallwey scores decreased significantly by 47%. Thus, in both groups, clinical responses after treatment did not correlate with changes in androgen levels. In the patients treated with both dexamethasone and spironolactone, serum androgen levels were not significantly different from the levels obtained from dexamethasone treatment alone, but the Ferriman-Gallwey scores improved markedly.

Conclusions.—Peripheral androgen metabolism may be the primary determinant of hirsutism in women. Measurement of serum androgen levels may not be helpful in predicting the response to therapy.

▶ Although I had not intended to select one of our own papers for comment, I decided to include this paper for a number of reasons. The study was not meant to be a demonstration of the effectiveness of treatment A versus treatment B for hirsutism. Nevertheless, 2 important points came out of this investigation. Point number 1 is that there is very poor correlation between serum markers of androgenicity and the clinical response. Therefore, in spite of beautiful normalization of androgen levels, the clinical response may vary considerably. The second point is that more and more data are emerging to suggest that it is really peripheral blockade of androgen metabolism that is important in the amelioration of hirsutism in women; therefore, as seen in this report, spironolactone was highly beneficial, despite a lack of reduction in ovarian and adrenal androgens.

These data therefore suggest that peripheral blockade should be part and parcel of all therapeutic regimens for suppression of androgen levels in the management of hirsutism. In a purer sense, I had always previously advocated normalizing androgen levels as a primary therapeutic approach in the treatment of hirsutism. These and other data begin to suggest that it is necessary to include peripheral blockade by some means to effectively remedy or ameliorate this difficult problem.—R.A. Lobo, M.D.

Comparison of Sequential Cyproterone Acetate/Estrogen Versus Spironolactone/Oral Contraceptive in the Treatment of Hirsutism

O'Brien RC, Cooper ME, Murray RML, Seeman E, Thomas AK, Jerums G (Austin Hosp, Heidelberg, Vic, Australia)

J Clin Endocrinol Metab 72:1008–1013, 1991 1–20

Background.—The antiandrogen drugs cyproterone acetate (CPA) and spironolactone are widely used to treat hirsutism. Both appear to act primarily by binding to the androgen receptor in target tissues. Both also decrease androgen biosynthesis. Cyproterone acetate is also strongly progestogenic. In a randomized study, the effects of CPA and spironolactone on hair growth and androgen levels were assessed in hirsute women.

Methods.—Forty-eight women received spironolactone, 100 mg daily, or CPA, 100 mg daily, on days 5–14 of their menstrual cycle. Twenty-six women completed 6 months of CPA therapy and 19 completed 6 months of spironolactone therapy. All but 10 women were given estrogen treatment concomitantly.

Results.—By objective measurement, the total hair diameter decreased by 17.1% with spironolactone and by 16.8% with CPA. The diameter of the hair medulla dropped by 17.8% and 31.7% in the 2 groups, respectively. The effect of the 2 drugs on hair diameter was not significantly different. Plasma testosterone levels also dropped significantly in both groups. Changes in the serum level of testosterone and in total hair diameter are shown in Figure 1–7. The frequency with which women performed cosmetic measures fell by 38% and 44.7% in the spironolactone-treated and CPA-treated groups, respectively. That difference was again nonsignificant. Side effects necessitated withdrawal of 1 women taking

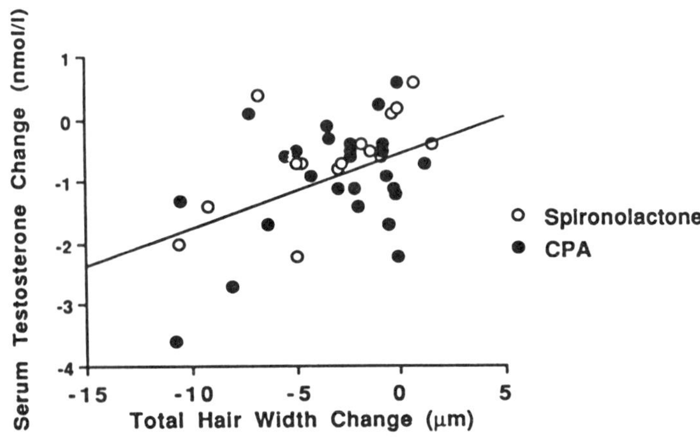

Fig 1–7.—The relationship between change in serum testosterone and change in total hair diameter for the whole study group. For each individual subject, the change in total hair diameter after 6 months of treatment is shown on the x axis, and the corresponding change in serum testosterone is shown on the y axis. R = .49, P = .001. (Courtesy of O'Brien RCC, Cooper ME, Murray RML, et al: *J Clin Endocrinol Metab* 72:1008–1013, 1991.)

CPA and 2 taking spironolactone. Milder side effects also occurred in 2 additional women in each group.

Conclusions.—Cyproterone acetate and spironolactone are effective in the treatment of hirsutism. Neither drug appears to have a particular advantage over the other.

▶ Hirsutism is an extremely frustrating problem, and there are no quick cures for it. This paper from Australia is the first to my knowledge randomizing 2 commonly used treatments for hirsutism, namely, CPA, which is widely used around the world, and spironolactone, which is used largely in the United States. Spironolactone is specifically approved in Australia for the treatment of hirsutism, as is CPA. There is no drug available that is specifically indicated for the treatment of hirsutism in the United States. Cyproterone acetate is not available here because it is deemed too difficult and too expensive for use in the necessary clinical trials. It has been used primarily in Europe, Canada, and other places in the world and has been shown to be efficacious.

Large doses are usually used, as in this study, 100 mg, and both spironolactone and CPA regimens included estrogen. With CPA, the reverse sequential regimen was used in which ethinyl estradiol was given after CPA. With spironolactone, oral contraceptives were used, primarily Triphasil. Birth control pills are added to the spironolactone regimen in the United States almost empirically and often to straighten out the menstrual disturbances that can occur.

The net result was not different with regard to the efficacy of these treatments, and both were beneficial (see Fig 1–7). This is not of tremendous surprise but is very reassuring for those of us who only have spironolactone and oral contraceptives available to treat this disorder. Cyproterone acetate and spironolactone are very similar; in fact, spironolactone causes greater inhibition of the androgen receptor in fibroblast cell culture. Another important point, as shown here is that at least 6 months are required before the true benefit is demonstrated. Many patients who have stopped using medications before 6 months will have thought that the treatment was inadequate.—R.A. Lobo, M.D.

Acanthosis Nigricans, Insulin Action, and Hyperandrogenism: Clinical, Histological, and Biochemical Findings

Dunaif A, Green G, Phelps RG, Lebwohl M, Futterweit W, Lewy L (Mount Sinai School of Medicine, New York)

J Clin Endocrinol Metab 73:590–595, 1991 1–21

Background.—Acanthosis nigricans (AN), a skin lesion that clinically appears brown, is characterized histologically by hyperkeratosis and papillomatosis. Patients often have variable hyperpigmentation. Acanthosis nigricans occurs in 5% to 50% of hyperandrogenic women and is associated with the presence and severity of hyperinsulinemia. The actual histologic prevalence of AN and its relationship to sex hormone levels and insulin action were studied.

Methods.—Groups of obese and lean healthy women and women with the polycystic ovary (PCO) syndrome were studied. Insulin-mediated glucose disposal was determined by the euglycemic clamp technique. Neck or axillary skin biopsy specimens were graded blindly for the presence and severity of AN in the women with PCO syndrome and their age-matched controls.

Results.—Acanthosis nigricans was found during clinical examination of 11 of 13 obese women with PCO syndrome and 3 of 6 lean women with PCO syndrome. It was also found in 4 of the 14 obese healthy women, but in none of the lean healthy women. Histologically, AN was present in all obese women with PCO syndrome and in 5 of 6 lean women with PCO syndrome. It was also present histologically in 13 of the 14 obese healthy women and in 1 of the 4 lean healthy women. The histologic severity of AN was most strongly correlated with insulin-mediated glucose disposal rather than fasting or glucose-stimulated insulin levels. Dehydroepiandrosterone sulfate was the only sex steroid correlated with histologic AN.

Conclusions.—Clinical skin examination appears to be insensitive for detecting AN. The best biochemical correlate of histologic AN is reduced insulin action. Acanthosis nigricans is a common epiphenomenon of insulin resistance. Its clinical presence should not be used as a criterion for stratifying hyperandrogenic women.

▶ Dunaif and others have characterized AN and its relationship to insulin resistance in a number of studies. An extension of this work, presented here, suggests that AN is extremely common, but clinically it is not always possible to discern its presence. On histologic examination, however, even obese "normal" women had evidence of AN. This suggests not only that it occurs with high frequency in a normal population, but also that it is highly correlated with insulin resistance, as suggested by the findings here using the euglycemic clamp. Of some interest also is that the only steroid that correlated with these responses was dehydroepiandrosterone sulfate, which, although it often shows a reciprocal relationship with insulin action, suggests further that adrenal androgen excess may be condition frequently associated with the findings of AN. Stressed in this paper and previously is that AN is an epiphenomenon that does not have prognostic significance and cannot by itself suggest the presence or absence of insulin resistance or other abnormalities related to hyperandrogenism.—R.A. Lobo, M.D.

Suppression of Circulating Δ^4-Androstenedione and Dehydroepiandrosterone Sulfate During Oral Glucose Tolerance Test in Normal Females

Hubert GD, Schriock ED, Givens JR, Buster JE (Univ of Tennessee, Memphis)

J Clin Endocrinol Metab 73:781–784, 1991 1–22

Background.—Increasing fasting insulin levels (>287 pmol/L) were associated with decreased dehydroepiandrosterone (DHEA) production in a recent study of women with polycystic ovarian syndrome and acanthosis nigricans. It was hypothesized that physiologic insulinemia after the oral administration of glucose suppresses circulating levels of DHEA, dehydroepiandrosterone sulfate (DHEA-S), and androstenedione (Δ^4A) in normal women.

Methods.—Seven normal-weight, ovulatory women were studied during the follicular phase of the menstrual cycle. The women were randomly assigned to receive either a standard 75-g glucose dose or sham (distilled water). Blood samples were obtained during the 3 hours after ingestion.

Results.—Oral glucose-induced insulinemia significantly suppressed DHEA-S levels below those in sham controls at 90 minutes and 120 minutes, and Δ^4A levels at 60, 90, and 120 minutes. Furthermore, there was a significant inverse linear relationship between insulin level and DHEA-S and Δ^4A levels. Neither DHEA, testosterone, nor cortisol levels were suppressed below sham levels at any time during the study.

Conclusion.—Endogenous insulinemia after oral glucose ingestion in normal women resulted in significant DHEA-S and Δ^4A suppression without testosterone and cortisol suppression. It is possible that, as serum insulin increases to very high physiologic or supraphysiologic levels, decreased adrenal androgen production and increased metabolic clearance suppress DHEA-S and Δ^4A levels.

▶ This interesting paper is abstracted just to bring the reader's attention to the reciprocal relationship that is found between insulin and DHEA. This paper shows that in normal women of normal body weight, an insulin increase results in a reduction in adrenal androgen secretion of DHEA and androstenedione. Previous studies in men have suggested that the administration of DHEA increases insulin sensitivity and reduces fasting insulin levels. This reciprocal relationship is somewhat perturbed in different types of hyperandrogenic patients (e.g., those with polycystic ovarian syndrome) who may have a dysregulation of this axis, although this is not a universal finding. However, DHEA is itself an extremely interesting steroid that has been thought to have both immunologic as well as metabolic effects that improve cardiovascular health. One of the ramifications of this work is that the metabolic consequences of insulin may be compensated for by a servo control mechanism via DHEA in normal individuals.—R.A. Lobo, M.D.

A Direct Effect of Hyperinsulinemia on Serum Sex Hormone-Binding Globulin Levels in Obese Women With the Polycystic Ovary Syndrome

Nestler JE, Powers LP, Matt DW, Steingold KA, Plymate SR, Rittmaster RS, Clore JN, Blackard WG (Med College of Virginia/Virginia Commonwealth Univ, Richmond, Madigan Army Med Ctr, Tacoma, Wash; Halifax Infirmary, Halifax, NS, Canada)

J Clin Endocrinol Metab 72:83–89, 1991 1–23

Background.—Polycystic ovary (PCO) syndrome, characterized by menstrual dysfunction, hirsutism, infertility, obesity, and polycystic ovaries, is poorly understood. The frequency of obesity is high, and insulin resistance with hyperinsulinemia occurs in both obese and nonobese women who have PCO syndrome. Hyperinsulinemia reduces serum sex hormone-binding globulin (SHBG) levels. Whether hyperinsulinemia can directly reduce serum SHBG levels in obese women with PCO syndrome was determined.

Methods.—Ovarian steroid production was suppressed in each of 6 women by the administration of 7.5 mg of leuprolide depot, a long-acting gonadotropin-releasing hormone agonist, 56 and 28 days before study and on the day the study was begun. While continuing leuprolide therapy, the women were given diazoxide, 300 mg/day orally for 10 days, to suppress serum insulin levels.

Results.—Initial leuprolide therapy resulted in substantial decreases in serum levels of testosterone, non–SHBG-bound testosterone, androstenedione, estrone, estradiol, and progesterone. There was no change in serum SHBG levels. Diazoxide therapy was associated with suppressed insulin release during a 100-g oral glucose tolerance test and glucose tolerance deterioration. Combined diazoxide and leuprolide treatment had no effect on the serum testosterone, androstenedione, estrone, estradiol, or progesterone levels. However, serum SHBG levels increased by 32% from 17.8 nmol/L on the first study day to 23.5 nmol/L on the tenth day. Primarily because of the rise in serum SHBG, serum non–SHBG-bound testosterone levels dropped by 43% from 19 pmol/L on the first day of the study to 11 pmol/L on the tenth day.

Conclusions.—Coupled with previous findings, these observations suggest that hyperinsulinemia can produce hyperandrogenism in obese women with PCO syndrome. It does this through dual mechanisms—stimulation of ovarian androgen production and a direct effect to reduce serum SHBG levels. Treatments aimed at reducing the magnitude of hyperinsulinemic insulin resistance in women with PCO syndrome may therefore ameliorate their hyperandrogenism. This may account for why weight loss is associated with a decrease in serum androgen levels and clinical manifestations of hyperandrogenism in patients with PCO syndrome.

▶ There used to be a theory that SHBG was central to the pathophysiology of PCO syndrome. The reduction in SHBG led to an increase in free androgen, heightening the hyperandrogenism of PCO syndrome and resulting in free estrogen, which contributes to the elevated level of luteinizing hormone. In this study the authors used diazoxide, a drug often given in treatment of malignant hypertension, to decrease insulin. The pharmacologic nature of this report makes any interpretation a little more tenuous. However, their use of diazoxide did not appear to affect other hormone levels. By lowering the insulin level in this way, the authors noted an increase in SHBG and a decrease in unbound testosterone of 43%. Although not specifically studied, probably a reduction in free estradiol occurred as well.

The authors point out the analogy between this type of approach and the successful results achieved by diet restriction. Not mentioned in this report is the close correlation between these types of interactions and changes in insulin-like growth factor-1 (IGF-1) and IGF-1 binding protein as studied by Kiddy. Acute dieting in women with PCO syndrome resulted not only in an increase in SHBG, as noted here, but also an increase in IGF binding protein, therefore attenuating the effects of IGF on ovarian androgen production. Clearly, dieting that achieves a lowering of the insulin level would be extremely important in patients with PCO syndrome. In hyperinsulinemia, insulin is also linked with tryglyceride and other lipoprotein abnormalities. However, until we can selectively decrease insulin pharmacologically or find an easy way for patients to diet, we will not observe these types of results.—R.A. Lobo, M.D.

Gestational Diabetes and Neonatal Macrosomia in the Polycystic Ovary Syndrome

Wortsman J, de Angeles S, Futterweit W, Singh KB, Kaufmann RC (Southern Illinois Univ, Springfield; Mount Sinai School of Medicine, New York; Louisiana State Univ, Shreveport)

J Reprod Med 36:659–661, 1991 1–24

Background.—The polycystic ovary (PCO) syndrome is a disorder of ovarian function characterized by menstrual irregularities, infertility, and androgenization. Peripheral resistance to insulin is common in patients with PCO syndrome, and they have higher insulin levels than normal, matched controls. During pregnancy, these patients may be at particular risk for gestational diabetes. The clinical records of patients with PCO syndrome who had successful pregnancies were reviewed with regard to gestational diabetes.

Methods.—The glucose tolerance in 53 pregnant patients with PCO syndrome from 2 centers was compared with that in a control population of 2306 consecutive normal pregnancies. Most of the patients with PCO syndrome had received fertility-promoting agents.

Findings.—The incidence of gestational diabetes among the patients was 7.5% compared to an incidence in the control population of 6.6%. The only congenital malformation observed in the group with PCO syndrome occurred in a patient who did not have gestational diabetes. The mean birth weight of the 57 neonates born to the patients with PCO syndrome was similar to that of the control infants. Neonatal macrosomia (birth weight ± 4,000 g at birth) was present in 7% of infants born to women with PCO syndrome, 12.4% in the control women with normal glucose tolerance tests, and 14.5% in control women with gestational diabetes. These differences were not statistically significant.

Conclusions.—Contrary to expected results, there was a normal incidence of gestational diabetes and/or neonatal macrosomia among pregnant women with PCO syndrome, regardless of the diabetogenic potential of their underlying disorder. The preexistence of polycystic ovaries does not increase the risk of gestational diabetes or neonatal macrosomia.

▶ Whereas this paper would seem to be reassuring, I need to raise a word of caution. Polycystic ovarian syndrome is extremely heterogeneous. There is no evidence that the patients in this report had insulin resistance. Insulin resistance is very prevalent in patients with PCO syndrome but varies depending on the patient population. The complications during pregnancy (e.g., preeclampsia and prematurity) and the stillborn rate are all increased in patients with PCO syndrome. Also, in some of these patients hyperinsulinemia is associated with hyperglycemia and frank glucose intolerance. Patients with glucose intolerance enter pregnancy in a prediabetic state to begin with. Screening of patients for this potential complication before pregnancy is imperative. Nevertheless, to patients who have no evidence of this, and specifically to those who do not have insulin resistance, this paper is reassuring and suggests that the incidence of complications related to gestational diabetes is no greater than that in other patients. However, one needs to individualize management because these patients are at risk for a number of complications of pregnancy.—R.A. Lobo, M.D.

Insulin Resistance: An Early Metabolic Defect of Turner's Syndrome

Caprio S, Boulware S, Diamond M, Sherwin RS, Carpenter TO, Rubin K, Amiel S, Press M, Tamborlane WV (Yale Univ)

J Clin Endocrinol Metab 72:832–836, 1991 1–25

Introduction.—Carbohydrate intolerance and non–insulin-dependent diabetes mellitus are common in women with Turner's syndrome. It is not clear whether the response to insulin is altered in young patients with Turner's syndrome and normal glucose homeostasis.

Study Design.—Two groups of nondiabetic patients with Turner's syndrome and age-matched normal controls were studied to assess whether insulin resistance is an early metabolic alteration of Turner's syndrome. Group 1 included 8 young children (mean age, 10 years) who had never received hormone therapy, and group 2 included 5 older patients (mean age, 17.6 years) who had been or were currently receiving estrogen therapy. Insulin sensitivity was assessed by using the euglycemic insulin clamp technique. Whole body glucose and lipid oxidation were assessed by indirect calorimetry. In addition, group 2 patients received [3-^{3}H] glucose during the euglycemic clamp to assess hepatic sensitivity to insulin.

Findings.—Despite comparable increases in plasma insulin levels during insulin infusion, glucose utilization was significantly reduced in both groups of patients with Turner's syndrome compared with controls. Insulin infusion produced a similar increase in the rate of oxidative glucose metabolism in the patients and in controls, but the rate of nonoxidative glucose disposal was profoundly impaired in the patients with Turner's syndrome. Insulin-induced suppression of hepatic glucose production and plasma free fatty acid was similar in the patients and controls.

Conclusion.—Insulin resistance appears to be a very early metabolic alteration in Turner's syndrome and apparently is not caused by estrogen replacement. The insulin resistance involves nonoxidative pathways of glucose metabolism and may likely predispose adults with Turner's syndrome to the subsequent development of non–insulin-dependent diabetes mellitus.

▶ Just as we have seen that there are alterations in bone mass in Turner's syndrome, this paper discusses the high incidence of type 2 or adult-onset diabetes in these patients. The finding of insulin resistance and type 2 diabetes is extremely important because of its associated excessive cardiovascular mortality as well as morbidity. This paper suggests that there is a tissue defect in patients with Turner's syndrome that makes them more vulnerable to the development of insulin resistance. The observation that this defect was not induced by estrogen replacement, which was used in some of the patients, is an old concept. Insulin resistance has not been shown to occur with moderate estrogen replacement. Indeed, there is evidence for the opposite—that there is improvement in glucose tolerance and improvement of insulin action with physiologic levels of estrogen replacement.

Nevertheless, high doses of estrogen that are supraphysiologic can induce a state of insulin resistance. These data clearly suggest, however, that a basic defect in the tissues of patients with Turner's syndrome makes them more vulnerable to insulin resistance, which again can be related to problems of insulin-like growth factor (IGF) and IGF binding protein, similar to the inherent problem of bone mass discussed in Abstract 1–30. The authors link this defect to the inherent genetic or chromosomal aberration of Turner's syndrome. Whereas this is, strictly speaking, most likely to be the case, other associated defects (e.g., deficiencies of growth hormone and the IGF system) could be specifically implicated as well. The take-home message here is that estrogen therapy in low to moderate doses is clearly indicated in these patients, and they should be followed closely to detect glucose intolerance.—R.A. Lobo, M.D.

Altered Testicular Hormone Production in Infertile Patients With Idiopathic Oligoasthenospermia

Scaglia HE, Carrere CA, Mariani VA, Zylbersztein CC, Rey-Valzacchi GJ, Kelly EE, Aquilano DR (Centro de Especialistas en Analisis Biologicos Distrito I; Inst of Andrology and Assisted Reproduction, La Plata, Argentina)

J Androl 12:273–280, 1991 1–26

Background.—Because little is known about the testicular hormone response to human chorionic gonadotropin (hCG) in men with idiopathic infertility, the dynamics of this response were assessed. Possible altered testicular hormone production was examined in patients with idiopathic oligoasthenospermia or asthenospermia.

Methods.—Sixty patients with oligoasthenospermia or asthenospermia and 10 healthy men participated in the study. The responses of testosterone, androstenedione, 17 OH-progesterone (17OHP), and estradiol were examined.

Findings.—The responses of testosterone, androstenedione, and 17OHP to hCG in the control group showed a biphasic pattern, with the first peak at 4 hours and the second after 24 hours. The estradiol response peaked once between 24 and 48 hours after hCG was administered. Patients had 2 types of testosterone responses. In 40 patients (group 1) there was no first peak; in 20 patients (group 2) the response pattern was normal. The androstenedione response was similar to the testosterone response; the estradiol response was normal in both groups. The 17OHP responses in group 1 were either high, low, or normal. However, the 17OHP response was normal in group 2. Aromatase inhibitor treatment in group 1 improved the acute testosterone response only in patients with a high or normal 17OHP response to hCG. The treatment had no effect in patients with a low 17OHP response. In group 2, aromatase inhibitors did not affect the testosterone response.

Conclusions.—Some patients with oligoasthenospermia or asthenospermia have altered testicular hormone production. Evidence of 2 enzyme blocks was found in this study: 1 at the 17,20 desmolase level, mediated by estradiol, and 1 at early biosynthetic steps, not mediated by estradiol.

▶ Most investigators have suggested that testicular hormone production is invariably normal in men with abnormal spermatogenesis of unknown etiology. This study presents data to show that this might not be the case. More studies are warranted.—C.A. Paulsen, M.D.

The Endocrine Effects of Long-Term Treatment With Mifepristone (RU 486)

Lamberts SWJ, Koper JW, de Jong FH (Erasmus Univ, Rotterdam)
J Clin Endocrinol Metab 73:187–191, 1991 1–27

Background.—Mifepristone (RU 486) has powerful progesterone activity, but it also has glucocorticoid receptor-blocking activity with no agonist effects on these receptors. The effect of RU 486 on the growth of meningiomas, which contain many high-affinity progesterone receptors but not estradiol receptors, have been studied previously. The endocrine effects of long-term RU 486 treatment in patients with meningioma were investigated.

Methods.—The patients were 7 women and 3 men with 1 or more meningiomas; only 1 of the women was premenopausal. Patients received RU 486, 200 mg/day, for 1 year. Prednisone, 7.5 mg/day, was added if side effects or signs of relative adrenocortical insufficiency developed. Patients were evaluated every 2 or 3 weeks for the first 3 months and every 2 months thereafter; hormone levels were measured at least 4 times during treatment.

Findings.—At the beginning of treatment, most patients had some nausea, vomiting, and/or tiredness, but this usually resolved after 2 weeks. Four patients needed prednisone to alleviate these side effects. These same patients also had the most rapid activation of the hypothalamic-pituitary-adrenal axis, as reflected by increased circulating cortisol levels and urinary cortisol excretion. The latter parameter doubled at 2 days, peaked at 3 weeks, and remained at peak levels for 12 months. In general, the hypothalamic-pituitary-adrenal axis was reset at a higher level. Patients' diurnal rhythm and responsiveness to corticotropin-releasing hormone were maintained, but they had diminished sensitivity to dexamethasone. Androstenedione and estradiol production increased significantly as a result.

Conclusions.—Mifepristone therapy induces partial cortisol receptor resistance, resulting in a variety of endocrine changes. Compensatory androgen overproduction, and resulting estrogen overproduction, might limit the usefulness of long-term RU 486 therapy as a single treatment for estrogen-dependent tumors.

▶ RU 486 has received much notoriety as of late because of its abortifacient effect in women. However, this very interesting compound is useful in a variety of other conditions. It has the propensity not only to bind the progestin receptor, but also the corticosteroid receptor. In this study the focus was on the long-term use of RU 486 for other medical indications. Indeed, for abortion induction doses of 400–600 mg are used; in this series, however, only 200 mg of RU 486 was given in the treatment of meningioma. It is not my intent to discuss meningiomas, which were targeted for treatment with RU 486 because they contain progestin receptors. Of interest here is the fact that because RU486 does have antiglucocorticord activity, it could be of benefit for patients with Cushing's syndrome as well as for women with breast cancer and those with premenstrual syndrome. All of these conditions require long-term treatment.

This year-long study noted that adrenal insufficiency occurred quite commonly, and that prednisone supplementation was needed both in men and women. A compensatory increase in the adrenocorticotropic hormone drive occurred, with an increase therefore of adrenal androgens, which were not blocked. The androgen is aromatized to estrogen, compounding the problem by the development of both androgen and estrogen excess along with glucocorticoid suppression, which required prednisone. These data suggest that long-term therapy is not without some complications. For breast cancer, if RU 486 therapy was deemed to be efficacious, it would be possible to add to the regimen an aromatase inhibitor such as 4-OH androstenedione. The final answer will come with the use of the next generation of compounds like RU 486, which have more specificity in terms of steroid receptors.—R.A. Lobo, M.D.

Successful Treatment of Severe Premenstrual Syndrome by Combined Use of Gonadotropin-Releasing Hormone Agonist and Estrogen/Progestin

Mortola JF, Girton L, Fischer U (Univ of California, San Diego, La Jolla)

J Clin Endocrinol Metab 71:252A–252F, 1991 1–28

Introduction.—The dosage of estrogen and progestin used in postmenopausal treatment appears to be sufficient to obviate the effects after gonadotropin-releasing hormone (GnRH) agonist treatment, and may be less than that needed to recreate symptoms of the premenstrual syndrome (PMS). The effects of estrogen/progestin replacements on the symptomatic improvement obtained with a GnRH agonist were investigated in 8 women with severe PMS.

Methods.—Using the Calendar of Premenstrual Experiences, the pa tients kept a daily record of their symptoms during the 9-month study period. After 2 cycles, which served as controls, the GnRH agonist Histrelin, 100 μg/day, was administered subcutaneously for 2 months. The GnRH agonist was given for an additional 4 months, during which exogenous steroids were replaced, respectively, by conjugated equine estrogen (CEE), .625 mg, on days 1–25; medroxyprogesterone acetate (MPA), 10 mg, on days 16–25; CEE on days 1–25; plus MPA on days 16–25; and

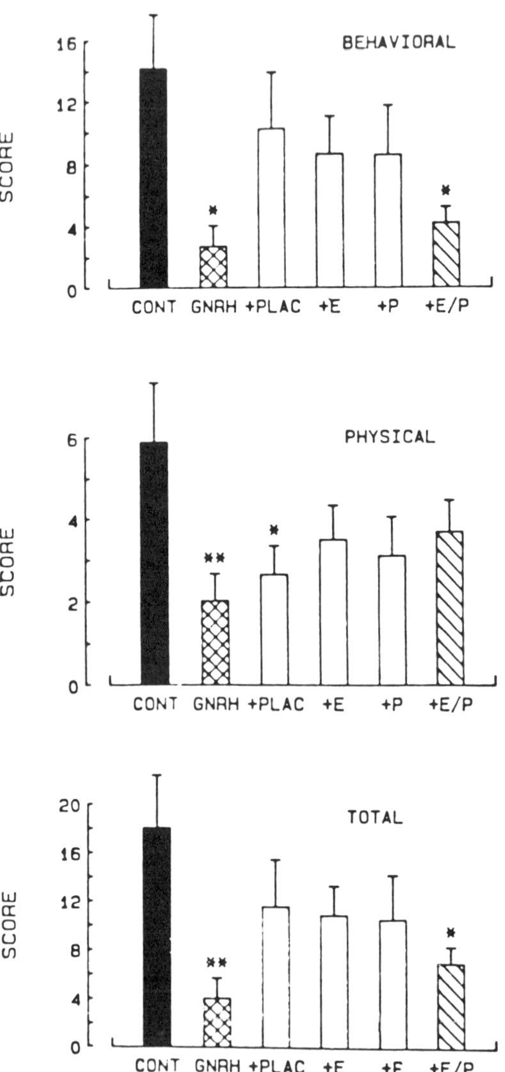

Fig 1–8.—Mean (±SE) daily luteal phase scores on the COPE for physical, behavioral, and total symptoms in 8 women with severe PMS during control months *(CONT)*, during the corresponding time interval of the second month of treatment with GnRH-a *(GNRH)* alone, and during months in which GnRH-a was simultaneously administered with placebo for both CEE and MPA *(PLAC)*, CEE (days 1–25) plus placebo for MPA *(E)*, placebo for CEE plus MPA (days 16–25; *P*), and the combination of CEE on days 1–25 and MPA on days 16–25 *(E/P)*. *, $P < .05$; **, $P < .01$. (Courtesy of Mortola JF, Girton L, Fischer U: *J Clin Endocrinol Metab* 71:252A–252F, 1991.)

placebo alone. The study was done in a randomized, double-blind, placebo-controlled, crossover fashion.

Results.—Unblinded administration of the GnRH agonist resulted in a 75% improvement in luteal phase symptom scores. When placebo was added, reductions in symptom scores were maintained, but behavioral symptom scores were not. The addition of either CEE or MPA did not change the scores significantly. The addition of both CEE and MPA improved simulated luteal phase scores by more than 60% of behavioral and total symptoms (Fig 1–8). There was a reduction in physical symptom scores with all treatments, with no significant differences among the various combinations.

Conclusion.—The GnRH agonist markedly reduces symptoms of PMS; however, the addition of placebo results in a return of behavioral symptoms. Neither replacement doses of CEE nor MPA induce symptoms in predisposed patients. The severity of total luteal phase symptoms continues to be reduced only when both CEE and MPA are added to the GnRH agonist. This regimen is the first safe and effective method to obtain the beneficial effects of a GnRH agonist in patients with PMS.

▶ Premenstrual syndrome is an extremely difficult condition to treat. Some of the problem arises in that not all symptoms encountered during the menstrual cycle reflect PMS. Careful detailed diaries have to be kept before the diagnosis can be made accurately. The approach in this report is something worth trying in patients with severe PMS. The GnRH agonist has proved to be extremely useful in this disorder. This small study by Mortola et al. shows that add-back therapy in terms of estrogen plus progestin reduces symptomatology substantially; also, luteal scores are reduced by 60% (Fig 1–8). Somewhat of a surprise to me was that, at least in this small study, the combination of estrogen and progestin was even better than estrogen alone. I would have thought that the use of estrogen alone would have been of benefit, and that adding progestin might worsen the symptomatology, which often is the case in postmenopausal women given such therapy. Obviously, this is a small study; larger series using different regimens are needed to confirm the findings. I would suggest that if sequential progestin therapy is used, small doses might be considered.—R.A. Lobo, M.D.

Lack of Bone Accretion and Amenorrhea: Evidence for a Relative Osteopenia in Weight-Bearing Bones

Warren MP, Brooks-Gunn J, Fox RP, Lancelot C, Newman D, Hamilton WG (St Luke's-Roosevelt Hosp, New York; Educational Testing Service, Princeton, NJ)

J Clin Endocrinol Metab 72:847–853, 1991 1–29

Introduction.—The role of estrogen deficiency in the development of osteopenia in bone stressed by activity and the potential for injury in this setting have not been evaluated. The effects of amenorrhea and exercise (dancing) on bone mineral density (BMD) were evaluated in young exercising amenorrheic girls to determine whether bone density is compromised and what changes are related to injury.

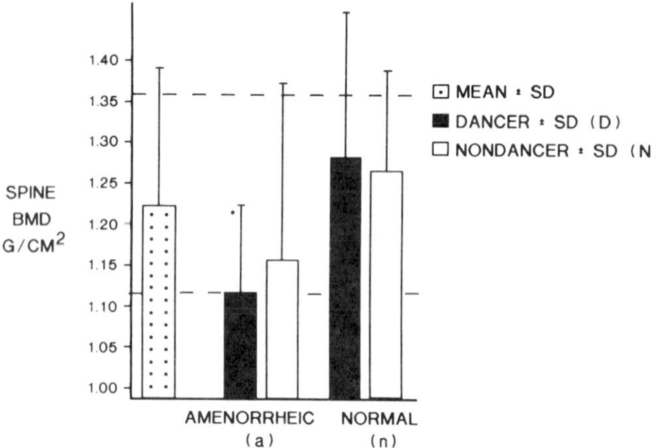

Fig 1–9.—Spine bone mineral densities in normal and amenorrheic subjects. Groups are divided into dancers and nondancers. Significance determined by ANOVA. $P < .05$. *Stippled bar,* mean of all values. Two-way ANOVA shows a significant effect of amenorrhea on BMD even when controlling for age but was eliminated by controlling for weight. (Courtesy of Warren MP, Brooks-Gunn J, Fox RP, et al: *J Clin Endocrinol Metab* 72:847–853, 1991.)

Study Design.—Enrolled in a cross-sectional study were 51 professional ballet dancers and 47 nondancers 9 (controls) whose mean age was 22 years. Dancers and controls were further subdivided into normally cycling and amenorrheic individuals.

Findings.—Amenorrhea significantly lowered the BMD in the spine, wrist, and metatarsal. All of these effects of amenorrhea were eliminated by controlling for weight; the effects on the wrist, but not on the spine and metatarsal, also were eliminated by age. There was significant interaction between amenorrhea and dancing on the BMD of the metatarsal, a weight-bearing bone (Fig 1–9). Dancing was associated with a further lowering of BMD; this interaction was eliminated after controlling for age but not after controlling for weight. Multiple comparisons of the groups showed that spine, wrist, and metatarsal BMD was significantly lower in amenorrheic dancers compared with normal dancers, even after controlling for age and weight in the metatarsal and for age in the spine. Estradiol levels correlated with BMD of the wrist and spine in both groups, but correlated with metatarsal density only in the dancers. Age at menarche was the only variable to predict stress fractures.

Conclusion.—Amenorrhea significantly affects BMD, but these effects are highly dependent on weight. The exercise-induced increase in bone mass in stressed bones (e.g., the metatarsal in dancers) is compromised in amenorrheic premenopausal women, even after controlling for weight. This effect may be age and estrogen dependent. A delay in menarche may affect the development of a normal skeletal mass, putting these individuals at risk for injury.

▶ This is a somewhat complex paper to interpret because of the multiple interactions that are operative. The importance of bringing this to the attention of readers is the fact that 40% of the skeletal mass in women is attained during adolescence. The age of menarche, if delayed, could potentially lead to problems in attainment of this peak bone mass, particularly if there are problems associated with bone remodeling at the time of adolescence. Bone mineral density was significantly affected by amenorrhea, yet this variable was also highly related to body weight. The greatest reduction in bone mass occurred in the amenorrheic dancers, who only had 87% of ideal body weight. If a bone is stressed by exercise, there is a compensatory increase in bone mass. Therefore, the metatarsal bones, which are stressed through ballet dancing, usually have an increased bone mass, but this was not the case for amenorrheic dancers (see Fig 1–9).

The real take-home message here is that, because peak bone mass in women occurs by about age 30, it is very important not to jeopardize the time of maximum bone mass attainment during adolescence; a low bone mass would lead subsequently to an increased risk of osteoporosis. Strategies to increase bone mass in athletic amenorrheic women are necessary. Two important variables that bring about an increased bone mass are increases in body weight and the individual's estrogen status. Weight gain may be something that athletes are not willing to accept; clearly, however, euestrogenism and attainment of a normal endocrine status could go a long way in preventing stress fractures and achieving more normal MBD.—R.A. Lobo, M.D.

Normal Bone Density of the Wrist and Spine and Increased Wrist Fractures in Girls With Turner's Syndrome

Ross JL, Long LM, Feuillan P, Cassorla F, Cutler GB Jr (Med College of Pennsylvania, Philadelphia; Natl Inst of Child Health and Human Development, Bethesda, Md)

J Clin Endocrinol Metab 73:355–359, 1991 1–30

Background.—Many skeletal abnormalities, including osteoporosis, are associated with Turner's syndrome. Girls with Turner's syndrome may have deficient bone density before the expected age of puberty.

Methods.—The bone mineral content of the wrist and lumbar spine in 78 girls with Turner's syndrome aged 4–13 years was compared with that of 28 normal prepubertal girls similar in age, bone age, body mass index, and height age. Bone mineral content was determined by both single-photon and dual-photon absorptiometry.

Results.—Single-photon absorptiometry values in the group with Turner's syndrome were lower than those in normal girls matched for age, bone age, and body mass index, but not for height age. Dual-photon absorptiometry values in the group with Turner's syndrome were lower than those in the controls matched for age and body mass index but not for bone age or height age. The annual incidence of wrist fracture among the girls with Turner's syndrome was significantly greater than that reported rate for normal children.

Conclusions.—Prepubertal girls with Turner's syndrome who are younger than age 13 years have normal bone density for their height age

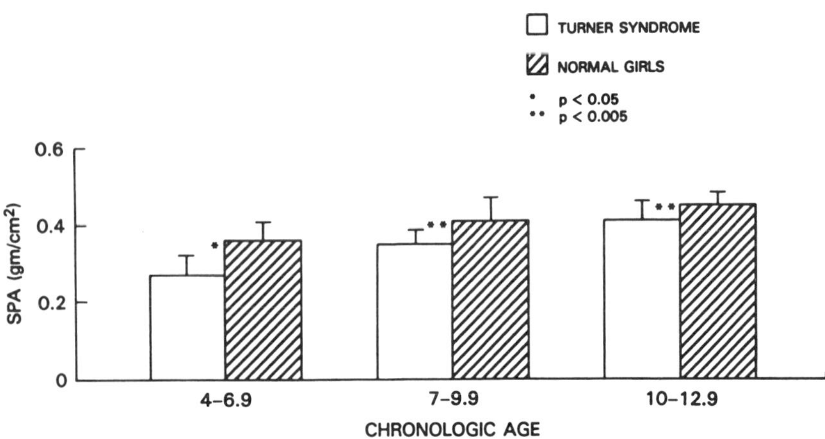

Fig 1–10.—Bone density of the wrist (SPA) in girls with Turner's syndrome and in age-matched prepubertal normal girls. (Courtesy of Ross JL, Long LM, Feuillan P, et al: *J Clin Endocrinol Metab* 73:355–359, 1991.)

but significantly reduced bone density of the wrist for chronological age, bone age, and body mass index (Fig 1–10). These girls also sustain significantly more wrist fractures than normal girls. Whether this is related to bone density is not clear.

▶ This title is somewhat deceptive. Bone mass was not actually normal in these individuals (see Fig 1–10). It was normal for height, which in Turner's patients is typically short, but the bone density was decreased for age and bone mass. There was clearly an increase in the wrist fracture rate, which was 9.1/1000 compared to 3.5/1000 in the general population. Also, there was a significant rate of scoliosis, occurring in 8 of 78 of these patients compared to 1 in 19 in a normal population. The interesting observation in this report, however, is the evidence of a dissociation between the findings of bone mass and the increased fracture rate. Therefore, the integrity of the bone is suspect. The integrity of bone in patients with Turner's syndrome may be somewhat different. This brings up issues of bone matrix and collagen support, which may be influenced by growth factors. This could be related to insulin-like growth factor-1, which has a direct effect on bone. Tissue defects in patients with Turner's syndrome is a concept that is explored further in Abstract 1–25. Clearly, the message in this report is that there are more subtle defects in Turner's syndrome that go beyond the known estrogen deficiency of these patients.—R.A. Lobo, M.D.

Vascular Resistance of Uterine Arteries: Physiological Effects of Estradiol and Progesterone

de Ziegler D, Bessis R, Frydman R (Hôpital A. Béclère, Clamart, France; Centre d'Echographie de l'Odéon, Paris)

Fertil Steril 55:775–779, 1991 1–31

Background.—Transvaginal pulsed Doppler and ultrasound imaging of pelvic structures has facilitated studies of uterine blood flow. Doppler studies of uterine arteries have detected a decrease in vascular resistance during early pregnancy. The exact role of physiologic levels of estrogen on the vascular resistance of human uterine arteries is unknown, but plasma estradiol (E_2) appears to have an effect. The role of reproductive hormones on the vascular resistance of uterine arteries was studied in 6 young women.

Methods.—The women, who had no or nonfunctioning ovaries, received transdermal E_2 and vaginal progesterone after a 28-day replacement regimen duplicating E_2 and progesterone levels seen in the menstrual cycle. Transvaginal pulsed Doppler and real-time imaging were used to evaluate vascular resistance of the uterine arteries before treatment and on days 13–14 and 26–27. The Doppler waveforms were analyzed by the pulsatility index (PI).

Results.—Baseline evaluation of the vascular resistance of uterine arteries showed narrow systolic Doppler flow waves with or without diastolic flow signal, indicative of elevated vascular resistance. On cycle day 13, the Doppler waveforms showed changes indicative of a profound decrease in vascular resistance, which was reflected by a significant decrease in the PI. Doppler measurements on days 26–27 showed no significant change.

Conclusions.—In the absence of ovarian hormone, uterine arteries have a high degree of vascular resistance, expressed by narrow systolic Doppler flow waves and high PI values. When plasma E_2 is elevated to menstrual cycle levels, modification of the Doppler flow pattern suggests a marked decrease in vascular resistance. At physiologic levels, E_2 affects the vascular resistance of uterine arteries. This estrogenic effect may be a valuable reflector of the biological efficacy of various estrogenic treatments.

▶ This is an extremely interesting study on the effects of estradiol on the systemic resistance of arteries in hypoestrogenic women. This study was conducted in young women primarily with premature ovarian failure. Although the age range was 27–36, we believe an analogy can be drawn between these patients and older postmenopausal patients. Also, this regimen was adopted for synchronizing uterine development for ovum donation and used high dosages of transdermal estrogen (from .1 mg to .4 mg), followed with physiologic replacement of vaginal progesterone. The PI, a marker of resistance, declined significantly, suggesting increased uterine blood flow. With estrogen therapy the PI went from 5.2 down to 1.3, a significant and important finding. Of interest, with natural progesterone and "physiologic" replacement in the late luteal phase, the PI increased slightly from 1.3 to about 1.7, suggesting that physiologic replacement of progesterone may not substantially attenuate blood flow. This has not been the experience with the use of more potent progestins in postmenopausal women. Also note that total estrogen delivery was higher than the normal replacement doses used in postmenopausal women. This study also illustrates the importance of the nonhepatic (lipoprotein-mediated) benefits of estrogen on the cardiovascular system.— R.A. Lobo, M.D.

Calcium Supplementation Reduces Vertebral Bone Loss in Perimenopausal Women: A Controlled Trial in 248 Women Between 46 and 55 Years of Age

Elders PJM, Netelenbos JC, Lips P, van Ginkel FC, Khoe E, Leeuwenkamp OR, Hackeng WHL, van der Stelt PF (Academisch Ziekenhuis Vrije Universiteit, Amsterdam; Academisch Centrum Tandhelelkunde Amsterdam; Bergwegziekenhuis, Rotterdam)

J Clin Endocrinol Metab 73:533–540, 1991 1–32

Background.—Calcium supplementation for the prevention of osteoporosis remains controversial. The effect of calcium supplementation on perimenopausal bone loss was further evaluated in a randomized clinical trial.

Methods.—A random sample of 295 women aged 46–55 years were assigned to a control group with no calcium supplementation, or to 1 of 2 supplementation groups receiving 1000 mg and 2000 mg, respectively, of elemental calcium per day for 2 years. Changes in the bone mineral density of the lumbar spine, as measured by dual-photon absorptiometry, combined metacarpal cortical thickness, and biochemical parameters were evaluated.

Outcome.—Lumbar bone loss was significantly reduced in both treatment groups compared with the control group. The mean lumbar bone loss was 1.3% in the group given 1000 mg of calcium and by .7% in the group given 2000 mg, compared with 3.5% in the control group. This treatment effect was significant only in the first year of supplementation, not in the second year. Calcium supplementation did not affect metacarpal cortical bone loss. There was no significant interaction between the menopausal status and the effect of calcium supplements. Calcium supplementation was associated with a significant increase in urinary calcium excretion and significant reductions in the urinary hydroxyproline/creatinine ratio, and serum levels of alkaline phosphatase, osteocalcin, and 1,25-dihydroxyvitamin D. Except for serum osteocalcin, these treatment effects remained significant at the end of the study.

Conclusion.—Calcium supplementation retards lumbar bone mineral loss in perimenopausal women by decreasing bone turnover during the first year of supplementation. The effect of lumbar bone loss after 1 year remains uncertain, although the effects on bone turnover remain apparent over a longer time span.

▶ There remains some controversy about the effectiveness of calcium in preventing bone loss in postmenopausal women, but it is clear that the average diet in the United States is deficient in calcium. Whereas studies have suggested that calcium alone in postmenopausal women is not beneficial for maintaining bone mass, calcium supplementation before the time of menopause may be of benefit if the calcium diet is deficient. Calcium is important for attainment of peak bone mass; the normal rate of bone loss, which occurs even before menopause, may be decreased by calcium supplementation. This study, which was conducted specifically to address this issue, suggests a substantial benefit with both 1000 mg and 2000 mg of supplemental calcium over placebo; the placebo group lost 3.5% of lumbar bone mass within a 2-year period.

Because attainment of peak bone mass and its maintenance are important to the outcome of osteoporosis and affect the fracture rate, it is necessary to ensure that adequate calcium supplementation is carried out. It may be of benefit, therefore, to start increasing calcium in the diet, to the tune of 1000 mg a day, in women in the perimenopausal age group. R.A. Lobo, M.D.

Contrasting Effects of Oral and Transdermal Routes of Estrogen Replacement Therapy on 24-Hour Growth Hormone (GH) Secretion, Insulin-Like Growth Factor I, and GH-Binding Protein in Postmenopausal Women

Weissberger AJ, Ho KKY, Lazarus L (St Vincent's Hosp, Sydney, Australia)

J Clin Endocrinol Metab 72:374–381, 1991 1–33

Introduction.—Estrogen deficiency may account for lower circulating growth hormone (GH) and insulin-like growth factor (IGF-I) concentrations in postmenopausal women. Because the liver is the major source of circulating IGF-1 and orally administered estrogens exert nonphysiologic effects on hepatic protein synthesis, the route of estrogen administration should be an important consideration in studies that test whether estrogen replacement therapy could restore the reduced GH and IGF-1 concentrations in postmenopausal women.

Study Design.—Serum GH over 24 hours and serum IGF-1 levels were measured in 12 postmenopausal women before and after 2 months of cyclical replacement therapy with either oral ethinyl estradiol (EE, 20 μg daily) or transdermal 17β-estradiol (E_2, 100-μg patches applied twice weekly). The results were compared with those in 7 premenopausal women. The extent of GH binding to its serum binding protein also was studied by measuring the percent specific binding of ^{125}I-labeled GH in serum.

Results.—The mean 24-hour serum GH and serum IGF-1 levels were significantly lower in postmenopausal women than in premenopausal women. Despite their comparable suppression in gonadotropins, oral and transdermal estrogen therapy had contrasting effects on the GH/IGF-1 axis. Oral estrogen therapy significantly increased the mean 24-hour serum GH level, mean pulse amplitude, and basal GH concentration, with values significantly exceeding those in premenopausal women. Oral doses of estrogen significantly suppressed circulating IGF-1, with a concomitant increase in the percent specific binding of ^{125}I-labeled GH in serum. However, the derived mean 24-hour free serum GH remained significantly greater than before treatment. In contrast, transdermal E_2 significantly increased serum IGF-1 to levels that were not significantly different from those of premenopausal women but without concomitant increases in the mean 24-hour serum level of GH and changes in the percent specific binding of ^{125}I-labeled GH. Transdermal E_2 restored circulating E_2 levels to the midfollicular range.

Conclusions.—The oral and transdermal routes of administering exogenous estrogen have totally dissimilar effects on the GH/IGF-1 axis. Oral estrogen inhibits hepatic IGF-1 synthesis and increases GH secretion through reduced feedback inhibition. Estrogen deficiency alone cannot account for the reduced GH secretion in postmenopausal women because GH secretion is not restored by attainment of physiologic E_2 concentrations by the transdermal route. The contrasting effects of these routes of estrogen administration on the GH/IGF-1 axis may have long-term therapeutic implications in the menopause (e.g., the effects on the musculoskeletal function and body composition).

▶ Could there be a bimodal effect of estrogen on IGF in postmenopausal women? This paper was selected because of the potential importance of GH and IGF in postmenopausal women with regard to muscular and skeletal support as well as bone mass. An important variable was to study differences between oral and transdermally administered estrogen because postmenopausal women have reduced levels and are perhaps deficient in both GH and IGF. As noted previously, GH is dependent on estrogen. How this relationship translates into biological activity of IGF is still not clear, however, because the circulating forms of IGF have specific binding proteins, both in serum and in various tissues. Nevertheless, if we can extrapolate the data concerning transdermally administered estrogen to suggest that physiologic replacement with natural estradiol increases IGF-1, this certainly correlates with improvement in bone mass in these patients, even though GH and IGF binding protein levels were not significantly altered. I think this is probably the normal effect of estrogen replacement. The other arm of the study used 20 μg of ethinyl estradiol, which I do not believe to be physiologic replacement; in fact, it may be supraphysiologic by about twofold or threefold. Given the consequences of this bolus effect on hepatic protein synthesis, what one notes is suppression of IGF and an increase in the percent of the specific binding. This resulted in an increase in GH as well. It would be interesting to determine whether lower doses of ethinyl estradiol given orally, perhaps 5 μg or perhaps .625 mg of conjugated equine estrogen, will produce the same results.—R.A. Lobo, M.D.

Effects of Postmenopausal Estrogen Replacement on the Concentrations and Metabolism of Plasma Lipoproteins

Walsh BW, Schiff I, Rosner B, Greenberg L, Ravnikar V, Sacks FM (Brigham and Women's Hosp, Boston; Harvard Med School)

N Engl J Med 325:1196–1204, 1991 1–34

Background.—Postmenopausal estrogen-replacement treatment may decrease the risk of cardiovascular disease, an effect that may be mediated partly by favorable changes in plasma lipid levels. The effects on plasma lipoprotein levels of postmenopausal estrogens in the low doses currently used have not been precisely established, nor is the mechanism of these effects known.

Methods.—Two randomized, double-blind, crossover trials were done. Participants were healthy postmenopausal women with normal lipid values at study entry. In the first study, 31 women received placebo and conjugated estrogens at 2 doses, each for 3 months. In the second study, 9 women were given placebo, orally administered micronized estradiol, and transdermally administered estradiol, each for 6 weeks.

Results.—In study 1, conjugated estrogen doses of .625 mg/day and 1.25 mg/day reduced the mean low-density lipoprotein (LDL) cholesterol level by 15% and 19%, respectively. These doses increased the high-density lipoprotein (HDL) cholesterol level by 16% and 18%, respectively. Very-low-density lipoprotein (VLDL) triglyceride levels also were raised by 24% and 42%, respectively. In study 2, orally administered estradiol raised the mean level of large VLDL apolipoprotein B by 30% through increasing its production rate by 82%. Most additional large VLDL was directly cleared from the circulation rather than being converted to small VLDL or LDL. Orally administered estradiol decreased LDL cholesterol levels by 14%, as LDL catabolism rose by 36%. Orally administered estradiol increased HDL cholesterol concentrations by 15%. No changes were associated with transdermally administered estradiol.

Conclusions.—The use of low-dose orally administered estrogens in postmenopausal women favorably affects LDL and HDL levels, which may protect such women against atherosclerosis. It also minimizes potentially adverse effects on triglyceride levels. Accelerated LDL catabolism is responsible for the reduction in LDL levels. The increased triglyceride levels result from higher production of large, triglyceride-rich VLDL.

▶ This extremely interesting and important paper really constitutes 2 studies that have been combined to unify the effects of oral and transdermally supplied estrogen on lipoproteins. This area is important because of the known cardioprotective effects of estrogen; such effects result in a reduction of about 50% in cardiovascular disease mortality in postmenopausal users. The predominant theory until recently has been that changes in the lipoproteins afforded by oral doses of estrogen are responsible for this benefit. It is more clear now that, whereas this benefit is important, there are direct arterial effects as well.

This study focuses on the various routes of administration as well as the mechanisms whereby estrogen alters lipoproteins. First it was noted, using conjugated equine estrogens, that doses of .625 and 1.25 mg produced nearly identical increments of HDL cholesterol. This is at variance with previous studies, which showed a dose-response relationship but were not carried out in a prospective controlled manner, such as the present study was. The second important point is that the triglyceride content of lipoproteins dramatically and significantly increases as the dose of estrogen increases. Because triglycerides may be an independent risk factor for cardiovascular disease, these data would suggest that levels of conjugate equine estrogen should remain at about .625 mg to achieve maximum benefit. Indeed, cardiovascular epidemiologic data would suggest that the cardioprotective benefit is not dose related.

Another important finding of this report is that the mechanism of the reduction in LDL cholesterol, which some view to be even more important than the elevation of HDL cholesterol, results from increased catabolism. This, in turn, is largely influenced by the oral route of administration, 2 mg of estradiol in this instance. Transdermally administered estrogen had no effect; of note, however, is the fact that this second study was only of 6 weeks' duration. Longer times of administration may be necessary to cause these changes with nonoral estrogens. Perhaps this mechanism is, in turn, not directly related to the hepatic degradation of LDL.—R.A. Lobo, M.D.

2 Epidemiology of Infertility

The Prevalence of Subfertility: A Review of the Current Confusion and a Report of Two New Studies

Greenhall E, Vessey M (Univ of Oxford, England)

Fertil Steril 54:978–983, 1990 2–1

Background.—Subfertility has been defined as failure to conceive after 1 year of unprotected intercourse or the occurrence of more than 2 consecutive natural miscarriages or stillbirths. There are few useful data on the incidence of this problem because of the inherent difficulties of measuring its prevalence. Two new approaches to measuring subfertility were examined.

Methods.—The first study included 872 women aged 25–44 years identified from a computerized age-sex register. Those who seemed to have unresolved subfertility were invited to an interview that included a detailed sexual and contraceptive history. The response rate was 78%. The second study involved 702 women aged 25–45 years who took part in a case-control study of breast cancer. Cases were married women treated for new breast cancer at 8 different hospitals; controls were married women admitted to the same hospitals for acute medical-surgical conditions. These women underwent a structured interview with specially trained nurses.

Findings.—In the general practice study, 403 of 683 women had no signs of subfertility. Of the 178 women with evidence of subfertility, 117 were interviewed and 102 others had evidence of resolved subfertility. The prevalence rates for unresolved primary subfertility were 3.4% in the general practice study and 3.2% in the hospital study. Other rates were as follows in the general practice and hospital groups, respectively: resolved primary subfertility, 7.3% and 12.8%; unresolved secondary subfertility, 7.7% and 4.2%; resolved secondary subfertility, 9.8% and 15%; any episode of primary subfertility in having or trying to have at least 1 child, 10.7% and 16%; any episode of secondary subfertility in having or trying to have more than 1 child, 16.2% and 18.7%; and any episode of subfertility in having or trying to have at least 1 child, 20.5% and 28%.

Conclusions.—About 25% of women who try to conceive have some episode of subfertility at some time during their reproductive life. This occurs in trying to conceive a first child in 1 of 8 cases and in trying to conceive a second child in 1 of 6 cases. Six percent of parous women could not have as many children as they wish, and 3% are involuntarily childless.

▶ Subfertility is usually defined as the inability to conceive after attempting to do so for at least 1 year. In this study, women with 2 or more successive miscarriages or stillbirths were also included in the definition. Nevertheless, because the incidence of recurrent miscarriage is less than 1%, the rate given in the abstract can be used to approximate the prevalence of infertility in the current population of British women. The results obtained from these 2 studies are in close agreement with those of several other British and American studies that indicate that a substantial proportion of women have difficulty becoming pregnant at some time in their life. More than 10% of women have difficulty conceiving their first child. These data can be used to counsel patients that infertility is common, despite the fact that many of their contemporaries become pregnant without difficulty.—D.R. Mishell, Jr., M.D.

Incidence and Main Causes of Infertility in a Resident Population (1,850, 000) of Three French Regions (1988–1989)

Thonneau P, Marchand S, Tallec A, Ferial M-L, Ducot B, Lansac J, Lopes P, Tabaste J-M, Spira A (Institut National de la Santé et de la Recherche Médicale, Centre Hospitalier Universitaire de Bicêtre; Centre Hospitalier Régional Universitaire de Tours; Observatoire Régional de la Santé des Pays de Loire; Centre Hospitalier Régional Universitaire de Limoges; Centre Hospitalier Régional Universitaire de Nantes, France)

Hum Reprod 6:811–816, 1991 2–2

Background.—A multicenter study was initiated in France in 1987 to assess the French infertility rate, risk factors, and different causes of infertility. The incidence and main causes of infertility in a resident population of 3 French regions were studied.

Methods and Findings.—All 1,686 couples in the 3 regions of the study who consulted a physician because of primary or secondary infertility from July 1988 to June 1989 were included. The infertility prevalence rate was 14.1%, meaning that 1 in 7 women in France will seek medical attention for an infertility problem during her reproductive life. The causes of female infertility were ovulation disorders in 32% and tubal damage in 26%. Male infertility was caused by oligo-terato-asthenozoospermia in 21%, asthenozoospermia in 17%, teratozoospermia in 10%, and azoospermia in 9%. Thirty-nine percent of both men and women had fertility disorders. Only the woman was infertile in 33% of the cases and only the man in 20%. Eight percent of the couples had unexplained infertility.

Conclusions.—These data provide a more precise definition of the level of infertility among French couples and of its main causes. Case-control studies of the same populations are currently under way.

▶ Adequate epidemiologic data in terms of infertility problems are lacking in many countries. This is particularly true for causal factors. In this study, the areas where defects were noted are well documented. It should be emphasized that in 30% of the couples, *both* partners demonstrated reproductive abnormalities. No surprise, but often overlooked in the clinics.—C.A. Paulsen, M.D.

Delaying Childbearing: Effect of Age on Fecundity and Outcome of Pregnancy

van Noord-Zaadstra BM, Looman CWN, Alsbach H, Habbema JDF, te Velde ER, Karbaat J (Toegepast Natuurwetenschappelijk Onderzoek Inst of Preventive Health Care, Leiden; Erasmus Univ, Rotterdam; Univ Hosp, Utrecht; Cryo Biological Labs, Bijdorp, Barendrecht, The Netherlands)

BMJ 302:1361–1365, 1991 2–3

Purpose.—Earlier studies suggested that reduced female fecundity starts during the age range of 31–35 years. Pinpointing this critical age is important to women who delay childbearing. Data were reviewed concerning a cohort of women scheduled for donor insemination, including the age of the start of the decline of fecundity (the critical age). The probability of a pregnancy leading to a healthy infant was examined, taking into account the woman's age to determine the age-dependent probability of conceiving a healthy child.

Methods.—Based on the criteria of being nulliparous, having an azoospermic husband, and never having received donor insemination, 751 women were selected. Outcome was measured by the number of cycles before pregnancy (a positive pregnancy test result), or stopping treatment and the result of pregnancy (successful outcome).

Results.—Of the 751 women, 555 became pregnant and 461 bore healthy infants. The probability of conception was about 95% at age 31 years but then fell by about 12% per cycle. The probability of having a healthy infant decreased by 3.5% yearly after the age of 30 years. By combining both of these age effects, a 35-year-old woman's chance of having a healthy infant was about 50% that of a 25-year-old woman (Fig 2–1).

Conclusions.—After the critical age of 31 years, a woman's probability of conception falls by about 12% per cycle. Treatment for longer than 12 cycles is recommended because the pregnancy rate increased in both

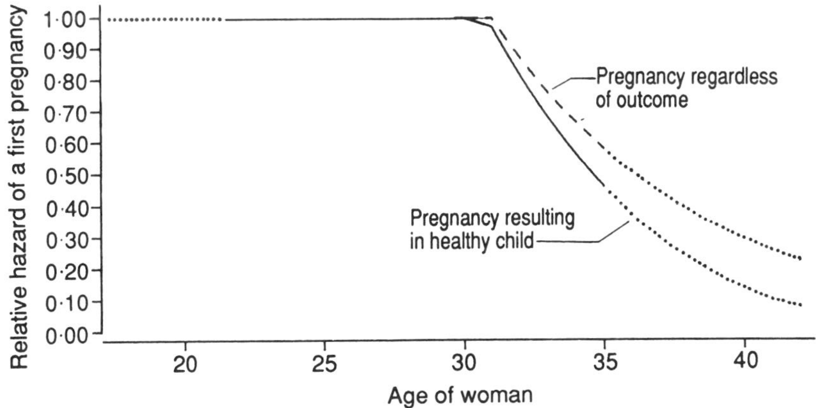

Fig 2–1.—Rate of pregnancy by age with regard to outcome. (Courtesy of van Noord-Zaadstra BM, Looman CWN, Alsbach H, et al: *BMJ* 302:1361–1365, 1991.)

older and younger women after 12 cycles. The probability of an adverse pregnancy outcome starts to increase at about the same age of 30 years, largely because of spontaneous abortion.

▶ The results of this well-done study are in agreement with those of several other reports showing that the monthly chance of conception and fecundity begins to decrease steadily after age 30. Thus it will take longer for women older than 30 to conceive than it will for younger women. Furthermore, when conception does occur, the incidence of spontaneous abortion increases after age 35. This incidence is attributable not only to an increased incidence of chromosomally abnormal conceptions, but also to an increased risk of abortion of chromosomally normal embryos after age 35. For these reasons, married childless couples who eventually wish to have children should be advised to start attempting conception before age 30. There are many valid reasons why couples delay childbearing—financial, sociologic, and need for education. However, for biological reasons it is not advisable to delay attempts to initiate pregnancy after age 30.—D.R. Mishell, Jr., M.D.

The Effect of Age on Female Fecundity
Stovall DW, Toma SK, Hammond MG, Talbert LM (Univ of North Carolina, Chapel Hill)
Obstet Gynecol 77:33–36, 1991 2–4

Introduction.—Although not supported by completed studies, many believe that female fecundity decreases with age. The effect of age on female fecundity was assessed in women who had no detectable infertility problem and who received therapeutic donor insemination.

Methods.—Participants included 210 women with no detectable factors for infertility. These women received 751 cycles of therapeutic donor

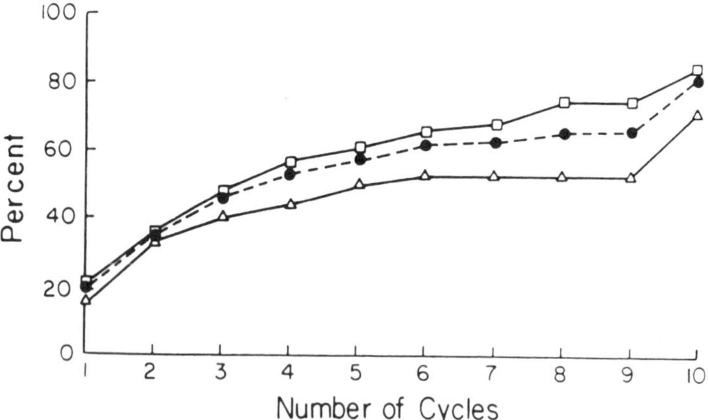

Fig 2–2.—Cumulative conception rates in women with no detectable infertility factors. *Closed circles* = all ages; *open squares* = younger than 35 years; *open triangles* = 35 to 45 years. (Courtesy of Stovall DW, Toma SK, Hammond MG, et al: *Obstet Gynecol* 77:33–36, 1991.)

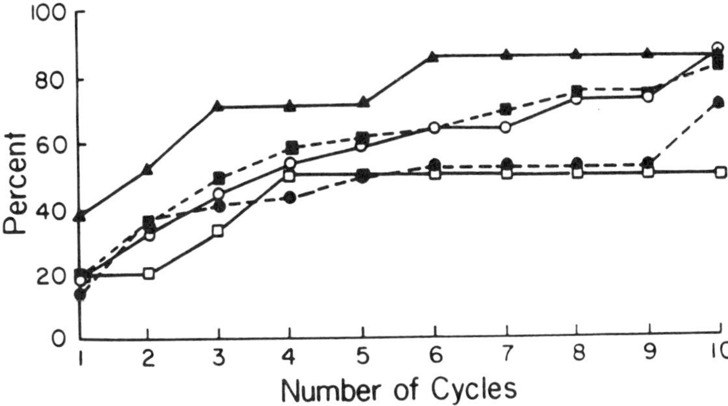

Fig 2–3.—Cumulative conception rates in women with no detectable infertility factors divided into 5 consecutive age groups. *Closed triangles* = 19 to 24 years; *closed squares* = 25 to 29 years; *open circles* = 30 to 34 years; *closed circles* = 35 to 39 years; *open squares* = 40 to 49 years. (Courtesy of Stovall DW, Toma SK, Hammond MG, et al: *Obstet Gynecol* 77:33–36, 1991.)

insemination. Semen donors comprised students from the University of North Carolina at Chapel Hill. Semen frozen using a 2-step nitrogen method was used in 92% of the cycles treated; in 8% of cycles fresh or fresh plus frozen semen was used.

Findings.—Women aged 35–45 years received semen in a total of 228 cycles, whereas those aged 19–34 years received semen in 523 cycles. The monthly fecundity outcome for all patients was 16% (Fig 2–2). The monthly fecundity results in women aged 19–34 years and 35–45 years differed significantly at 18.3% and 13%, respectively. The monthly fecundities for the 5 age groups assessed were 30% in the group aged 19–24 years; 18% in the group aged 25–29; 17% in the group aged 30–34; 13% in the group aged 35–39; and 14% in the group aged

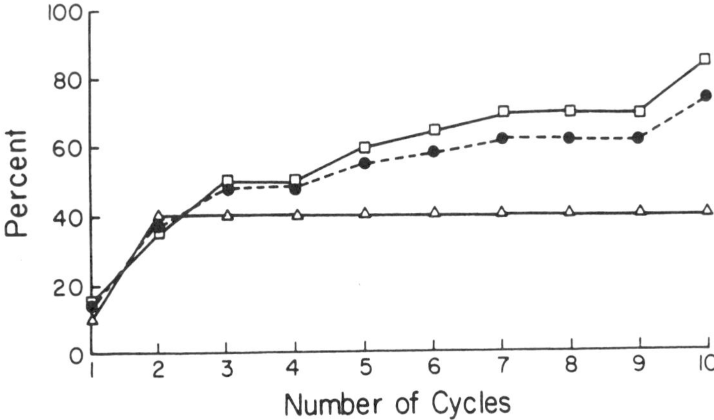

Fig 2–4.—Cumulative conception rates in women with no detectable infertility factors with laparoscopic confirmation. *Closed circles* = all ages; *open squares* = 19–34 years; *open triangles* = 35–45 years. (Courtesy of Stovall DW, Toma SK, Hammond MG, et al: *Obstet Gynecol* 77:33–36, 1991.)

40–45 (Fig 2–3). When considering these 5 groups, no significant differences were observed between successive age groups, but nonsuccessive age groups did differ significantly for fecundity. Thirty-eight women (186 cycles of therapeutic semen donation) underwent laparoscopy. The monthly fecundities for these women were 16.8% for those aged 19–34 years and 9% for those aged 35–45 years, but the difference between these 2 age groups did not reach significance (Fig 2–4).

Conclusions.—These findings support the concept of a progressive decrease in fecundity with age in a defined female population. In addition, the results indicate that frozen semen can produce acceptable rates of fecundity as long as the patient receives sufficient numbers of motile sperm during each procedure.

▶ The results of this study are in agreement with those of Abstract 2–3, indicating that the incidence of infertility increases steadily with increasing maternal age after ages 25–30. There are many social and economic reasons for postponing the age of childbearing, but clinicians should counsel their patients that as they grow older, the chances of conceiving decrease and the number of ovulatory cycles in their lifetime also steadily diminishes. For these reasons, it is best for women who wish to have a family to begin to attempt conception before the age of 30.—D.R. Mishell, Jr., M.D.

Poor Oocyte Quality Rather Than Implantation Failure as a Cause of Age-Related Decline in Female Fertility

Navot D, Bergh PA, Williams MA, Garrisi GJ, Guzman I, Sandler B, Grunfeld L (Mount Sinai Med Ctr, New York)

Lancet 337:1375–1377, 1991 2–5

Introduction.—The age-related decline in female fertility is a result of diminished oocyte quality and/or uterine-endometrial inadequacy. The results of ovum donation were evaluated.

Methods.—Ovum donation was from 29 young women undergoing in vitro fertilization. Recipients were 35 women aged 40 years or older who had experienced at least 3 years of infertility. Recipients had artificial endometrial cycles induced by sequential estrogen and progesterone, with 1 preparatory cycle before actual implantation.

Results.—The recipients conceiving with self-oocytes did not achieve viable pregnancies. Attempts with donated oocytes resulted in 28 pregnancies with evidence of implantation and 15 deliveries. There were significantly higher rates of implantation, pregnancy, and delivery after ovum donation compared to ovulation induction or in vitro fertilization in the same patients. Donors and recipients received oocytes from the same induced cohort, and pregnancy and delivery did not differ significantly between donors (33% and 23%) and older recipients (40% and 30%).

Discussion.—The age-related decline in female fertility results from oocyte quality rather than implantation failure. The good outcome in donation cycles is attributable to the higher pregnancy potential of oocytes from young donors. Previously held views on the negative effect of aging on the endometrial vasculature and uterine blood supply may be reevaluated in light of the fact that all of the viable ovum-donated pregnancies transpired after failure of conception with self-oocytes.

▶ The high rate of pregnancy, 56% in this group of older women with infertility and normal cycles who received donor oocytes, is remarkably similar to the 62% rate reported by Sauer et al. (see the 1991 YEAR BOOK OF INFERTILITY, p 216) in women with premature ovarian failure. Thus the findings of this study support the conclusion of Sauer et al. that the poor oocyte quality in older women, not aging of the uterus, is the reason for the markedly decreased rate of fertilization after age 40 and lower rates of success of in vitro fertility after age 40 compared to younger women. The use of donor oocytes can be offered to those women older than 40 years who fail to become pregnant after their own eggs have been fertilized in vitro.—D.R. Mishell, Jr., M.D.

Male Cigarette Smoking and Fecundity in Couples Attending an Infertility Clinic

Dunphy BC, Barratt CLR, von Tongelen BP, Cooke ID (Jessop Hosp for Women, Sheffield; John Radcliffe Hosp, Oxford, England)

Andrologia 23:223–225, 1991 2–6

Background and Methods.—Women who smoke have an increased risk of a poor pregnancy outcome. To determine whether there is also an association between male cigarette smoking and a reduced chance of conception, this relationship was examined in 330 couples attending an infertility clinic. Nearly 59% of the men did not smoke; 10% smoked between 1 and 5 cigarettes per day; 8% smoked between 6 and 10 cigarettes per day; 16% smoked up to a pack per day; and 7% smoked more than a pack per day. All semen analyses were performed by 1 technician.

Results.—The mean length of involuntary infertility before referral was 61 months. Of 138 apparently normal women, 19 conceived independent of treatment of either partner. There was no significant difference in the distribution of number of cigarettes smoked between the "normal" and "abnormal" female groups. There was no significant association between cigarette smoking and semen parameters. Nor was there a significant association between the number of cigarettes smoked and fertility outcome in either female group.

Conclusions.—Fertility outcome was apparently unrelated to the number of cigarettes smoked by the male partner. Smoking habits were self-reported, so there could have been some inaccuracies, or habits could have changed during the course of the study. However, the latter seems unlikely. Also, this study did not attempt to assess the effects of passive smoking.

Male Alcohol Consumption and Fecundity in Couples Attending an Infertility Clinic

Dunphy BC, Barratt CLR, Cooke ID (Jessop Hosp for Women, Sheffield, England)

Andrologia 23:219–221, 1991 2–7

Background and Methods.—Excessive alcohol consumption has been associated with poor reproductive function. Chronic alcoholism in men can cause testicular atrophy with decreased spermatogenesis or azoospermia secondary to endocrinologic consequences of hepatic compromise. Ejaculatory dysfunction can also result from chronic alcoholism. Whether the use of alcohol in lesser amounts affects reproductive function was examined in a study of male alcohol intake and fertility in 258 couples attending an infertility clinic.

Results.—The mean length of involuntary infertility before referral was 62 months. Women ranged in age from 20 to 46 years and men, 22–52 years. Sixteen of 110 women thought to be normal conceived independent of treatment of either partner. There was no significant difference in the distribution of number of units of alcohol consumed per week between women in the "normal" and "abnormal" groups. There was no significant association between male alcohol intake and semen parameters. Nor was there any significant association between the amount of alcohol men consumed weekly and fertility outcome in either female group.

Conclusions.—In this series there was no strong relationship between male alcohol intake and fertility outcome. Subjects may not have accurately assessed their alcohol intake. Although their habits could have changed during the course of the study, it is unlikely that drinking habits would have been altered appreciably.

▶ The 2 articles reviewed in Abstracts 2–6 and 2–7 were selected (despite the lack of proper controls) because of the attention paid by the media to these issues. It would have been nice if the investigators had examined men whose wives were attending a prenatal clinic as controls.—C.A. Paulsen, M.D.

A Study of the Effect of Perchloroethylene Exposure on Semen Quality in Dry Cleaning Workers

Eskenazi B, Wyrobek AJ, Fenster L, Katz DF, Sadler M, Lee J, Hudes M, Rempel DM (Univ of California, Berkeley; Lawrence Livermore Natl Lab, Livermore, Calif; California Dept of Health Services, Berkeley; Univ of California, Davis)

Am J Ind Med 20:575–591, 1991 2–8

Objective.—The effects of perchloroethylene (PCE) exposure, if any, on the quality of human semen were examined by comparing semen quality in 34 dry cleaners and 48 laundry workers. Seventeen semen parameters were related both to levels of PCE in expired air and to an index of exposure based on job tasks in the preceding 3 months. Nonvasectomized men aged 20–50 years were eligible to participate.

Findings.—Both groups of workers had average sperm concentrations that exceeded 80 million/mL, but about one fourth of each group were oligospermic. Proportions of abnormal forms were similar in the 2 groups, but sperm from the dry cleaners were more likely to be round rather than narrow. Motile sperm averaged just over 60% in both groups, with the sperm from dry cleaners tending to swim with a greater amplitude of lateral head displacement.

Conclusions.—Exposure to PCE at work apparently can have subtle effects on sperm quality, but further studies are needed to determine whether such effects can alter fertility. Subsequent studies should include men exposed to higher levels of PCE.

▶ This preliminary study evaluated the reproductive characteristics of men exposed to industrial toxicants. It incorporated a control population, but where are the data on fertility? This is a difficult issue, but in the long run, where potential toxicants in the work environment are concerned, industry will eventually recognize that prevention is not so expensive. Remember the DBCP scenario?—C.A. Paulsen, M.D.

Indirect Fertility Analysis in Painters Exposed to Ethylene Glycol Ethers: Sensitivity and Specificity

Welch LS, Plotkin E, Schrader S (George Washington Univ, Washington, DC; Yale Univ; Natl Inst for Occupational Safety and Health, Cincinnati)

Am J Ind Med 20:229–240, 1991 2–9

Introduction.—Collection and analysis of semen samples in a field setting can be problematic, but questionnaire-based methods of monitoring male fertility in such a setting avoid some of these difficulties. Using these methods, the rate of observed births for wives of workers can be compared with expected birth rates derived from United States fertility tables or unexposed workers. The sensitivity of the questionnaire method was compared with that of semen analysis in an assessment of reproductive function in men exposed to ethylene glycol ethers.

Methods.—Semen samples were obtained from and the questionnaire was distributed to 74 married painters exposed to ethylene glycol ethers and 51 married men not exposed to ethylene glycol ethers who worked at the same shipyard. The questionnaire elicited data on basic demographics, medical conditions, and personal habits known to affect semen parameters.

Results.—After adjustment for age, smoking, and abstinence, the mean sperm count and count per ejaculate were lower in the painters than in the controls. The proportion of men with a sperm count of less than 20 million was 13.5% in the exposed group and 5% in the control group. Among nonsmokers, exposed men had a greater rate of oligospermia. When the questionnaire data were analyzed, no effect of exposure on fertility was evident.

Conclusion.—Semen analysis showed a significant difference in the rate of oligospermia between nonsmoking men exposed to ethylene glycol ethers and unexposed men that was not found by the fertility questionnaire. The questionnaire method of assessing fertility appears to be less sensitive than semen analysis as a screening tool for male reproductive function.

▶ More precise epidemiological data are needed. In this instance, why didn't the questionnaire elicit the correlation? Perhaps it is more than just sensitivity.—C.A. Paulsen, M.D.

Stress From Infertility, Marriage Factors, and Subjective Well-Being of Wives and Husbands

Andrews FM, Abbey A, Halman LJ (Univ of Michigan; Wayne State Univ, Detroit)

J Health Soc Behav 32:238–253, 1991 2–10

Introduction.—The relationship between stress and fertility has received much attention anecdotally, but extensive empirical research on the psychological sequelae of infertility is lacking. Data derived from independent interviews of the wives and husbands of 157 white, middle-class couples experiencing infertility were examined. All had tried to conceive for at least a year but had not yet tried the more advanced treatments such as in vitro fertilization.

Model.—The general concepts used to analyze the interview data included stress linked with fertility, marital conflict, sexual self-esteem and dissatisfaction, frequency of intercourse, and subjective well-being. Well-being was estimated both from global life quality and also with respect to the self, the marriage, intimacy/sex/romance, and a health/appearance dimension.

Findings.—The wives reported higher levels of infertility-related stress than did their husbands. There were no marked differences in feelings about any aspect of life quality. Stress caused by the fertility problem related, as expected, to variables of marital and life quality; greater stress tended to correlate with more marital conflict, greater sexual dissatisfaction, and a lower quality of life. The marital partners sometimes experienced different levels of stress as related to infertility.

Interpretation.—Infertility has an overall negative effect on all aspects of life quality, on one's self-efficacy, and on health/appearance. Wives tend to experience a greater impact of infertility on their lives than do husbands, particularly in relation to the marriage and sexual satisfaction. Both the consequences of infertility and its treatment affect women more than men.

Suggestions.—One approach is to lower the stress itself through helping couples to better understand and cope with the problem. Another is to make concerted efforts to reduce marital conflict and to sustain each partner's sense of sexual attractiveness and adequacy.

▶ Although infertility is not a life-threatening disease, the emotional effects on mental health and quality of life, as noted in this abstract, are not trivial. Clinicians need to be aware of the emotional aspects of infertility and to readily suggest the use of trained psychological counselors to help treat the emotional problems associated with infertility.—D.R. Mishell, Jr., M.D.

3 Diagnostic Evaluation of the Female Partner

Gonadotropin, Steroid, and Inhibin Levels in Women With Incipient Ovarian Failure During Anovulatory and Ovulatory Rebound Cycles

Buckler HM, Evans CA, Mamtora H, Burger HG, Anderson DC (Hope Hosp, Salford, England; Prince Henry's Hosp, Melbourne, Australia)

J Clin Endocrinol Metab 72:116–124, 1991 3–1

Introduction.—In women approaching menopause, a monotropic rise occurs in the activity of follicle-stimulating hormone (FSH) as the first detectable endocrine manifestation of reproductive aging while regular menses continue. Thirteen women aged 27–38 years with infertility and regular menses with persistently raised FSH levels and probable incipient ovarian failure (IOF) were examined.

Methods.—Serum luteinizing hormone (LH), FSH, estradiol (E_2), and progesterone (P) levels, determined 3 times a week during 1 menstrual cycle, were compared to these levels in 60 infertile women with normal ovulatory cycles as determined by hormones and ultrasound scans (controls). In the group with IOF, hormone levels were also evaluated after attempts to suppress increased FSH levels with various estrogen progestogen preparations.

Findings.—In the group with IOF, the serum FSH level was significantly higher on all days of the cycle. It was raised on days 4 to 5 before and days 5–11 after the LH surge. Serum E_2 and P levels did not differ significantly from those of controls. Inhibin levels were significantly lower in the group with IOF, but displayed the same pattern over the cycle as that in the control group. Inhibin activity correlated inversely with the FSH level during the follicular and luteal phases and positively with the P level during the luteal phase. Ultrasound scanning showed failure of normal ovulation. In 11 women, amenorrhea and raised gonadotropin levels have developed since completion of the study. After 3 weeks of estrogen/progestogen treatment, LH and FSH levels fell to normal values. On withdrawal of suppression, ovulation occurred in 22 of 39 cycles in the presence of high FSH and low inhibin levels, but no pregnancies occurred (Fig 3–1).

Conclusion.—These findings suggest that inhibin deficiency may contribute to the elevated FSH levels of IOF, and that ovarian inhibin secretion may decline with IOF. Although rebound ovulation may occur after suppression of gonadotropins, this occurs in the presence of raised FSH and low inhibin levels; and the cycles still appear to be subfertile.

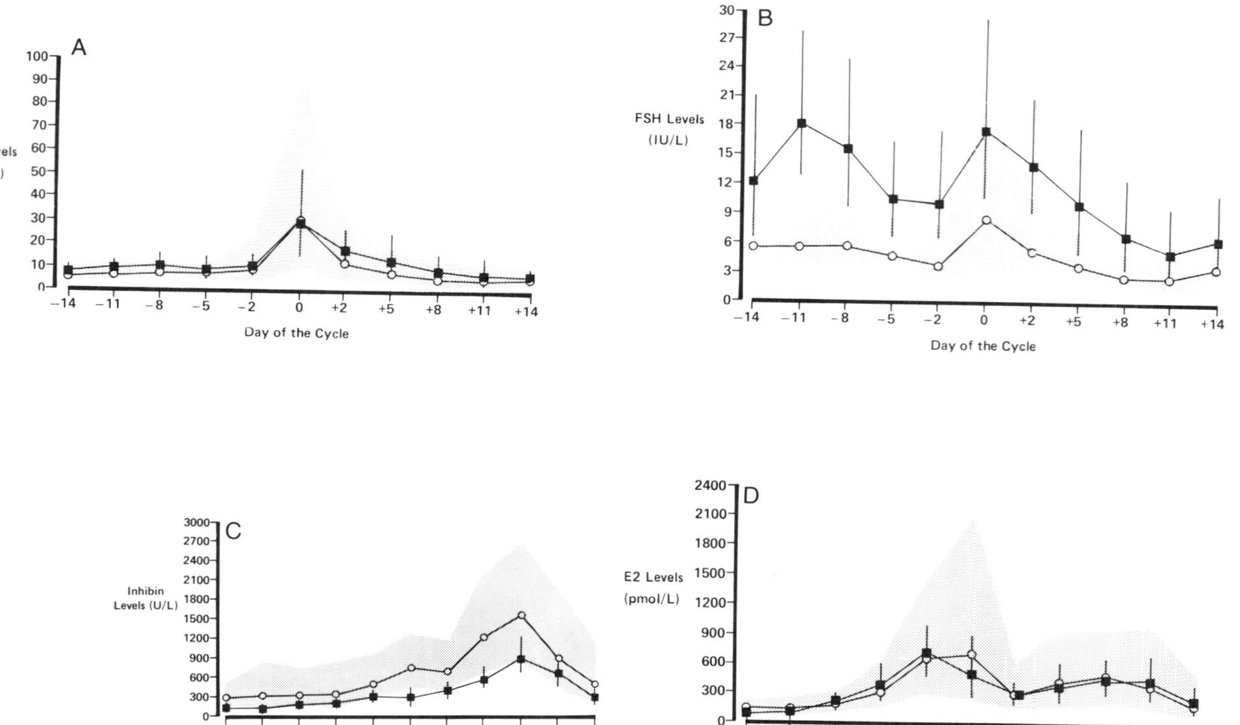

Fig 3–1.—LH (A), FSH (B), inhibin (C), E (D), and P (E) levels in ovulatory rebound cycles. The geometric mean and 95% confidence limits of the normal control group are shown in the shaded area. All data are log transformed. (Courtesy of Buckler HM, Evans CA, Mamtora H, et al: *J Clin Endocrinol Metab* 72:116–124, 1991.)

▶ The 13 women in this study ranged in age from 27 to 38, were infertile, and had regular menstrual cycles. Although they had normal luteal phase levels of serum progesterone, serial ultrasonographic scanning of the ovaries revealed a variety of abnormalities including abnormal follicular development and luteinized unruptured follicles. In the early follicular phase of the cycle, the mean FSH levels in these women were significantly elevated (Fig 3–1) and usually did not overlap with the normal range of ovulatory controls. The authors do not provide information about the frequency with which this entity occurs, but it may be worthwhile to measure the early follicular phase FSH level in women in this age group who have otherwise unexplained infertility to determine whether they have IOF.—D.R. Mishell, Jr., M.D.

Error in Histologic Dating of Secretory Endometrium: Variance Component Analysis

Gibson M, Lee KR, Badger GJ, Korson R, Byrn F, Trainer TD (Univ of Vermont, Burlington)

Fertil Steril 56:242–247, 1991 3–2

Background.—Histologic dating of secretory endometrium is the cornerstone of clinical evaluation of the luteal phase. The extent and sources of imprecision in endometrial histologic dating were characterized.

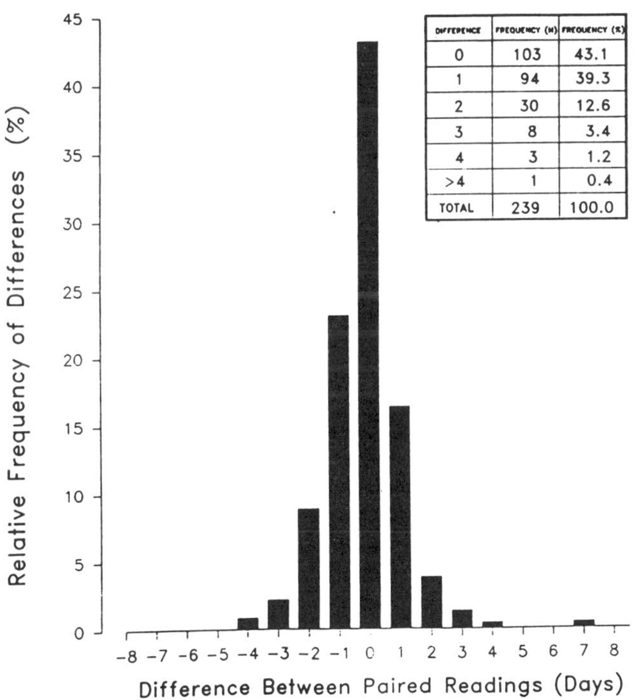

DIFFERENCE	FREQUENCY (N)	FREQUENCY (%)
0	103	43.1
1	94	39.3
2	30	12.6
3	8	3.4
4	3	1.2
>4	1	0.4
TOTAL	239	100.0

Fig 3–2.—Frequency distribution of differences between the dates assigned to endometrial biopsies on the first and second readings as performed by 5 evaluators reading 50 slides. *Inset table* shows this data numerically. (Courtesy of Gibson M, Lee KR, Badger GJ, et al: *Fertil Steril* 56:242–247, 1991.)

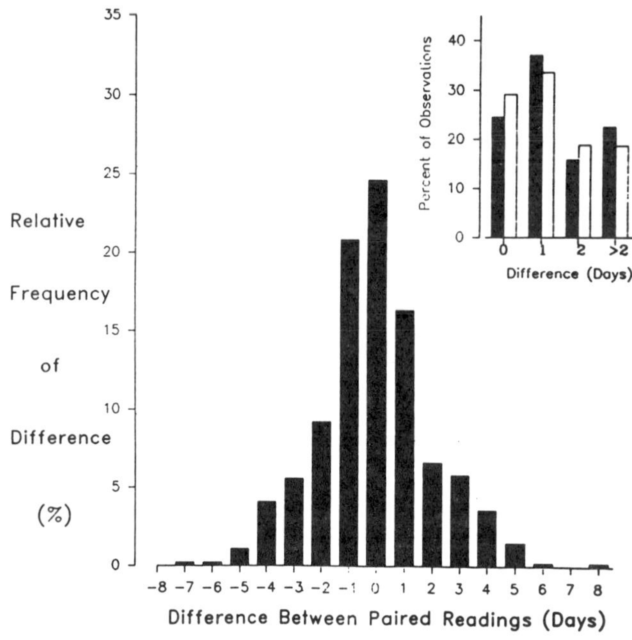

Fig 3–3.—Frequency distribution of all pair-wise differences between the 5 readers on the first reading of 50 slides (evaluable n = 467). Frequency difference in this study *(filled bar)* is compared with that reported by Noyes and Haman *(unfilled bar)* in the inset. (Courtesy of Gibson M, Lee KR, Badger GJ, et al: *Fertil Steril* 56:242–247, 1991.)

Methods.—Duplicate endometrial biopsy specimens were obtained on the same occasion from 25 women undergoing routine evaluation for infertility. Each of the 50 slides was studied by 5 evaluators on 2 separate occasions. Endometrial dates were assigned based on the criteria of Noyes et al. The evaluators had no previous formal teaching or consulting relationship concerning the dating of endometrial biopsy specimens. Estimates of intrauterine, intraevaluator, and interevaluator variability were determined by variance component analysis.

Results.—Duplicate readings of the same slide by the same evaluator were in agreement in 43.1% of the instances and were within 1 day of each other in 39.3% (Fig 3–2); only 5% were discordant by ≥3 days. The assignment of histologic days was in agreement in 25% of the readings, within 1 day of each other in 62%, and within 2 days in 78%; the other 22% of readings were discordant by >2 days (Fig 3–3). The mean histologic dates for the 2 biopsy specimens obtained at the same time agreed within 1 day in 56% of subjects and within 2 days in 95%. Variance component analysis indicated that interevaluator inconsistencies accounted for 65% of the observed variability, intraevaluator differences for 27%, and intrauterine inconsistencies for 8%.

Implication.—The data show an overall variance of 2.58 ($\hat{\sigma}$ = 1.61 days) associated with a single endometrial dating by a single reader. Assuming that the error is normal about the true histologic date, 12% of biopsy specimens will be mistakenly identified as lagging by ≥2 days. The overall error from intraevaluator, interevaluator, and intrauterine differences has the potential to result in a substantial false positive rate for diagnosis of a luteal phase defect.

▶ It has never been established whether the luteal phase defect, as diagnosed by out-of-phase endometrial dating, is a true cause of infertility. As shown by this and other studies, luteal insufficiency is greatly overdiagnosed because of the subjective means used to estimate dating of the endometrium based on morphometric imprecise criteria established more than 40 years ago. The inter- and intraobserver variation in dating, as well as the lack of precision in determining the true date of ovulation, contribute to overestimation of the diagnosis. Fortunately, the administration of progesterone is harmless and, combined with timed intercourse and increased duration of attempts to conceive, fertility rates will increase. Whether progesterone is superior to placebo has not been determined in randomized prospective trials.—D.R. Mishell, Jr., M.D.

A Clinical Comparison of Sonographic Hydrotubation and Hysterosalpingography

Mitri FF, Andronikou AD, Perpinyal S, Hofmeyr GJ, Sonnendecker EWW (Coronation Hosp; Johannesburg Hosp; Univ of the Witwatersrand, Johannesburg, South Africa)

Br J Obstet Gynaecol 98:1031–1036, 1991 3–3

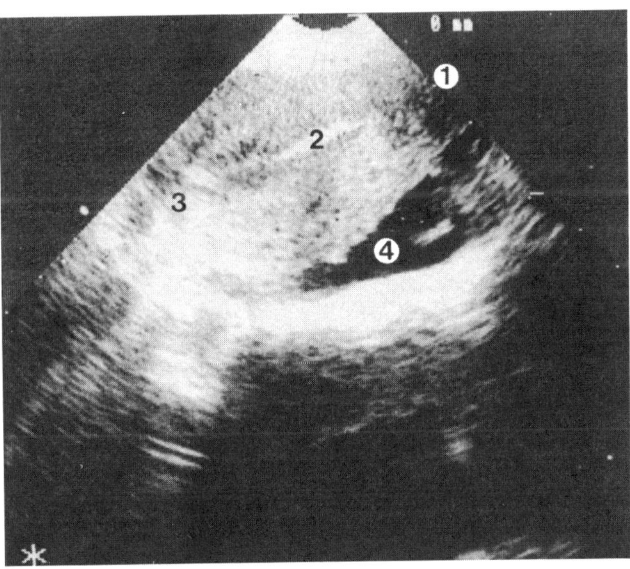

Fig 3–4.—Longitudinal section of uterus and tube showing hydrosalpinx. *1*, endocervix; *2*, endometrium; *3*, fundus; and *4*, hydrosalpinx. (Courtesy of Mitri FF, Andronikou AD, Perpinyal S, et al: *Br J Obstet Gynaecol* 98:1031–1036, 1991.)

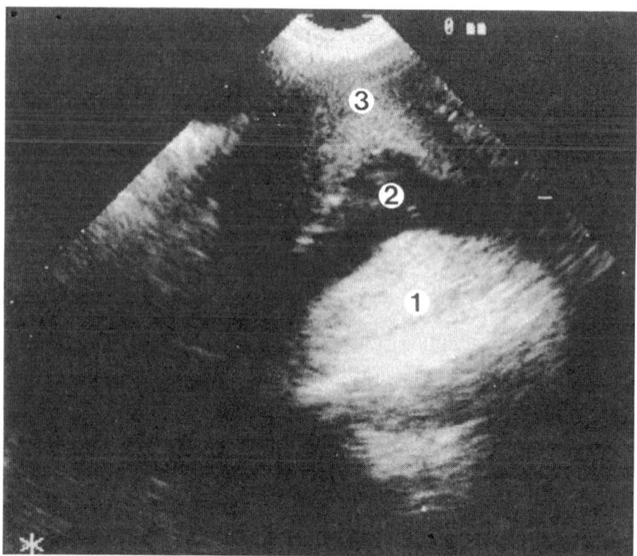

Fig 3–5.—Horizontal section showing intrauterine cavity of septate uterus *(2)* with fundus *(1)* pointing downward and cervix *(3)* at top of picture. (Courtesy of Mitri FF, Andronikou AD, Perpinyal S, et al: *Br J Obstet Gynaecol* 98:1031–1036, 1991.)

Background.—The value of hysterosalpingography (HSG) in infertile women who undergo laparoscopy is limited to demonstrating intrauterine and intratubal abnormalities. In addition, HSG is time consuming and labor intensive, and is associated with the risk of reaction to contrast media. The value of using vaginal sonographic hydrotubation as an alternative was investigated.

Methods.—Sixty women who were undergoing routine infertility testing participated in the prospective, blind, comparison study of HSG and sonographic hydrotubation. Within 4 weeks before or after HSG, sonographic hydrotubation was done. The uterus and tubes were identified by using a 5-MHz vaginal ultrasound probe; 10–20 mL of normal saline were injected into the uterine cavity through an endocervical catheter. The main outcome measures were the shape of the uterus and its cavity, the flow of saline through the tubes, the presence of hydrosalpinges before and after saline injection, and the presence of free fluid in the pouch of Douglas.

Results.—The findings at sonographic and HSG uterine assessment were comparable in 82% of the women. Tubal findings were comparable in 72%. In 7 women found to have bipolar tubal disease on sonography and cornual block on HSG, the sonographic diagnosis was confirmed at laparoscopy. Sonographic hydrotubation enabled a more certain diagnosis of a septate uterus in 3 cases (Figs 3–4 and 3–5).

Conclusions.—Sonographic hydrotubation is a simple office procedure that should be used in initial evaluation of the uterine cavity and fallopian tubes. The use of this technique decreases the need for HSG and, in some cases, for laparoscopy.

▶ Hysterosalpingography is a useful procedure to assist in the diagnosis of the cause of infertility. However, HSG is a cause of discomfort and is costly to perform. The technique of sonographic hydrotubation should result in less discomfort and be less expensive than HSG. The main advantage, however, appears to be its ability to diagnose the presence of both proximal and distal disease. With the use of HSG it is possible to detect only the presence of proximal disease because the dye does not fill the oviduct. In this study, in all 7 women (12%) with bipolar disease, the diagnosis was made by sonographic hydrotubation, and not by HSG. Once the diagnosis of bipolar disease is made, the patient should be advised to have in vitro fertilization and diagnostic laparoscopy need not be performed. The use of sonographic hydrotubation may shorten the time and expense of the infertility evaluation for some women.—D.R. Mishell, Jr., M.D.

Hysterosalpingography With Color Doppler Ultrasonography
Peters AJ, Coulam CB (Methodist Hosp of Indiana, Indianapolis)
Am J Obstet Gynecol 164:1530–1534, 1991 3–4

Objective.—Color Doppler flow ultrasonography and hysterosalpingography were carried out in 129 infertile women, 85 of whom also had x-ray hysterosalpingography and/or chromopertubation. Fifty-eight of these women underwent pelviscopic examination with chromopertubation.

Methods.—The ultrasonographic study was carried out by instilling 5–50 mL of saline transcervically into the endometrial cavity. Flow into and out of the tubes was monitored using an ATL Ultramark 9 color Doppler unit. Doppler scans were made transabdominally or transvaginally. Tubal occlusion was diagnosed when no fluid passed through the fallopian tubes, or when no fluid was seen entering the peritoneal cavity.

Findings.—Ultrasonography-hysterosalpingography indicated bilateral tubal patency in 66% of subjects, unilateral patency in 16%, and bilateral tubal occlusion in 18%. Comparison with x-ray examination and/or chromopertubation indicated agreement in 81% of instances. Ultrasonography-hysterosalpingography was falsely negative in 19% of cases and falsely positive in 6%. The corresponding figures for x-ray hysterosalpingography, compared with chromopertubation, were 45% and 18%.

Conclusion.—Accepting chromopertubation as the standard for diagnosing tubal occlusion, ultarsonography-hysterosalpingography is at least as accurate as x-ray hysterosalpingography. The method does not require anesthesia, antimicrobial administration, or contrast dye, and radiation exposure is avoided. It is an office procedure and is relatively inexpensive.

Hysterosalpingo-Contrast Sonography of the Uterus and Fallopian Tubes: Results of a Clinical Trial of a New Contrast Medium in 120 Patients
Schlief R, Deichert U (Schering AG, Berlin; Univ of Marburg, Germany)
Radiology 178:213–215, 1991 3–5

Background.—Fallopian tube occlusion often leads to female infertility. Hysterosalpingography and chromolaparoscopy are used as standard diagnostic imaging procedures for this condition. Diagnostic ultrasound techniques lack the necessary echogenic contrast medium to diagnose tubal patency and establish normal anatomy. A prospective study was done to evaluate the diagnostic efficacy of a new diagnostic method, hysterosalpingo–contrast sonography (HyCoSy), in 120 patients with suspected infertility. The average age was 29 years.

Methods.—The patients underwent Doppler ultrasound evaluation using the contrast agent SH U 454/Echovist, a galactose monosaccharide suspension. This echogenic suspension was prepared immediately before use. The patients reclined in the lithotomy position, the vagina was disinfected, and the transvaginal probe was inserted for imaging. The vaginal sonographic examination was performed, followed by repeat imaging with the cavity filled with the contrast medium.

Results.—Of the 120 patients, 106 underwent HyCoSy followed by a conventional control examination on the same day, with 79 being checked with B-mode scanning only, 17 having duplex scanning, and 10 undergoing color Doppler. Patency findings with the B-mode HyCoSy scanning agreed with the outcomes of the conventional methods. Sensitivity was 88% for the right tube and 90% for the left tube. Specificity was 100% for both tubes. The results of the total number of Doppler assessments compared with conventional studies indicated a sensitivity of 92% for the right tube and 91% for the left tube, and a specificity of 100% for both tubes. One of the 106 patients undergoing contrast-enhanced sonography experienced an increase in body temperature, and 1 of 7 patients examined without general anesthesia had severe transient pain.

Implications.—These findings indicate that HyCoSy offers high reliability in assessment of tubal patency. The procedure is appropriate for outpatient use, with a completion time of about 10 minutes. It also allows a reduction in radiation exposure and repeat procedures for patients with suspected infertility.

▶ These additional studies (Abstracts 3–4 and 3–5) comparing HyCoSy with x-ray hysterosalpingography demonstrate that the newer technique is as accurate as the older one and has the advantages of avoiding the use of contrast dye and radiation exposure, and also is less costly. The study by Schlief et al. indicates that it is unnecessary to use the expensive color Doppler ultrasonographic system instead of the more widely available office ultrasound unit with a vaginal probe.—D.R. Mishell, Jr., M.D.

Therapeutic Effect of Hysterosalpingography: Oil- Versus Water-Soluble Contrast Media—A Randomized Prospective Study

Rasmussen F, Lindequist S, Larsen C, Justesen P (Odense Univ Hosp, Odense, Denmark)

Radiology 179:75–78, 1991 3–6

Introduction.—Hysterosalpingography (HSG) has served as an important examination for female infertility and may provide some therapeutic effects. A randomized, prospective study was undertaken to compare the pregnancy rates after HSG using 4 different contrast media: the high-osmolar, ionic diatrizoate meglumine; the low-osmolar, nonionic iohexol; the low-osmolar, ionic ioxaglate; and ethiodized poppy seed oil.

Methods.—Patients included 507 consecutive women attending the outpatient clinic from 1985 to 1988 in Odense, Denmark. Spontaneous pregnancy was assessed by a 3-month waiting period before HSG. During this time, 40 of 50 patients became pregnant (7.9% of the 507). Four hundred patients underwent HSG, with 101 receiving iohexol, 102 receiving ioxaglate, 97 receiving diatrizoate, and 98 receiving ethiodized poppy seed oil. Five to 10 mL of contrast medium was injected slowly. The HSG procedure was performed at the end of menstrual bleeding and before the tenth day of the menstrual cycle.

Findings.—The 3-month postexamination pregnancy rate was 4% in the diatrizoate group, 6.9% in the ioxaglate group, 9.9% in the iohexol group, and 13% in the ethiodized poppy seed oil patients. Figure 3–6 demonstrates the number of pregnancies related to the ovulatory cycles after HSG. The overall pregnancy rates were 12%, 17.6%, 20.8%, and

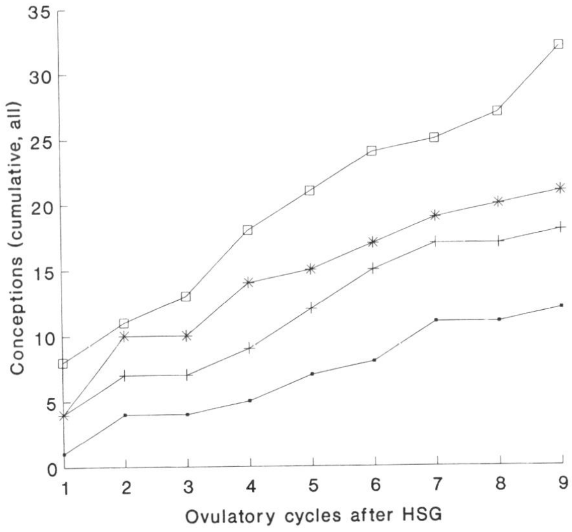

Fig 3–6.—Cumulative numbers of all conceptions vs. number of ovulatory cycles after HSG. *Squares* = ethiodized poppy seed oil; *asterisks* = iohexol; *plus signs* = ioxaglate; *dots* = diatrizoate. (Courtesy of Rasmussen F, Lindequist S, Larsen C, et al: *Radiology* 179:75–78, 1991.)

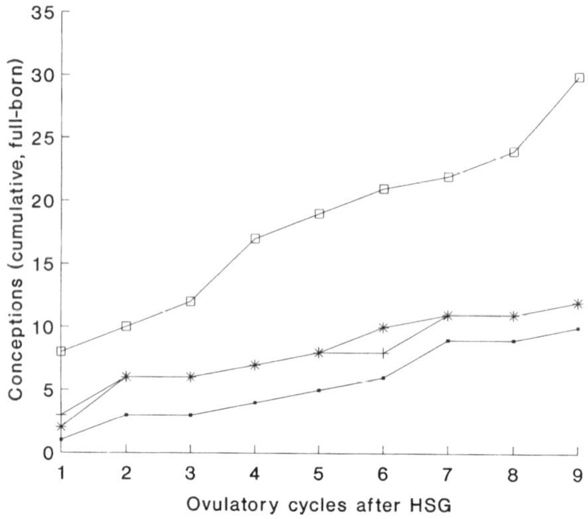

Fig 3–7.—Cumulative numbers of conceptions resulting in full-term childbirth vs. number of ovulatory cycles after HSG. *Squares* = ethiodized poppy seed oil; *asterisks* = iohexol; *plus signs* = ioxaglate; *dots* = diatrizoate. (Courtesy of Rasmussen F, Lindequist S, Larsen C, et al: *Radiology* 179:75–78, 1991.)

33% in the groups given diatrizoate, ioxaglate, iohexol, and ethiodized poppy seed oil, respectively. For intrauterine pregnancies leading to full-term births, the pregnancy rates were 10%, 11.8%, 11.9%, and 31%, respectively (Fig 3–7).

Conclusions.—These results indicate that significantly more patients had full-term childbirth after HSG with ethiodized poppy seed oil than with the other 3 contrast agents.

▶ It is controversial whether injecting oil-based contrast media through the oviducts has a therapeutic effect regarding pregnancy among infertile women. Previous studies have yielded conflicting results. In this large, prospective, randomized study there were no differences in the cause of or duration of infertility, patients' age, or findings on HSG among the 4 groups of randomized patients. Therefore, the conclusion indicating a therapeutic effect of the oil-based media appears valid. The progressive decline in pregnancy rates per cycle after the HSG lends further support to a cause-and-effect relationship. The reason for the therapeutic effect of the oil-based media on pregnancy needs to be determined in additional studies.—D.R. Mishell, Jr., M.D.

4 Diagnostic Evaluation of the Male Partner

▶ ↓ The next several abstracts focus on sperm antigens and antibodies. It has often been stated that the male reproductive system represents an immunologic jungle. For several decades investigators have worked on mapping the various sperm surface antigens with the hope that critical proteins whose function is "rate-limiting" in terms of the fertilization process can be identified. The consensus is that success may be near. In that regard, two contraceptive centers have been funded to accelerate that process. Dr. Herr heads the center at University of Virginia and Dr. Primakoff heads the center at University of Connecticut. Publications from these centers, as well as other investigators, should be followed closely for progress in this important field.—C.A. Paulsen, M.D.

Variation of Semen Quality in Normal Men

Mallidis C, Howard EJ, Baker HWG (Prince Henry's Inst of Med Research, Melbourne, Australia; Univ of Melbourne, Carlton)

Int J Androl 14:99–107, 1991 4–1

Background and Methods.—For many reasons, the sperm concentration in a given man can vary markedly from day to day. The proportion of within- and between-subject variation and seasonal changes in sperm concentration, ejaculate volume, percentage motility, and motility index were examined in 7 healthy men who provided from 61 to 205 specimens each for use in a donor insemination program. Paternity was not a requirement for selection, but all men fathered children either through the donor program or through marriage. Specimens were assessed for 72–324 weeks.

Results.—There were noticeable sample-to-sample variations. The largest proportion of overall variance was found within subjects. There was a 54% variance in sperm concentration, 59% variance in ejaculate volume, 96% variance in percentage motility, and 74% variance in motility index within subjects. There was no consistent trend, however, in variance over the year. There was no evidence suggesting that the differences resulted from changes in laboratory methods or changes in season.

Conclusions.—In most subjects, semen measurements changed over time, but there was no overall discernible pattern or trend. There appears to be no evidence that there is any intrinsic seasonal effect on semen quality in normal men living in Melbourne, Australia.

▶ Although only a small group was studied, the main issues in evaluating sperm in the ejaculate were examined. With respect to the wide variation, we would heartily agree with the authors. An example of our findings in a normal volunteer in our studies was depicted in Figure 1, presented in the *WHO, Laboratory Manual for the Examination of Human Semen and Semen-Cervical Mucus Interaction,* Press Concern, Singapore, 1980.—C.A. Paulsen, M.D.

Longitudinal Study of Semen Quality of Unexposed Workers: Sperm Motility Characteristics

Schrader SM, Turner TW, Simon SD (Natl Inst for Occupational Safety and Health, Cincinnati)

J Androl 12:126–131, 1991 4–2

Introduction.—Sperm motility characteristics are used routinely to assess male reproductive toxicants, but the variability of these characteristics within individuals over time is uncertain. To obtain information on the population stability and variability of sperm motility, the variations in sperm motility characteristics within an ejaculate, between ejaculates from the same man, and between healthy men without known exposure to reproductive toxicants were evaluated.

Methods.—The sperm motility assessments were part of a previously described longitudinal study of human semen characteristics in which 45 men provided monthly semen samples for 9 months. Motility characteristics were assessed by computer-assisted sperm analysis; variability was calculated using a nested analysis of variance.

Results.—The percentage of motile sperm seemed largely repeatable

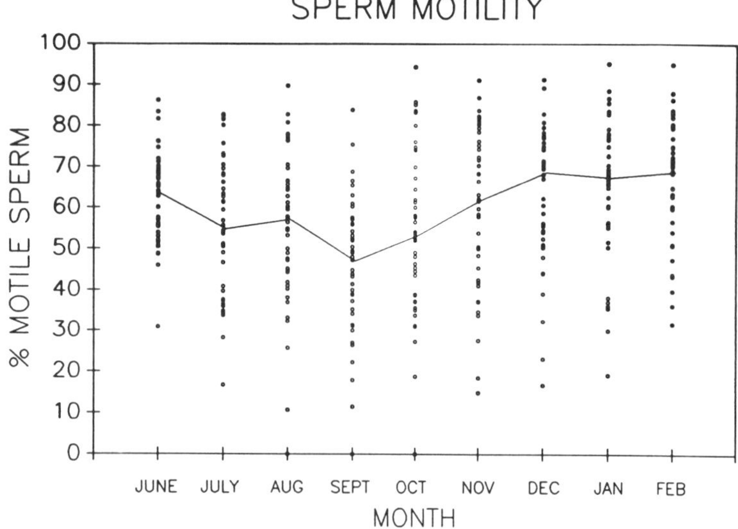

Fig 4–1.—Percent motile sperm. *Open circles* represent the sample distribution for each month. Only 1 circle is shown for each value even if more than 1 sample had that value. *Solid line* represents the median value for each month. (Courtesy of Schrader SM, Turner TW, Simon SD: *J Androl* 12:126–131, 1991.)

(Fig 4–1), but single measurements were too variable to fairly represent either an individual or a population. In contrast, curvilinear velocity, straight line velocity, linearity, amplitude of lateral head displacement, and beat-cross frequency had low variability. For all measurements, variation between cells accounted for 90% to 95% of the total variation. Variation between men accounted for only 1% to 4% of the total variation compared with 3.2% to 7.1% variation between samples from the average man.

Conclusion.—This statistical analysis suggests that percent motile sperm measurements are relatively imprecise. In contrast, single measurements of sperm velocity measurements seem to be sufficiently precise to characterize either populations or individuals.

▶ This study represents an extension of the previous authors' study (Abstract 4–1) namely, the variation in semen characteristics found in healthy men, to establish guidelines that may be used when examining a control population compared to "toxicant"-exposed males.—C.A. Paulsen, M.D.

Computer-Assisted Assessment of Human Sperm Morphology: Comparison With Visual Assessment

Wang C, Ng V, Leung A, Lee K-F, Tsoi W-L, Chan SYW, Leung J (Univ of Hong Kong, Cedars Sinai Med Ctr, Los Angeles)

Fertil Steril 55:983–988, 1991 4–3

Introduction.—Interobserver, intraobserver, and laboratory variations vary greatly when sperm morphology is analyzed by visual assessment methods. Morphological parameters (e.g., sperm head length, width, area, circumference, and ratio of length to width) can be assessed using computer-assisted semen analysis.

Methods.—Sperm head morphology from 50 semen samples from men attending an infertility clinic were analyzed by computer-assisted semen analysis with software for image analysis and morphometry (Morpholo-

TABLE 1.—Coefficients of Variation of Sperm Morphology Assessment by Manual and Morphologizer Methods

Sperm head morphology classification	Manual		Morphologizer	
	Mean	CV	Mean	CV
Normal	69.8	5.7	64.8	6.1
Small	13.8	53.5	19.4	25.1
Big	2.5	84.4	4.3	54.3
Tapered	1.7	122.9	5.5	60.9
Amorphous	8.4	62.8	5.4	50.7

Note: Calculated from assessment of 5 slides each analyzed 6 times by the same technician. Values are percents.

(Courtesy of Wang C, Ng V, Leung A, et al: *Fertil Steril* 55:983–988, 1991.)

TABLE 2.—Comparison of Results of Morphology Classification by Manual Method and the Morphologizer

	Manual method	Morphologizer	Significance of paired differences	Mean differences between paired measurements
Normal	72.4 ± 1.6 *	72.3 ± 1.3	P = 0.956	0.75 ± 1.50
	(32 to 89)	(37 to 89)		(−30 to 23)
Small	9.2 ± 0.9	9.9 ± 1.0	P = 0.450	−0.72 ± 0.95
	(0 to 26)	(1 to 26)		(−20 to 11)
Big	2.7 ± 0.5	4.9 ± 0.5	P = 0.004	−2.17 ± 0.72
	(0 to 13)	(0 to 14)		(−14 to 11)
Taper	3.7 ± 0.6	6.5 ± 0.7	P = 0.000	−2.80 ± 0.65
	(0 to 15)	(1 to 22)		(−12 to 5)
Amorphous	7.7 ± 0.9	6.0 ± 0.6	P = 0.071	1.71 ± 0.93
	(0 to 26)	(1 to 22)		(−20 to 20)

*Values are means ± SE with range in parentheses.
(Courtesy of Wang C, Ng V, Leung A, et al: *Fertil Steril* 55:983–988, 1991.)

gizer II) and the standard visual method. Sperm head morphology were classified as normal (oval), small oval, big oval, taper, and amorphous.

Results.—The coefficient of variations for normal head morphology was 5.7% for the manual method and 6.1% for the morphologizer method. The coefficient of variations for assessment of abnormal head morphology, however, was large, varying from 25% to 123% (Table 1). The mean percentage of normal, small, and amorphous head forms did not differ significantly between the 2 methods, but the percentages of big oval and taper forms were significantly greater with the morphologizer. The differences between paired values obtained by the 2 methods were highly variable, ranging from −20% to +20% (Table 2). Analysis with the statistical method of Bland and Altman showed only a small difference between the 2 methods, but the 95% range of difference was large. In contrast, the variations in the morphometric analyses between samples were small.

Conclusion.—The morphologizer has no advantage over the standard visual method in assessment of human sperm morphology. The percentage of sperm with normal morphology can be accurately assessed visually and by computer-assisted methods, but large variations exist between the 2 methods when classifying abnormal sperm morphology.

▶ What do you know! An automated system for morphology does not appear to improve the assessment of this parameter.—C.A. Paulsen, M.D.

Correlation of Motile Sperm Density and Subsequent Pregnancy Rates in Infertile Couples

Check JH, Nowroozi K, Bollendorf A (Univ of Medicine and Dentistry of New Jersey, Camden; Cooper Hosp/Univ Med Ctr, Camden)
Arch Androl 27:113–115, 1991 4–4

Objective.—Men with subnormal motile sperm density values may be capable of fathering a child, whereas others with normal findings may be subfertile. Whether men with motile sperm density levels above the lower normal limit achieve higher fertility rates than those with lower values was investigated.

Methods.—Samples were acquired from 281 consecutive men of infertile couples among whom the female partner initially had an infertility factor. Two semen analyses obtained 48–72 hours after the last ejaculation were averaged.

Findings.—The conception rate was 36% when the motile sperm density was less than 4×10^6/mL and 81% when it was at least 5×10^6/mL. The difference in pregnancies was significant when couples with motile sperm density values below and above 2.5×10^6/mL were compared.

Conclusion.—It appears that motile sperm density does not distinguish between fertile and subfertile men, except possibly when the motile sperm density is less than 2.5×10^6/mL.

▶ These 3 reports (Abstracts 4–2, 4–3, and 4–4) serve to emphasize the point that present studies of sperm "biology," even when carefully performed, fall far short in terms of solving the infertility problems of couples when male factors are considered causal.—C.A. Paulsen, M.D.

Effect of Spermatozoa Selection on a Simplified Percoll Gradient in Case of Asthenozoospermia

Mathieu C, Mein M, Lornage J, Li JG, Guerin JF (Laboratoire de Biologie de la Reproduction, Lyon, France; Institut de Biologie de la Reproduction-Université Médicale no. 2 de Shanghai, République Populaire de Chine)

Andrologia 22:467–471, 1990 4–5

Objective.—Centrifugation on a Percoll gradient is an efficient method of selecting motile spermatozoa, but it requires more time than swim-up migration or simple resuspension after washing. The efficiency of a sim-

TABLE 1.—Sperm Characteristics in 21 Oligoasthenospermic Patients

	Mean ± SEM	Range
Concentration ($\times 10^6$/ml)	11.98 (± 1.45)	2.26-29.4
Motility (%)	19.19 (± 1.54)	5.99-29.53
Curvilinear Velocity (μm/s)	39.49 (± 1.87)	21.44-57.54
Linearity index	4.92 (± 0.19)	3.13-6.18
ALH* mean (μ)	2.64 (± 0.13)	1.52-4.05
ALH* max (μ)	3.32 (± 0.14)	1.86-4.87

**Abbreviation: ALH*, amplitude of lateral head displacement.
(Courtesy of Mathieu C, Mein M, Lornage J, et al: *Andrologia* 22:467–471, 1990.)

TABLE 2.—Sperm Characteristics in 21 Patients Regarding the Result of Swim-Up Migration

	Failure of migration N=9 (mean ± SEM)	Migration N=12 (mean ± SEM)
Concentration (x 10^6/ml)	10.87 (± 2.67) NS†	12.81 (± 1.63)
Motility (%)	19.90 (± 1.95) NS	18.67 (± 2.31)
Curvilinear Velocity (μm/s)	39.15 (± 2.66) NS	39.74 (± 2.70)
Linearity index	4.52 (± 0.31) NS	4.68 (± 0.23)
ALH* mean	2.59 (± 0.17) NS	2.67 (± 0.19)
ALH* max (μ)	3.21 (± 0.19) NS	3.39 (± 0.21)

Abbreviation: ALH, amplitude of lateral head displacement.
†NS = Student's t-test.
(Courtesy of Mathieu C, Mein M, Lornage J, et al: *Andrologia* 22:467–471, 1990.)

plified Percoll gradient for preparing semen in patients with asthenozoospermia was studied to determine whether it is possible to use this method for intrauterine insemination.

Methods.—In 21 patients with asthenozoospermia (motile forms ≤30%) (Table 1), semen preparation was performed with the swim-up migration or centrifugation on a 2-step density (40% and 70%) Percoll gradient. Sperm characteristics were studied by automated videomicrographic analysis.

Results.—Swim-up migration failed in 9 patients, whereas centrifugation on a Percoll gradient failed in only 1; the difference was significant.

TABLE 3.—Characteristics of the Fractions Obtained After Sperm Treatment by Swim-Up Migration and Centrifugation on a Simplified Percoll Gradient

	Migration N=12 Mean ± SEM	Percoll N=12 Mean ± SEM
Concentration (x 10^6/ml)	3.67 (± 0.62) NS	5.98 (± 0.85)
Motility (%)	22.26 (± 2.89) NS	26.04 (± 4.38)
Curvilinear Velocity (μm/s)	53.5 (± 3.25) †	47.60 (± 3.21)
Linearity index	5.82 (± 0.4) NS	5.16 (± 0.40)
ALH* mean (μ)	3.03 (± 0.25) NS	2.83 (± 0.27)
ALH* max (μ)	3.70 (± 0.29) NS	3.59 (± 0.29)

Abbreviation: ALH, amplitude of lateral head displacement.
† = $P < .01$ pair-test.
(Courtesy of Mathieu C, Mein M, Lornage J, et al: *Andrologia* 22:467–471, 1990.)

TABLE 4.—Characteristics of Sperm Movement After a 24-Hour Incubation

	Migration	Percoll
Total number	0/12	13/20
		(Mean ± SEM)
Motility (%)	0	17.85 (±2.98)
Curvilinear Velocitiy (μm/s)	-	42.55 (±2.52)
Linearity index	-	4.06 (±0.31)
ALH* mean	-	3.36 (±0.19)
ALH* max	-	4.14 (±0.20)

Abbreviation: ALH, amplitude of lateral head displacement.
(Courtesy of Mathieu C, Mein M, Lornage J, et al: *Andrologia* 22:467–471, 1990.)

Except for the higher curvilinear velocity after swim-up migration, there were no other significant differences in sperm parameters between the 2 groups (Tables 2 and 3). Survival of spermatozoa after 24 hours was undoubtedly better after centrifugation on a Percoll gradient, with two thirds of the motile spermatozoa at the initial time still motile at 24 hours (Table 4), although the characteristics of motility were modified.

Discussion.—Centrifugation on a 2-step Percoll gradient is more efficient than swim-up migration for selecting spermatozoa. With this method, preliminary results with intrauterine insemination are rather encouraging. Six pregnancies were achieved in 27 couples in which the male had oligozoospermia and/or asthenozoospermia, for a pregnancy rate per couple of 22% and a pregnancy rate per cycle of 11.54%.

Relationship Between Morphology and Motion Characteristics of Human Spermatozoa in Semen and in the Swim-Up Sperm Fractions

Oehninger S, Acosta R, Morshedi M, Philput C, Swanson RJ, Acosta AA (Jones Inst for Reproductive Medicine, Norfolk, Va; Eastern Virginia Med School, Norfolk)

J Androl 11:446–452, 1990 4–6

Purpose.—To determine the morphological patterns and motion characteristics of human spermatozoa, studies were made before and after swim-up preparation.

Methods.—A group of 57 patients who were undergoing fertility evaluation were divided into 2 morphologically different groups based on the percentage of normal sperm forms. Of the 36 patients with a sperm concentration of >20 × 10^6/mL and a progressive motility of >30%, 25 had ≥4% normal sperm forms [good prognosis pattern (G group)] and 11 had <4% normal forms [poor prognostic pattern (P group)]. Of the 16 oligoasthenozoospermic patients, 8 belonged to the G group and 8 were in the P group. Before and after the double-wash swim-up prepara-

TABLE 1.—Sperm Parameters in the Original Samples in Both Groups

	"Good" prognosis pattern (n = 25)	"Poor" prognosis pattern (n = 11)	P value
Volume (ml)	3.0 ± 0.2	2.9 ± 0.2	0.7
Concentration (× 10^6/ml)	90.6 ± 9.8	81.5 ± 16.7	0.6
% normal forms	8.8 ± 0.6	1.8 ± 0.3	0.0001*
% slightly abnormal forms	28.6 ± 1.3	19.2 ± 1.4	0.0002*
% severely amorphous heads	41.8 ± 2.4	54.6 ± 3.2	0.005*
% severely amorphous necks	12.4 ± 2.0	10.6 ± 2.5	0.6
% tail defects	5.6 ± 1.0	5.7 ± 1.1	0.9
% other defects	2.8 ± 0.7	8.1 ± 2.3	0.01
% motility	62.6 ± 3.2	50.4 ± 6.1	0.06
velocity (μm/sec)	44.7 ± 1.0	36.9 ± 2.4	0.001*
% cells velocity >80 (μm/sec)	5.5 ± 0.9	4.4 ± 1.1	0.4
% cells velocity >50 (μm/sec)	41.8 ± 2.5	28.5 ± 5.5	0.01
linearity	5.7 ± 0.1	5.7 ± 0.2	0.8
% cells linearity >8	26.4 ± 2.9	26.7 ± 4.8	0.9
% cells linearity >5	66.1 ± 2.7	62.5 ± 4.0	0.4

*Significant differences.
(Courtesy of Oehninger S, Acosta R, Morshedi M, et al: *J Androl* 11:446–452, 1990.)

tion, the morphology was assessed by 2 independent observers using the criteria of Kruger et al. Motile characteristics were analyzed by a computerized semen analyzer with constant parameter settings.

Results.—In patients with an acceptable sperm concentration and percentage of motility, there were no significant differences between the G and P groups in semen volume, percentage of neck and tail defects, semen concentration, or percentage of motility and linearity before swim-up (Table 1). However, the P group had significantly lower percentages of normal forms and slightly abnormal forms, and higher percentages of severe head defects with lower mean velocity. After swim-up, the C group had a higher percentage of motility and total number of motile cells, and a higher recovery rate, compared with the P group (Table 2). The inci-

TABLE 2.—Sperm Parameters After Swim-Up Separation in Both Groups

	"Good" prognosis pattern	P value (compared to original)	"Poor" prognosis pattern	P value (compared to original)	P value (comparing "good" vs. "poor" after swim-up)
% morphology	13.2 ± 0.6	0.00001*	4.0 ± 0.6	0.005*	0.00001*
% motility	89.2 ± 1.3	0.0001*	76.1 ± 2.2	0.0001*	0.0001*
velocity (μm/sec)	61.5 ± 2.0	0.0001*	55.1 ± 2.5	0.0001*	0.05
% cells velocity > 80 (μm/sec)	23.6 ± 3.5	0.0001*	15.3 ± 3.3	0.009*	0.1
% cells velocity > 50 (μm/sec)	70.4 ± 3.1	0.0001*	62.0 ± 4.8	0.0002*	0.1
linearity	6.6 ± 0.2	0.002*	5.8 ± 0.4	0.7	0.07
% cells linearity > 8	38.5 ± 4.4	0.02	26.0 ± 6.0	0.9	0.1
% cells linearity > 5	77.2 ± 3.1	0.01	62.6 ± 8.0	0.9	0.04
Total motile recoverable/ejaculate (× 10^6)	76.6 ± 15.0	—	41.3 ± 16.5		0.00001*
Recovery rate (%)	42.0 ± 4.0	—	18.0 ± 2.8		0.00001*

*Significant differences.
(Courtesy of Oehninger S, Acosta R, Morshedi M, et al: *J Androl* 11:446–452, 1990.)

TABLE 3.—Sperm Parameters Before and After Swim-Up Separation in Patients With Oligoasthenoteratozoospermia and in Patients With Oligoasthenozoospermia

	Oligoasthenoteratozoospermia (n = 8)	Oligoasthenozoospermia (n = 8)
Original sample		
% normal forms	1.7 ± 0.4	6.5 ± 0.9
% slightly abnormal forms	22.3 ± 2.9	25.6 ± 3.1
% severely amorphous heads	47.8 ± 5.4	40.8 ± 18.0
% motility	25.7 ± 4.1	22.5 ± 4.6
velocity (μm/sec)	37.8 ± 3.7	41.4 ± 2.2
linearity	6.3 ± 0.4	4.1 ± 0.4
Concentration motile ($\times 10^6$/ml)	4.7 ± 0.4	9.0 ± 3.3
Post swim-up		
% normal forms	4.0 ± 0.4*	9.7 ± 0.7
% motility	47.9 ± 5.4*	66.7 ± 4.7*
velocity (μm/sec)	58.3 ± 3.0*	62.6 ± 3.3*
Total motile/ejaculate ($\times 10^6$)	1.6 ± 0.5	3.2 ± 1.9
Recovery rate (%)	12.4 ± 3.1	20.9 ± 6.9

*Significant differences compared to original.
(Courtesy of Oehninger S, Acosta R, Morshedi M, et al: *J Androl* 11:446–452, 1991.)

dence of severe head defects correlated negatively with the percentage of cells having a velocity of >80% μm/sec. Similar results were obtained in the oligoasthenozoospermic patients, with recovery rates being lower than those in patients with G pattern and good concentration and motility after swim-up, indicating dramatic impairment of sperm function (Table 3).

Conclusion.—The percentage of motility and velocity improves substantially after swim-up, but the recovery rates and percentage of motility are lower in the P group. Those patients with a high incidence of sperm head defects have impaired initial velocity; swim-up selects for velocity, as well as for normal forms and motility.

Male Infertility Due to Asthenozoospermia and Flagellar Anomaly: Detection in Routine Semen Analysis

Marmor D, Grob-Menendez F (Hôpital Saint-Antoine, Paris)

Int J Androl 14:108–116, 1991 4–7

Background.—Sperm tail anomalies that affect the length and/or thickness of the sperm tail can be recognized by light microscopic analysis. A morphological classification was used in routine semen analysis that permitted recognition of major monomorphous teratozoospermia caused by flagellar structural anomalies associated with asthenozoospermia and infertility.

Methods.—Semen samples were obtained from 4,231 infertile men, all of whom provided a complete history and underwent a physical examination. Sperm mobility and forward motility were measured at 1 hour and 4 hours after ejaculation. One hundred sperm were examined under high magnification and classified according to each abnormality. Absent, short, thick, irregular diameter, coiled, and multiple sperm tail anomalies were recorded. In vitro sperm penetration tests into human cervical mucus also were performed.

Results.—Of 4,231 patients, 69 had major monomorphous teratozoospermia. Flagella were either absent or very short in 16 cases, shortened and of irregular thickness in 18 cases, and of normal length but with diameter abnormalities in 8 cases. These syndromes were always associated with poor forward motility, but mobility and penetration into human cervical mucus were sometimes only partially impaired. A trained observer and good sperm smears made it possible to make the diagnosis without using electron microscopy. All affected patients were sterile, and several had syndromes that could have been transmitted genetically.

Conclusions.—There is no present treatment for sperm tail structural anomaly, but sperm with abnormal tails can undergo acrosome reaction and penetrate zona-free hamster ova. Therefore, it is likely that these men could benefit from the new techniques of in vitro fertilization using sperm microinjection under the zona pellucida.

▶ A practical suggestion comes from this extensive study. An electron microscope is not necessary to detect the most frequent flagellar anomalies in sperm from infertile men.—C.A. Paulsen, M.D.

Evaluation of Human Sperm Hyperactivated Motility and Its Relationship With the Zona-Free Hamster Oocyte Sperm Penetration Assay

Wang C, Leung A, Tsoi W-L, Leung J, Ng V, Lee K-F, Chan SYW (Univ of Hong Kong, Queen Mary Hosp, Hong Kong; Cedars-Sinai Med Ctr, Los Angeles)

J Androl 12:253–257, 1991 4–8

Introduction.—Capacitation, the final maturation of spermatozoa, usually occurs in the female reproductive tract before oocyte interaction. It is characterized by spermatozoa undergoing the acrosome reaction and developing hyperactivated motility (HA). Assessing HA may be a means of evaluating capacitation.

Methods.—The HA characteristics of human spermatozoa were studied in 50 samples from patients attending an infertility clinic. The relationship of HA to the results of zona-free hamster oocyte sperm penetration assays (SPA) of the semen samples was investigated. Hyperactivated motility was assessed in the seminal plasma and after swim-up preparation of spermatozoa at 1, 3, and 24 hours of incubation in capacitation media.

Results.—Hyperactivated motility peaked at 1 hour and plateaued at 3 hours. The group with no penetration in the SPA had a significantly lower percentage of spermatozoa in seminal plasma with star-spin hyperactivated motility. Characteristics of HA were not different in groups with or without penetration. According to correlation analysis, there was no significant relationship between the HA parameters and SPA score.

When HA characteristics were compared in samples with normal and abnormal semen analysis, the total percentage of spermatozoa with HA and the proportion with star-spin at 3 hours were significantly reduced in the group with abnormal semen analysis.

Conclusion.—Lower HA of spermatozoa was found in patients with a score of 0 for SPA and in those with abnormal semen analysis. Although the results of SPA and HA were not directly correlated, assessing HA may nevertheless be a useful early indicator of capacitation abnormalities in human spermatozoa not measured by SPA.

▶ The need to use human sperm hyperactivated motility does not appear to be very important.—C.A. Paulsen, M.D.

Relationship Between Hypoosmotic Swelling Test, Semen Analysis, and Zona-Free Hamster Ovum Test

Fuse H, Kazama T, Katayama T (Toyama Medical and Pharmaceutical Univ, Toyama, Japan)

Arch Androl 27:73–78, 1991 4–9

Introduction.—Routine semen analysis cannot demonstrate the functional capacity of a sample. The zona-free hamster ovum sperm penetration test (ZSPT) is time consuming and complex. An alternative is the hypoosmotic swelling test (HOST), a relatively simple means of determining the integrity of the sperm membrane.

Study Plan.—Semen samples from 54 patients aged 20–45 years with infertility of unknown origin were evaluated by routine analysis, the HOST, and the ZSPT.

Findings.—Swollen sperm were significantly more prevalent in samples having normal routine parameters than when the sperm concentration and/or percentage of motile sperm were abnormal. Sperm concentration correlated with the percent of swollen sperm, as did the percent of motile sperm. The percent of swollen sperm correlated only weakly with the percent of sperm penetration.

Conclusion.—The HOST cannot be used as an alternative to the ZSPT for assessing the competency of fertilization.

Hypoosmotic Swelling Test of Sperm

Takahashi K, Uchida A, Kitao M (Shimane Med Univ, Izumo, Japan)

Arch Androl 25:225–242, 1990 4–10

Introduction.—Experience with standard semen analysis has shown that this technique cannot be relied upon to accurately determine the potential of sperm for fertilization. In view of the recent advances and increased application of in vitro fertilization methods, a simple and more accurate sperm fertility test for predicting pregnancy outcome is needed. The hypoosmotic swelling test (HOST) is used to test sperm fertility func-

Semen Analysis and Hypoosmotic Swelling Test of Infertile Men, Fertile Men, and Patients Who Achieved Pregnancy by Artificial Insemination-Husband

	Total Sperm Concentration ($\times 10^6$/ml)	Motility (%)	Motile Sperm Concentration ($\times 10^6$/ml)	HOS Test Total Swollen (%)	HOS Test g-Type Swollen (%)
Infertile men (n = 74)	29.7 ± 20.3^a	44.6 ± 20.4^a	13.0 ± 10.6^a	40.6 ± 14.3^a	14.3 ± 8.0^a
AIH men (n = 7)	38.3 ± 11.1^c	65.2 ± 11.7^c	25.0 ± 8.5^a	53.5 ± 7.7^d	21.5 ± 8.4^d
Fertile men (n = 10)	115.6 ± 47.0^b	78.3 ± 12.7^b	86.0 ± 26.4^b	57.6 ± 7.9^b	23.8 ± 5.0^b

$^{a\text{-}b}P < .001$.
$^{b\text{-}c}P < .01$.
$^{b\text{-}d}P < .05$.
(Courtesy of Takahashi K, Uchida A, Kitao M: *Arch Androl* 25:225–242, 1990.)

tions. The usefulness of the HOST in predicting sperm potential for fertilization was evaluated.

Method. To perform the HOST, a small quantity of semen is suspended in hypoosmotic solution, incubated for 60 minutes at 37° C, and then immediately examined at 400× magnification under a phase-contrast microscope. The morphological changes in the cell membrane of the sperm tails are classified into groups a – g. At least 100 spermatozoa are counted and the percentage of g-type swollen sperm, considered to be an effective index of fertility, is determined.

Study Design.—Standard semen analysis and the HOST were performed on sperm samples obtained from 74 infertile men, 7 men who achieved pregnancy by artificial insemination-husband, and 10 fertile men. A comparison between standard semen analysis and the HOST showed a positive weak correlation between total sperm concentration, percent motility, and motile sperm concentration, and percentages of total swollen sperm and g-type swollen sperm (table). Although a previous study found that the HOST and the hamster test correlated strongly for normal sperm, no correlation was observed here between the percentages of sperm penetration using the hamster test and total swollen sperm using the HOST, but a weak correlation existed with the percentage of g-type swollen sperm. However, these 2 tests appear to reflect different aspects of sperm function. When sperm motility and swollen sperm rates were compared after sperm adjustment using the swim-up/washing method, there were no differences in sperm motility between normal and abnormal sperm groups, but significant differences between the groups persisted for swollen sperm (Fig 4–2). The HOST not only evaluates sperm motility; it also reflects other functions involved in infertility. Overall, the results of the HOST showed high values when pregnancy was achieved. Thus it may be the most effective predictor of the results of therapy for male infertility.

Conclusion.—The HOST appears currently to be the most practical test for predicting the potential of sperm for fertilization in couples treated for male infertility.

▶ These 2 reports (Abstracts 4–9 and 4–10) underscore the difficulty of using

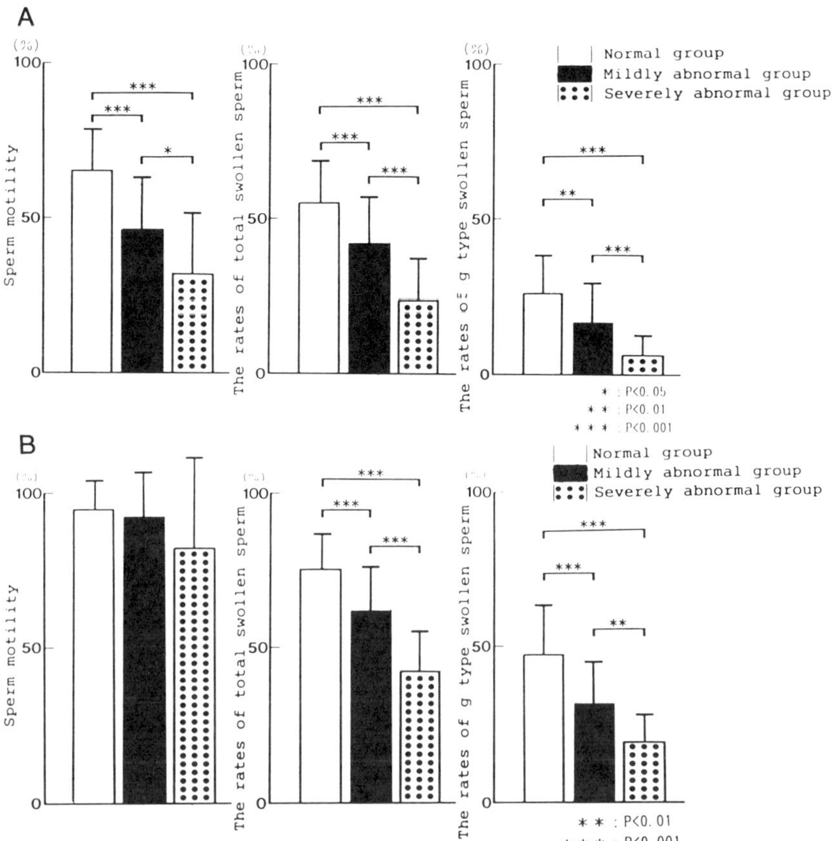

Fig 4–2.—Comparison of sperm motility and swollen sperm rates of semen sample from the normal abnormal groups (mean ± SD). **A,** original sperm. There were significant differences between the groups in sperm motility and swollen sperm rates of the original sperm sample. **B,** adjusted sperm. After sperm adjustment, there were significant differences among the groups in the swollen sperm. There were no significant differences in sperm motility. (Courtesy of Takahashi K, Uchida A, Kitao M: *Arch Androl* 25:225–242, 1990.)

results obtained from hypoosmotic swelling as an assessment of normalcy.— C.A. Paulsen, M.D.

Defining the Valid Hemizona Assay: Accounting for Binding Variability Within Zonae Pellucidae and Within Semen Samples From Fertile Males
Franken DR, Oehninger SC, Coddington CC, Kruger TF, Burkman LJ, Hodgen GD, Oosthuizen WT (Tygerberg Hosp, Parow, South Africa; Eastern Virginia Med School, Norfolk)
Fertil Steril 56:1156–1161, 1991 4–11

Background.—The hemizona assay (HZA) is a bioassay for assessing sperm performance. Its optimal use will depend on a better understanding of the variables that affect data interpretation and clinical correlations. The variability of sperm binding capacity within and between fertile controls was studied.

Methods.—Semen were collected from proven fertile men and 1 subfertile man. The variability of sperm binding capacity during 90 days, variability of sperm binding using different oocytes, and the lower limits of the number of sperm bound from the fertile control in 2 laboratories were determined. The main outcome measure was the number of sperm bound tightly to the hemizona.

Findings.—In the 6 fertile men a similar degree of variability was observed in zona binding during 90 days. The average individual sperm binding ranged from 68 to 127. Three of the 15 simultaneous assays showed very low numbers of sperm bound, indicating that 20% of the zonae had poor binding. In 18 men with 0% fertilization in an in vitro fertilization system using mature oocytes, the HZA indicated poor sperm binding. The 95% confidence interval was 20 sperm bound.

Conclusions.—Within the limitations of this research, the HZA is able to control for the intrinsic variability in zona pellucida binding capacity because it uses the matching halves of a single egg. With these guidelines, HZA applications can be made with more reassurance of a valid bioassay of sperm fertilizing potential.

▶ Careful definition as the lower percent binding shown by fertile men when HZA is used.—C.A. Paulsen, M.D.

Functional Aspects of Human Sperm Binding to the Zona Pellucida Using the Hemizona Assay

Coddington CC, Franken DR, Burkman LJ, Oosthuizen WT, Kruger T, Hodgen GD (Eastern Virginia Med School, Norfolk; Tygerberg Hosp, Parow, South Africa)

J Androl 12:1–8, 1991 4–12

Objective.—The hemizona assay (HZA) facilitates investigation of factors that influence sperm binding to the zona pellucida. Three studies were conducted to examine the relationship between hyperactivated sperm motility and HZA binding, to assess the binding kinetics and efficiency of sperm from subfertile men, and to determine the effects of the freeze/thaw procedure on binding capacity.

Methods. Semen was obtained from 7 subfertile men who failed to achieve fertilization in an in vitro fertilization program and from 7 men proved to be fertile. A general HZA protocol was adopted (Fig 4–3), and the hemizona index was calculated for each experimental and control hemizona. The effects of the frozen/thaw procedure on zona binding kinetics were evaluated by comparing thawed sperm specimens with fresh sperm preparation from the same fertile man.

Results.—The mean number of bound spermatozoa and the incidence of hyperactivated motility were significantly greater for sperm samples

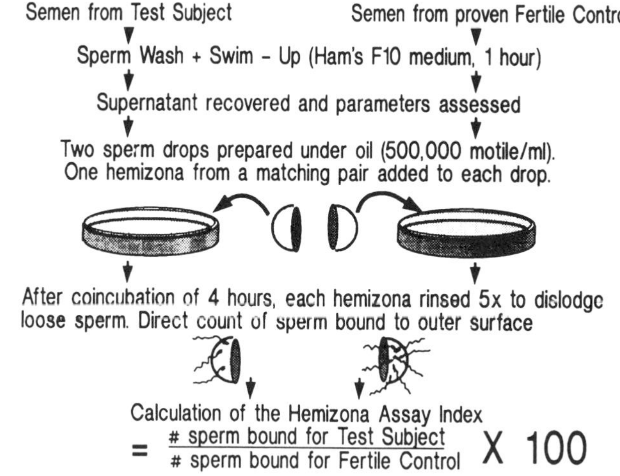

Fig 4–3.—Flow diagram of the general procedure for the hemizona assay. (Courtesy of Coddington CC, Franken DR, Burkman LJ, et al: *J Androl* 12:1–8, 1991.)

from proved fertile men than for those from subfertile men (table). There was a significant positive correlation between hyperactivated motility and the efficiency of tight binding to the zona pellucida. The kinetics of sperm binding was optimal at 4 hours in both the fertile and subfertile groups, and longer incubations did not increase binding. Although the kinetics of the hemizona binding curves were parallel in the fertile and subfertile groups, the magnitude of binding was severely reduced in the latter. Compared with matched fresh sperm, the frozen-thawed sperm showed HZA binding efficiency reduced by as much as 30% (Fig 4–4). However,

Incidence of Hyperactivated Motility, Binding to the Hemizona at 4 Hours, and Sperm Morphology for Proved Fertile and Subfertile Men (Series 1)

	Fertile men			Subfertile men		
Exp. no.	Hyper. (%)	Bound* (no.)	Normal morphology (%)	Hyper. (%)	Bound* (no.)	Normal morphology (%)
1	13.3	16	18	18.8	10	3
2	45.0	15	7	19.0	4	0
3	30.0	64	20	17.5	20	0
4	20.0	28	8	10.0	17	2
5	19.2	17	9	5.9	0	1
6	34.0	35	19	11.1	3	1
7	40.0	44	28	25.0	2	5
Mean ± SEM	30.44† ± 4.18	36.67‡ ± 8.54	16.4† ± 2.7	15.33 ± 2.48	6.56 ± 2.47	1.44 ± 0.6

*Smaller number of sperm bound here are the result of original HZA methodology, which employed 250,000 sperm/mL. All subsequent data were generated with 500,000 motile sperm/mL, which would make these numbers approximately twofold larger.

†Mean is significantly greater than the value for subfertile men ($P < .05$).

‡Mean is significantly greater than the value for subfertile men ($P < .001$).

(Courtesy of Coddington CC, Franken DR, Burkman LJ, et al: *J Androl* 12:1–8, 1991.)

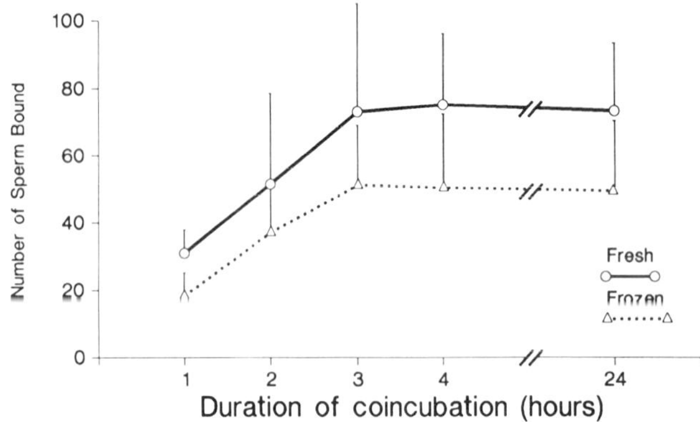

Fig 4–4.—Kinetics of zona binding by fresh vs. frozen-thawed spermatozoa from proved fertile men. Coincubation was carried through 24 hours, with brief interruptions for sperm counting at 1, 2, 3, and 4 hours (mean ± 1 SD; series 3). (Courtesy of Coddington CC, Franken DR, Burkman LJ, et al: *J Androl* 12:1–8, 1991.)

the kinetics of hemizona binding curves for the fresh and thawed sperm remained parallel.

Conclusion.—Hyperactivated sperm motility correlates positively with zona binding capacity. The deficient zona binding capacity of sperm from subfertile men results from markedly reduced sperm binding. The process of freezing and thawing spermatozoa impairs their capacity to binding to the zona pellucida.

▶ Another study showing that present methods for freezing and thawing sperm are not adequate. It is hoped that new methods will be developed to solve this pressing problem now that the use of "fresh" semen for donor insemination is prohibited.—C.A. Paulsen, M.D.

Staining of the Inner Acrosomal Membrane of Human Spermatozoa With Concanavalin A Lectin as an Indicator of Potential Egg Penetration Ability

Holden CA, Trounson AO (Monash Med Ctr, Clayton, Victoria, Australia)

Fertil Steril 56:967–974, 1991 4–13

Background.—A newly developed method of assessing the acrosomal status of human spermatozoa involves the specific binding of fluorescein-labeled concanavalin A (FITC-ConA) to the inner acrosomal membrane. Loss of the acrosomal cap is clearly visualized and, when combined with viability staining, the method distinguishes between true and degenerative acrosomal loss.

Objective.—The sensitivity of the FITC-ConA staining method in evaluating acrosomal status was examined by estimating acrosomal loss after 4 hours and 10 hours of incubation. Penetration of zona-free human eggs then was determined 16 hours after reinsemination.

Findings.—Acrosomal loss increased significantly when human spermatozoa were incubated in strontium- or lanthanum-based medium, or in T6 plus 10% maternal serum supplemented with cyclic guanosine monophosphate and imidazole for 4 hours before transfer to fresh T6 plus 10% maternal serum for 6 hours more (compared with T6 plus 10% serum for a total of 10 hours). Increased acrosomal loss correlated well with the increased development of pronuclei in zona-free human eggs.

Conclusions.—The FITC-ConA staining method is a simple means of evaluating acrosomal status and the penetrating ability of human spermatozoa. The method should prove useful both clinically and in research on sperm fertilizing ability.

Determination of Neutrophil Concentration in Semen by Measurement of Superoxide Radical Formation

Kovalski N, de Lamirande E, Gagnon C (Royal Victoria Hosp, Montreal; McGill Univ, Montreal)

Fertil Steril 56:946–953, 1991 4–14

Objective.—An attempt was made to develop an inexpensive, rapid, quantitative, and functional test of neutrophil concentration that is applicable to semen. To be suitable for an infertility clinic, such a test would necessarily be technically simple and easy to interpret.

The Assay.—The nitroblue tetrazolium (NBT) assay measures the functional capacity of neutrophils in seminal fluid. Because it is reduced by superoxide anion to yield blue formazan, the NBT can serve as an indicator of reactive oxygen species produced by neutrophils.

Observations.—The NBT assay clearly detects neutrophils at concentrations as low as $.5 \times 10^6$/mL in semen, independent of the sperm concentration. Only 10 minutes of preparation time are required. The intensity of the derived blue color is proportional to the concentration of active neutrophils. Only 2 of 67 infertile men with round cells in the ejaculate had positive assay findings of at least $.5 \times 10^6$/mL.

Conclusions.—The NBT assay should prove helpful in determining whether neutrophil function is a better indicator of genital infection than concentration per se. The assay may be applicable to vaginal and cervical secretions.

▶ Reasonable suggestion. Because many normal fertile men have significant numbers of neutrophils in their ejaculate, tests for determining the "potency" of these cells should be developed.—C.A. Paulsen, M.D.

Evaluation of Human Sperm Morphology Using Strict Criteria After Diff-Quik Staining: Correlation of Morphology With Fertilization In Vitro

Enginsu ME, Dumoulin JCM, Pieters MHEC, Bras M, Evers JLH, Geraedts JPM (Univ of Limburg, Maastricht, The Netherlands)

Hum Reprod 6:854–858, 1991 4–15

Objective.—Because simple assessment of the proportion of abnormal spermatozoa in human semen remains subject to considerable debate in the context of male infertility, strict criteria were used in evaluating sperm morphology after Diff-Quik staining. Morphological scores were correlated with fertilization in 64 men who participated in an in vitro fertilization program. All had a sperm concentration of 20 million/mL or higher and progressive motility exceeding 30%.

Findings.—When 4% or fewer sperm appeared normal on strict criteria, the fertilization rate per oocyte was 23%. In contrast, a fertilization rate of 77% was found if 11% or more of the sperm had normal morphology. With 4% to 11% of normal sperm, the fertilization rate per oocyte was 49%. Classic semen parameters did not differ significantly in these groups except for the morphology evaluation using WHO criteria.

Conclusion.—Diff-Quik staining with very strict criteria for assessing sperm morphology is a useful means of predicting the outcome of in vitro fertilization for individual couples. Each laboratory should establish its own cutoff levels for predicting fertilization rates.

▶ Before this editor capitulates *(supra vidae),* it will be necessary to see data on clinical pregnancy and "take-home baby" comparisons.—C.A. Paulsen, M.D.

Use of Aniline Blue to Assess Chromatin Condensation in Morphologically Normal Spermatozoa in Normal and Infertile Men

Hofmann N, Hilscher B (Heinrich-Heine Univ Düsseldorf; Medical Inst of Environmental Hygiene, Düsseldorf, Germany)

Hum Reprod 6:979–982, 1991 4–16

Introduction.—Condensation of chromatin is critical for normal sperm function in carrying the paternal genome. The degree of condensation can be demonstrated by acidic aniline blue staining, which distinguishes between lysine-rich histones on one hand, and arginine- and cysteine-rich protamines on the other.

Study Plan.—Semen samples were acquired from 107 patients with fertility disorders who attended an andrological clinical and from 56 others who had failed to respond in assisted fertility programs.

Findings.—Chromatin condensation was abnormal not only in malformed, but also in morphologically normal, spermatozoa. About 25% of morphologically normal sperm were immature and exhibited uptake of aniline blue dye. Stained spermatozoa formed up to 78% of the total where repeated attempts at in vitro fertilization had failed.

Implication.—A prospective study is in order to determine the value of acidic aniline blue staining of spermatozoa in assisted fertilization programs.

▶ This report shows again that normal appearing sperm are not necessarily biologically normal regardless of which strict criteria are used or whether swim-up or other "harvesting" procedures are employed. (The study in Abstract 4–17 refutes my comments.)—C.A. Paulsen, M.D.

Ejaculatory Duct Obstruction in Subfertile Males: Analysis of 87 Patients
Pryor JP, Hendry WF (Inst of Urology, London)
Fertil Steril 56:725–730, 1991 4–17

Objective.—Ejaculatory duct obstruction is considered to be rare. The diagnosis may be suspected clinically from seminal analysis. The finding of a small volume of acid semen which does not contain fructose, in a patient with azoospermia or severe oligozoospermia in whom the vasa are palpable is virtually pathognomonic. The clinical picture may be complicated, however, by the obstruction being unilateral, partial, or functional. The diagnosis can be confirmed only by vasography.

Patients.—Ejaculatory duct obstruction was found in 87 men who underwent scrotal exploration and concomitant vasography under general anesthesia. Obstructing cystic congenital lesions in the region of the verumontanum were treated by incision of the verumontanum with the optical urethrotome. Ductal obstruction was treated by resection of the verumontanum. Coexisting epididymal obstruction was treated by epididymovasostomies when indicated.

Results.—Sixty-seven of the 87 patients had azoospermia, 17 had very severe oligozoospermia, 1 had oligozoospermia, and 2 had normal sperm concentrations. A small volume of ejaculate with acid pH and low or absent fructose content was found in 89% of the 75 men for whom this information was available. In 17 men, vasography revealed single midline müllerian duct cysts, ranging from 1 to 2 cm in diameter. Endoscopic incision of the cyst improved the seminal quality in 10 of 12 men with adequate follow-up data, and 5 female partners subsequently became pregnant. In 19 men with wolffian malformations, surgical treatment was

Number of Patients Successfully Treated/Number With Adequate Follow-Up in the Various Groups

Group	Patency	Reservoirs	Pregnancies produced
Congenital			
Müllerian (n = 17)	10/12		5
Wolffian (n = 19)	1/6	1/3	1
Traumatic (n = 15)	2/6	4/4	1
Postinfective (n = 19)	4/6	1/4	2
Tuberculous (n = 8)			1
Megavesicles (n = 8)	1/1	1/1	
Neoplastic (n = 1)			
Total (n = 87)	18/31	7/12	10

(Courtesy of Pryor JP, Hendry WF: *Fertil Steril* 56:725–730, 1991.)

largely unsuccessful as patency was restored in only 1 of them. Fifteen men had traumatic obstructions from previous operations, and 19 men had a history of previous genital, urinary, or tuberculous infection. Patency was restored in 4 patients with previous infections, and 1 partner subsequently became pregnant. In all, patency was restored in 25 of 43 men with adequate follow-up, and 10 partners became pregnant (table). Treatment was primarily surgical in 31 men, of whom 18 achieved patency and 6 produced pregnancies in their partners. Reservoirs were inserted in 12 men, spermatozoa were obtained in 7, and 2 of them produced pregnancies.

Conclusion.—Ejaculatory duct obstruction in subfertile men is not as rare as previously thought. Surgical intervention may restore fertility in some patients. Routine vasography is recommended to avoid overlooking this diagnosis.

▶ Although ejaculatory duct obstruction is a rare condition, if the male partner of an infertile couple has azoospermia or severe oligozoospermia the clinician should perform the appropriate diagnostic studies to determine whether this condition is present. If so, it is one of the few causes of azoospermia that can be treated successfully.—D.R. Mishell, Jr., M.D.

5 Pathophysiology of Male Infertility

Testicular Function After Unilateral Bacterial Epididymo-Orchitis

Osegbe DN (Lagos Univ Teaching Hosp, Surulere, Lagos, Nigeria)

Eur Urol 19:204–208, 1991 5–1

Introduction.—Infection is not typically associated with male infertility, and studies on this subject are lacking. A link between male infertility and bacterial gonadal infection was investigated in 45 men aged 18–50 years who had unilateral bacterial epididymo-orchitis.

Methods.—All of the men had scrotal pain and had been treated with some form of antibiotic for preliminary urethritis. Fertility was evaluated by paternity history, repeated semen examinations, serum follicle-stimulating hormone (FSH) determinations, and testicular biopsy. Cefotaxime treatment and analgesics were continued on an outpatient basis. Semen was analyzed at 1, 3, 6, and 12 weeks, and then every 3 months. The FSH was determined again at 6 months. Clinical response to treatment was assessed at 1 week and 2 weeks, and then monthly.

Results.—Testicular pain abated between 5 days and 7 days after initiation of cefotaxime therapy in all subjects. Tenderness and swelling lasted somewhat longer. Fourteen men had proved their fertility before infection. Two years after infection, only 21% of those fathers produced semen considered adequate for conception, and 60% of all subjects had semen concentrations inadequate for conception. Unilateral infection of the testis and its epididymis resulted in severe oligospermia and azoospermia in many men, with biopsy specimens indicating bilateral gonadal damage.

Discussion.—Delayed or inappropriate treatment for bacterial gonadal infection causes testicular loss and subsequent failure of the testis to regain spermatogenic function. Gonadal bacterial infection can cause infertility, and prompt, aggressive treatment must be administered to avoid resultant azoospermia or permanent oligospermia.

► An interesting article from a geographical area where almost an epidemic of infertility, secondary to genital tract infections in both men and women, plays an important etiologic role.—C.A. Paulsen, M.D.

Testicular Dysfunction in Hodgkin's Disease Before and After Treatment

Viviani S, Ragni G, Santoro A, Perotti L, Caccamo E, Negretti E, Valagussa P, Bonadonna G (Istituto Nazionale Tumori, Milan; Univ of Milan, Italy)

Eur J Cancer 27:1389–1392, 1991 5–2

Background.—Treatment of Hodgkin's disease with mechlorethamine, vincristine, procarbazine, prednisone (MOPP) or similar drug combinations produces testicular damage in perhaps 90% of patients. It has been suggested that hypogonadism in untreated patients may result not simply from primary testicular failure, but from a complex abnormality involving the hypothalamic-pituitary axis.

Study Plan.—Testicular function was examined in 92 males with Hodgkin's disease before treatment, and studies were repeated in 77 patients who were in complete remission after alternating therapy with MOPP and combined doxorubicin, bleomycin, vinblastine, and dacarbazine (ABVD protocol).

Findings.—Pretreatment studies suggested impaired fertility in two thirds of the patients despite normal basal levels of gonadotropins, testosterone, and prolactin. Nearly 90% of those in remission after chemotherapy were azoospermic; only 4% were normospermic. Spermatogenesis recovered in 40% of 42 patients who were reassessed after a median of 27 months. Gonadotropin levels rose significantly after chemotherapy, but testosterone and prolactin levels did not change significantly. The FSH levels remained high in 8 of 10 patients who recovered testicular function.

Conclusions.—Young men with Hodgkin's disease have underlying gonadal dysfunction apart from the effects of chemotherapy. Cryopreservation of semen may not be the answer. An alternative is to design new treatment regimens that produce minimal gonadal toxicity.

▶ Another look at an important problem. The main finding was the abnormalities observed in these men before chemotherapy.—C.A. Paulsen, M.D.

Comparison of the Incidence of *Ureaplasma urealyticum* in Infertile Men and in Donors of Semen

de Jong Z, Pontonnier F, Plante P, Perie N, Talazac N, Mansat A, Chabanon G (Rangueil Univ Hosp, Toulouse, France; Hosp La Grave, Toulouse)

Eur Urol 18:127–131, 1990 5–3

Introduction.—The role of the genital mycoplasmas in human infertility has not been established.

Methods.—The frequency of *Ureaplasma urealyticum* in semen specimens from fertile and infertile men was investigated in 569 infertile and 75 fertile men studied from 1985 to 1987. The fertile men were semen donors who had at least 1 child and normal semen characteristics.

Results.—*Ureaplasma urealyticum* was found in the semen samples from 40 infertile men (7%) and from 4 fertile men (5.3%). The difference between these frequencies was not statistically significant. Infertile men with *U. urealyticum* in semen specimens had an average period of infertility of 4 years; 35 of these men had primary and 5 had secondary infertility. When the results of routine semen analysis in the 40 infertile men with *U. urealyticum* were compared with those in infertile uninfected men, no significant differences were found between the 2 groups. Of the infertile men with *U. urealyticum* treated with doxycycline, 100 mg twice a day for 28 days, treatment was successful in 77.5%.

Conclusions.—*Ureaplasma urealyticum* appears to be as frequent in fertile men as in infertile men.

▶ Several studies now have concluded that the incidence of genital mycoplasmas has very little to do with infertility, but studies such as this are needed to convince the clinicians.—C.A. Paulsen, M.D.

Andrological Investigations in Men Treated With Acitretin (Ro 10-1670)

Parsch E-M, Ruzicka Th, Przybilla B, Schill W-B (Dermatologische Klinik und Poliklinik d Ludwig-Maximilians-Universität München, Germany)

Andrologia 22:479–482, 1990 5–4

Introduction.—Acitretin, the free acid of etretinate, is a dermatologic preparation used in the treatment of psoriasis and other keratinization disorders. Its effects on spermatogenesis and the hypothalamic-pituitary-gonadal axis in men were assessed.

Methods.—Ten men were treated with orally administered acitretin (Ro 10-1670), 25–50 mg daily for 3 months. The group included healthy men and men with psoriasis. Semen and blood analyses were performed before, during, and after treatment to evaluate the effects of acitretin on spermatogenesis and the hypothalamic-pituitary-gonadal axis.

Results.—Compared with pretreatment values, the sperm concentration, sperm morphology, total sperm motility, ejaculate volume, and the seminal plasma fructose concentration remained unchanged during and

TABLE 1.—Semen Parameters of 10 Male Probands Treated With Acitretin (Ro 10-1670)

Semen parameters	Before treatment (mean of 2 pretreatment values)	Treatment 4 weeks	Treatment 12 weeks	After treatment 1 - 3 months
sperm count (Mio/ml)	96.9 ± 64.9	88.7 ± 86.6	112.8 ± 96.3	94.3 ± 89.8
total sperm motility (%)	48.3 ± 12.1	45.0 ± 9.7	46.1 ± 12.2	45.4 ± 15.9
sperm morphology (% normal shaped)	48.1 ± 13.4	43.3 ± 14.5	43.3 ± 13.0	42.2 ± 11.9
ejaculate volume (ml)	3.0 ± 1.5	3.3 ± 1.5	3.7 ± 1.7	3.4 ± 1.4
seminal plasma fructose concentration (mg/ml)	2.7 ± 1.2	2.8 ± 1.1	3.0 ± 0.9	2.5 ± 0.9

Mean values (±SEM) of various semen criteria are given before, after 4 weeks, at the end of a 3-month treatment period, and 1–3 months after withdrawal of medication.

(Courtesy of Parsch E-M, Ruzicka Th, Przybilla B, et al: *Andrologia* 22:479–482, 1990.)

TABLE 2.—Serum Hormone Levels of 10 Men Treated with Acitretin (Ro 10-1670) Over a Period of 3 Months

Hormones	Pretreatment value	After 4 weeks	After 12 weeks	After treatment 1 - 3 months
FSH (mIU/ml)	5.0 ± 1.5	5.4 ± 1.3	5.0 ± 0.9	5.2 ± 1.1
LH (mIU/ml)	7.3 ± 1.5	6.4 ± 3.5	6.3 ± 1.7	6.7 ± 2.3
Testosterone (ng/ml)	5.8 ± 2.4	6.0 ± 1.9	5.6 ± 1.2	4.2 ± 2.4

Mean values (±SEM) are given.
(Courtesy of Parsch E-M, Ruzicka Th, Przybilla B, et al: *Andrologia* 22:479–482, 1990.)

after treatment in men with normal pretreatment spermatogenesis and those with preexisting sperm abnormalities (Table 1). There were no significant changes in serum concentrations of major gonadal hormones during or after treatment, compared with pretreatment values (Table 2).

Conclusion.—Prolonged acitretin treatment in therapeutic doses apparently does not adversely affect male reproductive function.

▶ This article contains important negative data on a new preparation being used to treat psoriasis. The known adverse effect of certain retinoids were not observed in these men.—C.A. Paulsen, M.D.

Human Preovulatory Oocytes Have a Higher Sperm-Binding Ability Than Immature Oocytes Under Hemizona Assay Conditions: Evidence Supporting the Concept of "Zona Maturation"

Oehninger S, Kruger TF, Veeck L, Acosta AA, Franken D, Hodgen GD (Eastern Virginia Med School, Norfolk; Tygerberg Hosp, Tygerberg, South Africa)

Fertil Steril 55:1165–1170, 1991 5–5

Background.—Research involving a primate model showed an association between nuclear oocyte maturation and the ability of the zona pellucida for tight sperm binding under hemizona assay conditions. The sperm-binding potential of human oocytes was assessed at different stages of nuclear maturation under these conditions.

Methods.—In a prospective, blinded study, surplus oocytes donated by patients having in vitro fertilization after gonadotropin stimulation were analyzed. All assays used semen from a fertile donor. Five groups of oocytes were studied: immature, prophase 1 oocytes; metaphase 1 oocytes; metaphase 2 oocytes; inseminated, unfertilized metaphase 2 oocytes; and immature, prophase 1 oocytes matured in vitro to metaphase 2. Tight binding of sperm to the zona pellucida under hemizonal assay conditions was analyzed after gametes were coincubated for 4 hours.

Results.—The oocytes in metaphase 2 had significantly higher binding than those in the other groups. The mean value of the difference between the 2 halves was nonsignificant, indicating a small intra-assay variation for oocytes in all maturational stages.

Conclusions.—Maturation of the zona pellucida of human oocytes advances along with nuclear maturation in vivo. These processes appear, however, to be more independent when immature oocytes are cultured in vitro.

▶ Binding of sperm to the zona pellucida is an essential step in the process of fertilization. These investigators sought to determine whether the nuclear maturation of the oocyte in humans influences binding of the zona to sperm. This was shown previously in the monkey model. The hemizona assay is an excellent model to determine the relative binding efficiency of the zona pellucida because using half of each egg allows controls to be run at the same time. In essence, these results confirm the monkey data showing that nuclear maturation correlates well with the ability for tight binding of sperm to the zona pellucida, suggesting that only the mature oocytes have the ability to bind well.

The potential weakness of this work is that this observation pertains only to spare oocytes or donated oocytes from in vitro fertilization. This study would otherwise have been difficult to do because human material is used. These sparing oocytes may not necessarily have been the more healthy looking; more specifically, the oocytes used were obtained from patients who had received stimulation and therefore pharmacologic manipulation of follicular development. The authors do allude to this, however, and suggest that there may be actual differences between stimulated oocytes and natural cycle oocytes. Even with more immature oocytes they found better binding in unstimulated compared to stimulated cycles. If this pans out, it would suggest that stimulation by various methods may actually detract from the ability of sperm to bind adequately under certain circumstances. Clearly, we will have to watch for further developments in this new field.—R.A. Lobo, M.D.

Epididymal Secretory Function in Men With Asthenoteratozoospermia

Purvis K, Brekke I, Tollefsrud A (Natl Hosp, Oslo)

Hum Reprod 6:850–853, 1991 5–6

Background.—The epididymis has some role in conferring fertilizing ability on spermatozoa and in the development of progressive movement. α-Glucosidase was used to evaluate epididymal secretory function in the seminal plasma of men with normozoospermia and asthenoteratozoospermia.

Methods.—The series included 121 men with normozoospermia and 74 men with asthenoteratozoospermia undergoing routine semen analysis. Both groups had sperm concentrations of more than 35×10^6/mL. Twenty-eight men who had had a vasectomy and 59 men with oligo- or asthenoteratozoospermia with sperm concentrations of less than 10×10^6/mL also were studied. Sperm motility and other parameters were measured in semen samples, as well as in an assay of seminal plasma α-glucosidase.

Results.—Enzyme activity was significantly related to sperm count in men with normozoospermia but not in men with asthenoteratozoospermia. Men who had had a vasectomy had about 20% the enzyme levels of normal men. There was no difference between the 2 groups in the total quantity of enzyme secreted into the ejaculate. Men with asthenoterato-zoospermia with normal sperm counts had a significantly greater total enzyme content than men with severe oligoasthenoteratospermia. The low-sperm-count group had a higher incidence of epididymal occlusion or dysfunction. When enzyme quantities were expressed per million sperm cells, they were unrelated to extremes of progressive motility or abnormal morphology in men with normozoospermia.

Conclusions.—If α-glucosidase is a reliable index of epididymal secretory function, then the poor sperm quality seen in asthenoteratozoospermia cannot be explained by variation in secretory function. This parameter does not appear to be useful in investigating the mechanisms of male infertility, except in distinguishing between testicular failure and epididymal obstruction in azoospermia.

▶ A good negative study, but the data on the marker α-glucosidase does not entirely rule out epididymal dysfunction in these patients.—C.A. Paulsen, M.D.

Evidence for Altered Receptor-Binding Activity of Serum Follicle-Stimulating Hormone in Male Infertility

Buch JP, Lipshultz LI, Smith RG (Baylor College of Medicine, Houston)

Fertil Steril 55:358–362, 1991 5–7

Background.—The clinical evaluation of infertile men requires assessment of the integrity of the hypothalamic-pituitary-testicular axis. This has generally been accomplished by analyzing serum follicle-stimulating hormone (FSH) levels by radioimmunoassay (RIA). The immunologic activity of serum FSH has been assumed to be identical to the molecule's biological activity. The validity of this assumption was tested.

Methods.—Serum samples were collected from 11 fertile men and from 35 selected infertile men. The samples were evaluated by standard RIA and by radioreceptor assay (RRA). Results were analyzed in terms of the ratio of binding (RRA) to immunologic (RIA) activity × 100%. The result, called the B/I%, was based on data from the RRA and RIA, respectively, for each subject.

Results.—The B/I% for fertile men ranged from 44% to 113% (mean, 80%). The B/I% in 11 infertile men with normal FSH levels by RIA did not differ significantly from the B/I% in the 11 fertile men. There was a statistically significant decrease in B/I%, however, in the 24 hypergonadotropic infertile men with RIA levels of serum FSH of less than 300 ng/mL. In this group the B/I% ranged from 7% to 35% (mean, 18%).

Conclusions.—Because there were significant differences between receptor-binding and immunologic activities of serum FSH, using RIAs alone may not be a valid method for the endocrine evaluation of infertile men with elevated serum FSH levels. Use of other parameters may help to identify men with remediable endocrine-based infertility who were not previously recognizable.

▶ More studies in this important area. Previous reports of measurement of FSH and luteinizing hormone have generally suggested that B/I ratios remain unchanged in men whose testicular function is impaired, but these investigators suggest otherwise.—C.A. Paulsen, M.D.

Comparative Study of the Fertility Potential of Men With Only One Testis

Ferreira U, Netto NR Jr, Esteves SC, Rivero MA, Schirren C (State Univ of Campinas Med School, Brazil; Military Hosp of Buenos Aires, Argentina; Univ of Hamburg, Germany)

Scand J Urol Nephrol 25:255–259, 1991 5–8

Background.—Cryptorchidism lowers germ cell function, and the fertility of these patients is in doubt. Most patients undergoing unilateral orchidectomy for cancer have reduced spermatogenesis. The fertility potential of men with a single testis was evaluated.

Patients.—Fifty-four men aged 19–42 years underwent unilateral orchidectomy, retaining a single testis of normal volume and consistency. Unilateral cryptorchidism was the most common indication for orchidectomy (Table 1). Nearly 90% of patients were pubertal or postpubertal at the time of operation. The median follow-up interval was 5 years.

Outcome.—Testes of more than 25 mL in volume were considered to be hypertrophic (Table 2). Although only 25% of specimens had a perfectly normal sperm volume, all values were within the reference range. Hormonal profiles showed no significant differences regardless of the indication for orchidectomy.

Conclusions.—Patients who undergo orchidectomy for various reasons have similar fertility potential. Reduced potential could reflect a quantitative loss of terminative epithelium secondary to unilateral orchidectomy.

▶ This is an important study. It would have been nice if the authors had documented the fertility history in these men, or at least in those men who had the opportunity.—C.A. Paulsen, M.D.

TABLE 1.—Reasons for Orchidectomy

Group	Diagnosis	Number of patients
I	Unilateral cryptorchism	19
II	Testicular torsion	14
III	Testicular cancer	12
IV	Accidental (injury to spermatic cord during hernia repair)	9
Total		54

(Courtesy of Ferreira U, Netto NR Jr, Esteves SC, et al: *Scand J Urol Nephrol* 5:255–259, 1991.)

TABLE 2.—Median Volume of the Remaining Testes and Percentage of Testicular Hypertrophy in the 4 Groups According to the Reason for Orchidectomy

Group	Testicular volume (ml)	Testicular hypertrophy (%)
I (*n*=19)	25	47
II (*n*=14)	25	43
III (*n*=12)	20	8
IV (*n*=9)	25	44
Total (*n*=54)	25	37

(Courtesy of Ferreira U, Netto NR Jr, Esteves SC, et al: *Scand J Urol Nephrol* 25:255–259, 1991.)

Testis Volumes, Semen Quality, and Hormonal Patterns in Adolescents With and Without a Varicocele

Haans LCF, te Velde ER, Laven JSE, Wensing CJG, Mali WPTM (Univ Hosp, Utrecht, The Netherlands)

Fertil Steril 56:731–736, 1991 5–9

Objective.—A prospective study was undertaken in 67 male patients aged 17–20 years who had varicocele and 21 others who formed a control group. Semen samples were collected at an interval of 1 week to 3 months, after at least 3 days of sexual abstinence.

Findings.—The mean volume of the left testis was significantly smaller in patients with either grade II or grade III varicocele than in controls. Adolescents with the most marked testicular growth failure had a reduced number of spermatozoa, but sperm concentration, motility, and morphology were unaffected. All groups had normal levels of gonadotropins, testosterone, and prolactin.

Implications.—Testicular growth failure associated with a varicocele does not seem to be clearly associated with reduced semen quality in adolescents. It is not clear, however, whether testicular growth failure continues and can disturb fertility in adult life.

▶ This study focuses indirectly on a controversial point, namely, whether prophylactic varicocele ligation should be performed in young men in whom a varicocele is found on routine physical examination. It will be difficult to obtain a definitive answer, but studies such as this are useful in establishing a foundation for therapeutic decisions. Also, check a previous study that included details of fertile men with varicocele in the patient comparisons (1).—C.A. Paulsen, M.D.

Reference

1. Nagao RR, et al: *Fertil Steril* 46:930, 1986.

Levels of Transferrin, β_2-Microglobulin, and Albumin in Seminal Plasma

Group	Transferrin	Probability[b]	β_2-microglobulin	Probability[b]	Albumin	Probability[b]
	mg/mL		*mg/L*		*mg/L*	
Normal (n = 50)	51.5 ± 35	<0.001	56.8 ± 25.6	0.214	795 ± 418	<0.001
Azoospermia (n = 31)	18.6 ± 10.4	—	49.8 ± 18	—	552 ± 422	—
Oligospermia (n = 49)	26.2 ± 18	0.029	46.3 ± 16	NS[c]	614 ± 306	0.104
Polyzoospermia (n = 10)	88.4 ± 60.1	<0.001	70.9 ± 34.2	0.019	1,293 ± 725	<0.001
Vasectomized (n = 31)	20.1 ± 12.4	NS[c]	48.8 ± 14.8	NS[c]	507 ± 192	NS[c]

[a]Values are means ± SD.
[b]Probability of a significant difference from the results in individuals with azoospermia (Mann-Whitney U-test).
[c]*Abbreviation: NS,* not significant.
(Courtesy of Chard T, Parslow J, Rehmann T, et al: *Fertil Steril* 55:211–213, 1991.)

The Concentrations of Transferrin, β_2-Microglobulin, and Albumin in Seminal Plasma in Relation to Sperm Count

Chard T, Parslow J, Rehmann T, Dawnay A (St Bartholomew's Hosp, London)
Fertil Steril 55:211–213, 1991

5–10

Purpose.—Previous studies have shown a direct relationship between transferrin levels in seminal plasma and sperm count. To clarify further, the relationship of sperm count to seminal plasma transferrin levels as well as to 2 unrelated plasma proteins, albumin and β_2-microglobulin, was studied.

Methods.—The levels of transferrin, β_2-microglobulin, and albumin were measured in 171 seminal plasma samples from 50 men with normal sperm counts, 31 with azoospermia, 49 with oligozoospermia, 10 with polyzoospermia, and 31 who had been vasectomized.

Findings.—All 3 proteins were related to sperm count (table). The highest levels were found in men with polyzoospermia and the lowest in those with azoospermia.

Conclusion.—There is a direct relationship between seminal plasma transferrin levels and sperm count. The same relationship also applies to the unrelated proteins, β_2-microglobulin and albumin. There probably is a nonspecific relationship between seminal plasma proteins and sperm numbers in general; certain products of the sperm may control the entry of plasma proteins into seminal plasma.

▶ The hypothesis needs further study. To me, the different values for transferrin are more convincing than the unrelated proteins these authors studied.—C.A. Paulsen, M.D.

Tail Stump Spermatozoa: Morphogenesis of the Defect: An Ultrastructural Study of Sperm and Testicular Biopsy

Barthelemy C, Tharanne MJ, Lebos C, Lecomte P, Lansac J (CHU Bretonneau, Tours, France)
Andrologia 22:417–425, 1990

5–11

Objective.—The ultrastructural features of testes biopsy specimens and immotile spermatozoa obtained from a supposed secondary infertile man were examined.

Case Report.—Man, 33, was seen for investigation of secondary infertility. The most striking feature on semen analysis was the total absence of motility in all samples. Light and electron microscopic studies of the sperm showed that all air-dried samples had the same profile, with mainly tail disturbances (Fig 5–1). The flagellum was absent in 21% to 33%, short-tail spermatozoa were present in 14% to 29%, and coiled tails were seen in 11% to 26%; there was an abnormal proportion of spermatids, spermatocytes, and cytoplasmic residues. Most sperm heads were abnormally shaped, the nucleus exhibiting a high degree of maturity with a well-condensed karyoplasm. Light and electron microscopic examination

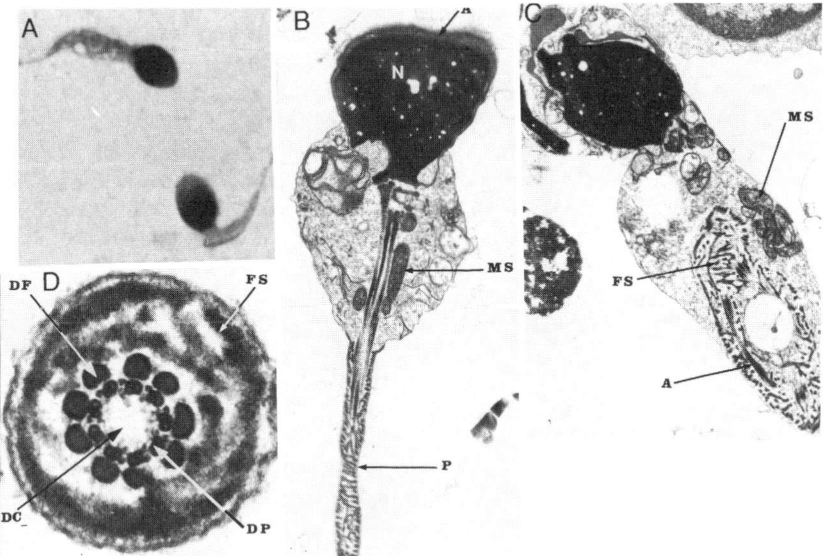

Fig 5–1.—Electron and light microscopy of sperm. **A,** aspect of Schorr staining sperm cells in light microscopy showing short tail spermatozoa (5,000). **B,** longitudinal section of spermatozoon (TEM): acrosome *(A)* on an irregular head (15,000), nucleus with a normal degree of condensation *(N)*, disorganized mitochondrial sheath *(MS)*, short principal piece *(P)*. **C,** longitudinal section of a spermatozoon: principal piece with a complete derangement of axoneme *(A)*, mitochondria *(MS)*, and fibrous sheath *(FS)* (13,500). **D,** transversal section of axoneme with a thickened fibrous sheath *(FS)*, 9 dense fibers *(DF)* and 9 peripheral doublets *(DP)* of the central complex *(DC)* (90,000). (Courtesy of Barthelemy C, Tharanne MJ, Lebos C, et al: *Andrologia* 22:417–425, 1990.)

of the testes showed markedly impaired spermatogenesis, more precisely during spermiogenesis at the latest stages during flagellum elongation in spermatids (Fig 5–2). At these stages, the spermatid tails were replaced by stumps having different shapes. In the tubular lumen, spermiation showed stump spermatozoa, tailless spermatozoa, and many cytoplasmic residues.

Conclusion.—Electron microscopic analyses are important in evaluation of male infertility. Complete asthenozoospermia with ultrastructural perturbations of flagellum structures could confirm male infertility definitively.

▶ Is electron microscopy necessary in situations such as described?—C.A. Paulsen, M.D.

Effects of Subchronic Treatment With Cis-Platinum on Testicular Function, Fertility, Pregnancy Outcome, and Progeny

Seethalakshmi L, Flores C, Kinkead T, Carboni AA, Malhotra RK, Menon M (Univ of Massachusetts Med Ctr, Worcester)

J Androl 13:65–74, 1992 5–12

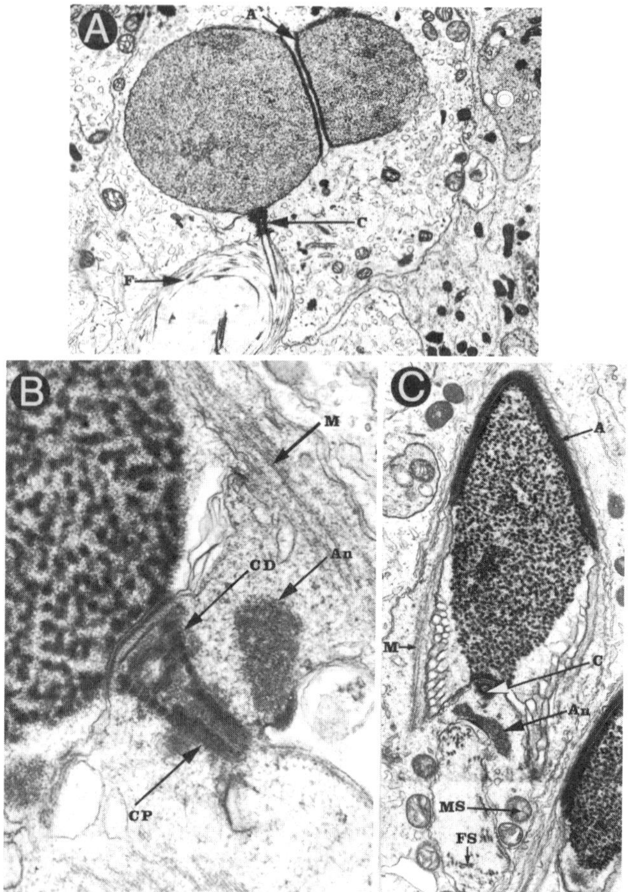

Fig 5–2.—Electron microscopy (TEM) testicular biopsy specimen. **A**, binucleated spermatid step 2 showing a centered acrosome *(A)* with a not yet aligned coiled flagellum *(F)*. Implantation fossa are seen on the nucleus and centrioles *(C)* (7,500). **B**, spermatid at step 5: detail of the neck; centrioles distal *(CD)* and proximal *(CP)*, annulus *(An)* and microtubules of the manchette *(M)* (37,500). **C**, spermatid step 5: nucleus *(N)* with chromatin condensed in coarse granules, acrosome *(A)* elongated by microtubules of the manchette *(M)* showing centriole *(C)*, annulus *(An)* still near nucleus, and a disorganized flagellum fibrous sheath *(FS)* and mitochondria *(MS)* (12,000). (Courtesy of Barthelemy C, Tharanne MJ, Lebos C, et al: *Andrologia* 22:417–425, 1990.)

Background.—Chemotherapy that includes cis-platinum impairs spermatogenesis, but the effects of paternal treatment on the progeny are not clear. Cis-platinum was given intraperitoneally in a dose of .5 mg/kg daily for 9 weeks to sexually mature male rats, which were mated at intervals with females in proestrus.

Findings.—Animals exposed to cis-platinum failed to grow. The weights of reproductive organs decreased, as did sperm counts, and sperm motility was lowered. Both circulating and testicular levels of testosterone decreased after 3 weeks of treatment, whereas levels of follicle-stimulating hormone were unchanged. The serum level of luteinizing hormone declined from week 3. The pituitary response to gonadotropin-releasing hormone remained intact. Fertility was not compromised in treated animals, but pre- and postimplantation fetal losses were increased. Relatively fewer males were observed after treatment. A significant number of offspring of treated rats were growth-retarded or malformed.

Conclusions.—Low-dose cis-platinum treatment can substantially alter the outcome of pregnancy in rats. A prospective study is needed to assess the pregnancy outcome when human males are treated with cis-platinum.

▶ Clear demonstration that certain toxic substances may affect the DNA of sperm, subsequently leading to fetal problems.—C.A. Paulsen, M.D.

Techniques for Selection of Normal-Chromatin Sperm Preparations

Wang FN, Hong CY, Chou TS, Hsiung CHC, Karow WG, Pesic MC (Cathay Gen Hosp, Taipei, Taiwan; Southern California Fertility Inst, Los Angeles; Inst for Immunology/Thymus Research, Bad Harzburg, Germany)

Arch Androl 27:87–92, 1991 5–13

Introduction.—Detection of sperm chromatin heterogeneity often is neglected, but the ability of sperm nuclear chromatin to resist denaturation is associated with male fertility potential. Twenty human semen samples from normal donors and patients attending an infertility clinic were examined by the acridine orange fluorescence test (AOT).

Observations.—Untreated semen contained an average of 58% green sperm in the AOT. After treatment with Wang's tube system the proportion of green sperm was 99%. The respective values for the Percoll gradient and swim-up techniques were 78% and 72%. Specimens prepared with Wang's tube method contained significantly more normal chromatin structure than those treated by the other methods.

Conclusion.—The Wang tube technique is the preferred method of separating sperm and of selecting highly motile, morphologically normal sperm for use in artificial insemination and in vitro fertilization.

▶ As mentioned in Abstracts 4–4, 4–9, and 4–6, the harvesting of so-called normal sperm should be equated with a seminal biological method of validation. These authors then need to establish the significance of their method.—C.A. Paulsen, M.D.

Nature of the Inhibitory Effect of Complex Saccharide Moieties on the Tight Binding of Human Spermatozoa to the Human Zona Pellucida

Oehninger S, Clark GF, Acosta AA, Hodgen GD (Eastern Virginia Med School, Norfolk)

Fertil Steril 55:165–169, 1991 5–14

Introduction.—Fucoidin and heparin sulfate inhibit human sperm binding to the human zona pellucida in hemizona assay (HZA) conditions. The HZA was used to investigate tight sperm binding with or without preincubation of the sperm with other sulfated and nonsulfated glycoconjugates and charged polymers.

Methods.—Two fertile men who had fathered children within the preceding 2 years provided 8 semen samples. Sugars and charged polymers were tested uniformly. The number of tightly bound sperm in the HZA and control substances were compared.

Results.—Fucoidin significantly inhibited binding compared with control values, even when sperm were washed after preincubation with the saccharide. Dextran sulfate also significantly inhibited tight binding in the HZA, although to a lesser degree. The HZA results for the other common saccharides tested indicated that dextran, heparin, chondroitin sulfate, chondroitin sulfate B, and hyaluronic acid had no significant effect on tight binding. Sodium sulfate and polyglutamic acid did not affect HZA results. Polyphosphates produced moderate inhibition.

Conclusion.—The potent inhibitory effect of fucoidin and dextran is probably of the receptor-ligand type. The lack of significant effects of simple charged molecules indicates that the degree of sulfation may not be crucial to its inhibitory action.

▶ This article concerns further refinement to the use of the hemizona assay. Much more data are needed before the importance of these various substances can be placed into proper perspective.—C.A. Paulsen, M.D.

Expression of D-Mannose Binding Sites on Human Spermatozoa: Comparison of Fertile Donors and Infertile Patients

Tesarik J, Mendoza C, Carreras A (Institut National de la Santé et de la Recherche Médicale, Clamart, France; Univ of Granada, Granada, Spain)

Fertil Steril 56:113–118, 1991 5–15

Background and Methods.—Defective expression of D-mannose binding sites has been hypothesized to be related to male infertility. This hy-

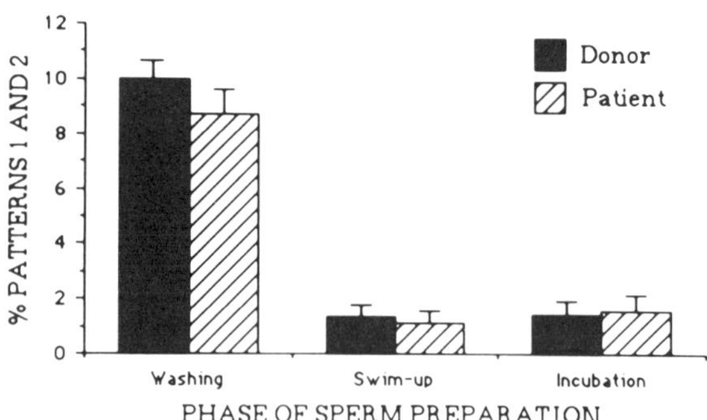

Fig 5–3.—Cumulative percentages of spermatozoa from fertile *(filled column)* and infertile *(striped column)* men showing patterns 1 and 2 of D-mannosylated albumin binding at different phases of sperm preparation for in vitro capacitation. Values are means ± SE of 5 replicates, each including spermatozoa from 2–3 individuals. (Courtesy of Tesarik J, Mendoza C, Carreras A: *Fertil Steril* 56:113–118, 1991.)

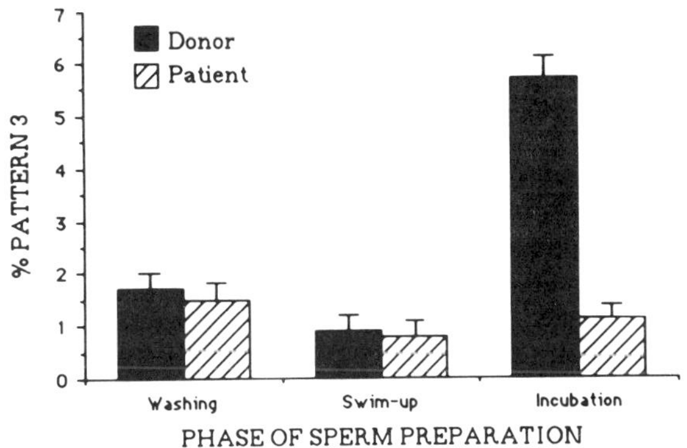

Fig 5–4.—Percentages of spermatozoa from fertile *(filled column)* and infertile *(striped column)* men showing pattern 3 of D-mannosylated albumin binding at different phases of sperm preparation for in vitro capacitation. Values are means ± SE of 5 replicates, each involving spermatozoa from 2–3 individuals. (Courtesy of Tesarik J, Mendoza C, Carreras A: *Fertil Steril* 56:113–118, 1991.)

pothesis was tested in a comparison of sperm samples obtained from fertile and infertile men. The fertile group consisted of healthy sperm donors; the infertile group included patients seen at 1 center. Fluorescence microscopy with a mannosylated neoglycoprotein probe was used to visualize D-mannose binding sites.

Results.—The percentages of spermatozoa showing patterns 1 and 2 of D-mannosylated albumin binding did not differ between groups at any step of sperm preparation for in vitro capacitation (Fig 5–3). Similar values in sperm samples from the 2 groups also were seen for pattern 3 in washed and swim-up sperm populations (Fig 5–4). When spermatozoa from infertile men were incubated for in vitro capacitation, however, there was no significant increase of spermatozoa showing pattern 3 of D-mannosylated albumin binding, unlike in the fertile group. In addition, pattern 3A was rarely found in the incubated samples of patient spermatozoa. The size of this subpopulation did not exceed 10% of pattern 3 spermatozoa in any case.

Conclusions.—In this study, sperm from fertile men showed a characteristic pattern of changes in the expression of D-mannose binding sites during in vitro capacitation that sperm from infertile men did not. If the relationship between defective D-mannose binding site expression and reduced sperm fertilizing ability is confirmed by parallel tests of sperm-zona binding, it may be used to create chemical tests to replace current ones that use human zonae pellucidae.

▶ This article concerns another modification for validating normal or abnormal sperm. This information might be useful to those centers where hemizona binding is not available and the clinician desires to examine this dimension of semen analysis.—C.A. Paulsen, M.D.

Epidermal Growth Factor (EGF) Is Not an Index of Seminiferous Tubular Function

Delgado SR, Ramirez K, Mallea E (Instituto Nacional de Endocrinologia, Havana, Cuba)

Andrologia 23:241–243, 1991 5–16

Background and Methods.—Epidermoid growth factor (EGF) has been identified in male reproductive tissues and fluids. Human Sertoli cells in culture produce a growth factor that binds to EGF receptors with high affinity. Whether EGF levels in human seminal plasma could serve as indices of seminiferous tubular function was investigated. Concentrations of EGF and amounts per ejaculate were determined in 162 infertile and 50 fertile men who served as controls. Men in the infertile group had varying degrees of gonadal dysfunction.

Results.—There were no significant differences in plasma EGF concentrations or amounts per ejaculate between the groups overall. Nor were there any significant differences between them when the infertile men were subdivided according to sperm count. The EGF concentrations were not correlated either to sperm count, motility, viability, or normal morphology.

Conclusions.—That EGF in seminal plasma is unrelated to seminiferous tubule function may reflect the fact that growth factor with EGF-like activity produced by Sertoli cells differs from actual EGF in certain characteristics. Most of the EGF found in seminal plasma is probably produced by the prostate. In that event, measuring the growth factor in seminal plasma has no value in assessing seminiferous tubule function.

▶ These studies, although important, do not refute the experiments of Tsutsumi et al. (1). The latter authors removed the sialomandibular gland in adult mice, which resulted in a marked decrease in EGF with an associated reduction in epididymal sperm. Administration of EGF appears to be important to spermatogenesis, at least in mice. It may be that the biochemical defect(s) present in the patients studied here may not be responsive to EGF levels or be the origin of EGF.—C.A. Paulsen, M.D.

Reference

1. Tsutsumi O, et al: *Science* 233:975, 1986.

Lymphocyte Subset Distribution and Natural Killer Cell Activity in Men With Idiopathic Hypogonadotropic Hypogonadism

Kiess W, Liu LL, Hall NR (Natl Insts of Health, Bethesda, Md; Univ of South Florida, Tampa; Children's Hosp, Munich, Germany)

Acta Endocrinol (Copenh) 124:399–404, 1991 5–17

Introduction.—Gonadal hormones in men may influence certain immune responses, e.g., lymphocyte subset distribution in peripheral blood

Lymphocyte Subset Distribution and Natural Killer Cell Activity in Men With Idiopathic Hypongonadotropic Hypogonadism Before and After Treatment

	Without treatment	After treatment	(Standard range)†	N
T-cells (CD3+)	77±1	75±1	(75±7)	15 (31)
	NS			
T-helper cells (CD4+)	53±2	47±2	(45±10)	15 (31)
	(p<0.05)			
T-suppressor cells (CD8+)	22±2	26±2	(28±9)	15 (31)
	NS			
CD4+/CD8+ ratio	2.7±0.3	2.1±0.3		15 (31)
	NS			
NK cells (CD16+)	6±1	11±1	(15±7)	15 (31)
	(p<0.001)			
NK cell activity	31±5	41±5	(33±4)	18 (39)
	NS			

Note: Lymphocyte subset distribution is expressed as % of total peripheral mononuclear cells expressing the indicated phenotype. Natural killer *(NK)* activity is expressed as lytic units. Values represent mean ± SEM. N = the number of individuals tested, number in parentheses = total number of determinations. NS = not significant.

†in normal men.

(Courtesy of Kiess W, Liu LL, Hall NR: *Acta Endocrinol (Copenh)* 124:399–404, 1991.)

and natural killer cell function. To investigate further, 18 men with idiopathic hypogonadotropic hypogonadism (IHH) were studied before treatment and after hormonal treatment had normalized plasma testosterone levels.

Methods.—Lymphocyte subset distribution and the natural killer cell activity of peripheral mononuclear cells were measured before and after at least 4 weeks of treatment with testosterone, gonadotropin, or gonadotropin-releasing hormone designed to normalize plasma testosterone levels.

Findings.—All patients with IHH had significantly low plasma testosterone levels before treatment. Plasma testosterone levels normalized after hormonal treatment. The percentage of peripheral CD3+ lymphocytes, CD8+ cells, the CD4+/CD8+ ratio, and natural killer cell activity before treatment in patients with IHH did not differ from those percentages in normal healthy adults and remained unchanged after hormonal treatment had normalized plasma testosterone levels. In contrast, the percentage of the T-helper cell phenotype CD4+ was significantly higher before treatment, compared with that in normal adults and after hormonal treatment (table). The percentage of peripheral CD16+ cells (non-T-non-B cells) was significantly lower before treatment in IHH patients than in normal controls, and it increased significantly after hormonal treatment restored plasma testosterone levels to normal (Fig 5–5). In ad-

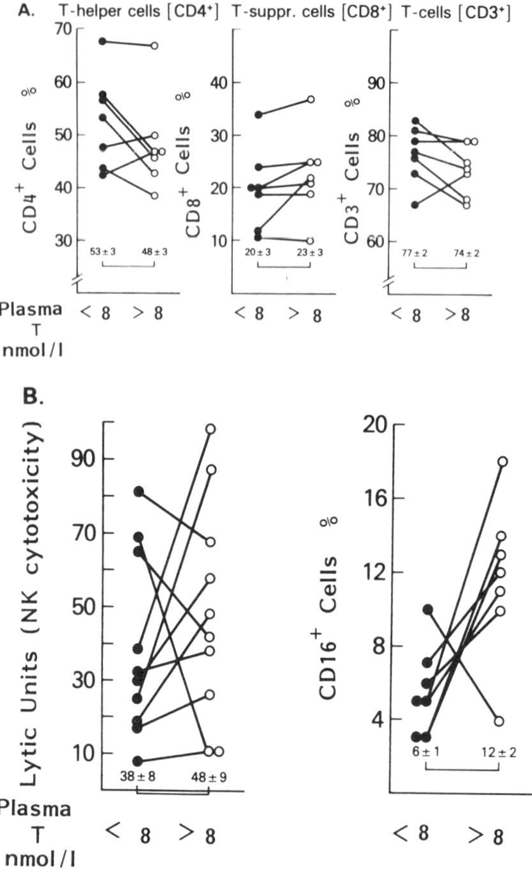

Fig 5–5.—Distribution of lymphocyte subsets and natural killer *(NK)* cell activity in 7 patients with idiopathic hypogonadotropic hypogonadism measured before *(filled circle)* and after *(open circle)* hormonal treatment in the same patient. The percentage of CD16+ cells was significantly higher after normalization of plasma testosterone levels ($P < .05$). (Courtesy of Kiess W, Liu LL, Hall NR: *Acta Endocrinol (Copenh)* 124:399–404, 1991.)

dition, the percentage of peripheral CD16+ cells correlated significantly with the plasma testosterone levels in patients with IHH.

Conclusion.—The percentage of peripheral CD4+ and peripheral CD16+ cells are related to plasma testosterone levels in men with IHH, suggesting that in vivo human immune cells may be under the regulatory influence of endogenous sex steroids.

▶ Years ago when immature male rats were used for the bioassay of gonadotropins, testosterone, and the like, we carefully removed the thymus as part of the assessment. It was quite clear that endogenously produced testosterone or exogenously administered testosterone and other androgens reduced the thymus gland dramatically. The line of investigation reported by these authors deserves more attention.—C.A. Paulsen, M.D.

Hypogonadism Caused by a Single Amino Acid Substitution in the β Subunit of Luteinizing Hormone

Weiss J, Axelrod L, Whitcomb RW, Harris PE, Crowley WF, Jameson JL (Massachusetts Gen Hosp, Boston)

N Engl J Med 326:179–183, 1992 5–18

Introduction.—Luteinizing hormone (LH) is a glycoprotein hormone, consisting of a common α subunit and a specific β subunit, that confers specificity for receptors in the target organ. A family was encountered in which the defect appeared limited to LH, suggesting a structural change in either the coding sequence of the β subunit (LHβ) or in its posttranslational processing.

Findings.—Studies of the proband, seen at age 17 years with pubertal delay, identified a mutation in the coding sequence of the LHβ gene that eliminates the ability of LH to bind to its receptor. The patient was given testosterone for 2 years but had no evidence of spontaneous puberty afterward. His serum immunoreactive LH level was twice normal, whereas the serum testosterone level was low. Testicular biopsy showed arrested spermatogenesis and no Leydig cells. Long-term treatment with human chorionic gonadotropin led to normal virilization.

Genetic Studies.—The mutation causes a substitution of arginine for glutamine in amino acid 54 of the LHβ subunit. The alteration in the LHβ gene sequence appears to have arisen as a spontaneous mutation. Transfection studies showed that the absence of biological activity in the mutant LH resulted from an inability to bind to receptors. No serum LH was detected in the proband's radioreceptor assay despite the elevated levels observed on radioimmunoassay.

Interpretation.—It is not clear whether this mutation identifies a contact site with the receptor, or whether it causes a structural change that interferes secondarily with receptor binding.

▶ Very interesting report. It would be important to evaluate the Leydig cell response to gonadotropin-releasing hormone in terms of biologically active LH.—C.A. Paulsen, M.D.

Young's Syndrome (Obstructive Azoospermia and Chronic Sinobronchial Infection): A Quantitative Study of Axonemal Ultrastructure and Function

Wilton LJ, Southwick GJ, Teichtahl H, Burger HG, Temple-Smith PD, de Kretser DM, Johnson JL (Prince Henry's Hosp, Melbourne, Vic, Australia)

Fertil Steril 55:144–151, 1991 5–19

Objective.—Young's syndrome is characterized by male infertility (obstructive azoospermia) and chronic sinopulmonary infection. The ultrastructure and function of nasal cilia and sperm tails in 23 men with Young's syndrome were compared to data collected previously from 10 normal men.

Data Analysis.—There were no obvious structural anomalies in the ultrastructure of sperm tail and ciliary axonemes in patients with Young's

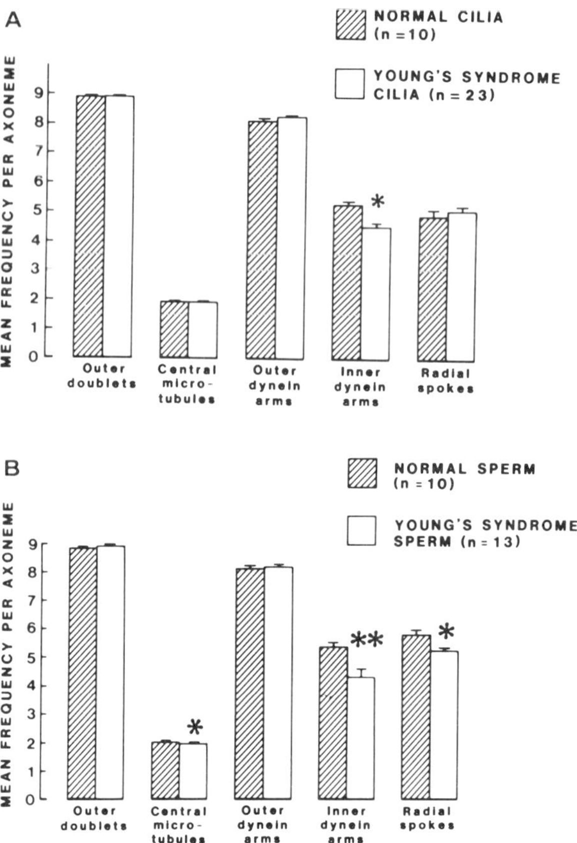

Fig 5–6.—**A**, ultrastructural analysis of Young's syndrome cilia. Significantly fewer inner dynein arms were found in cilia from patients with Young's syndrome compared with normal men ($P < .01$). There was no significant difference in any other axonemal structures. **B**, ultrastructural analysis of Young's syndrome sperm. Significantly fewer central pair microtubules ($P < .01$), inner dynein arms ($P < .001$), and radial spokes ($P < .01$) were found in Young's syndrome sperm compared with normal sperm. No statistical difference was found between outer doublet microtubules or outer dynein arms in sperm from normal men or men with Young's syndrome. Values represent mean ± SE; *, $P < .01$; **$P < .001$. (Courtesy of Wilton LJ, Southwick GJ, Teichtahl H, et al: *Fertil Steril* 55:144–151, 1991.)

syndrome. However, quantitative analysis showed that ciliary and sperm tail axonemes from these patients were structurally deficient compared with those of normal subjects. There were significantly fewer central pair microtubules, radial spokes, and inner dynein arms in the sperm tails, and fewer inner dynein arms in the cilia from patients with Young's syndrome than in the axonemes of normal subjects (Fig 5–6). There were no significant differences between groups in the incidence of sperm tail axonemes with outer doublet microtubule defects and compound axonemes, but the incidence of central microtubule defects in cilia and sperm tail axonemes and the percentage of compound cilia were significantly increased in patients with Young's syndrome compared with normal subjects (table). The in vitro ciliary beat frequency in patients with Young's

Comparison of the Incidence of Axonemes With Microtubular Defects and Compound Axonemes in Young's Syndrome Patients and Normal Men

	Central microtubule defects	Outer doublet microtubule defects	Compound axonemes
		%	
Cilia			
Young's syndrome (n = 23)	7.2 ± 4.2	5.9 ± 3.9	2.25 ± 2.60
Normal (n = 10)[b]	2.4 ± 1.4[c]	4.1 ± 1.7	0.40 ± 0.64[d]
Sperm			
Young's syndrome (n = 13)	4.9 ± 3.2	5.5 ± 3.4	0.69 ± 1.44
Normal (n = 10)	3.0 ± 0.8[e]	9.9 ± 4.8[d,f]	0.13 ± 0.43

Note: Values are means ± SD.
[b]Normal data taken from Wilton LJ, Teichtahl H, Temple-Smith PD, et al: *J Clin Invest* 75:825, 1985.
[c]$P < .0001$.
[d]$P < .05$.
[e]$P < .005$.
[f]One male in control group had a very high level of outer doublet defects. (Courtesy of Wilton LJ, Teichtahl H, Temple-Smith PD, et al: *J Clin Invest* 75:825, 1985.) If this subject is excluded, there is no significant difference between patients with Young's syndrome and the control group.
(From Wilton LJ, Southwick GJ, Teichtahl H, et al: *Fertil Steril* 55:144–151,1991.)

syndrome did not differ significantly from normal. Twelve patients with Young's syndrome had normal mucociliary clearance. The remaining 11 had markedly abnormal nasal mucociliary clearance in vivo, but the structural components per axoneme and ciliary beat frequency did not differ significantly between patients with normal or abnormal nasal mucociliary clearance.

Conclusion.—Minor structural abnormalities exist in the ciliary and flagellar axonemes of patients with Young's syndrome. These abnormalities may constitute a common factor in both the reproductive and respiratory tract features of this disorder. Although these structural abnormalities may not be sufficient to affect ciliary function in vitro, they may cause defective ciliary function in an abnormal in vivo mucus environment.

Young's Syndrome: Report of Two Japanese Cases

Matsuda T, Horii Y, Nishimura K, Amitani R, Matsui Y, Yoshida O (Kyoto Univ, Kyoto, Japan)

Urol Int 47:53–56, 1991 5–20

Introduction.—Young's syndrome is characterized by azoospermia caused by bilateral epididymal obstruction in association with chronic sinobronchial disease. The incidence of Young's syndrome in patients with obstructive azoospermia ranges from 50% to 67% in Caucasians, but only a few cases in mongoloids have been reported.

Case Reports.—Two Japanese men, 34 and 30, were seen because of primary infertility. Both patients had markedly reduced tracheobronchial mucociliary clearance. Semen analysis showed azoospermia, but analysis of a testicular biopsy

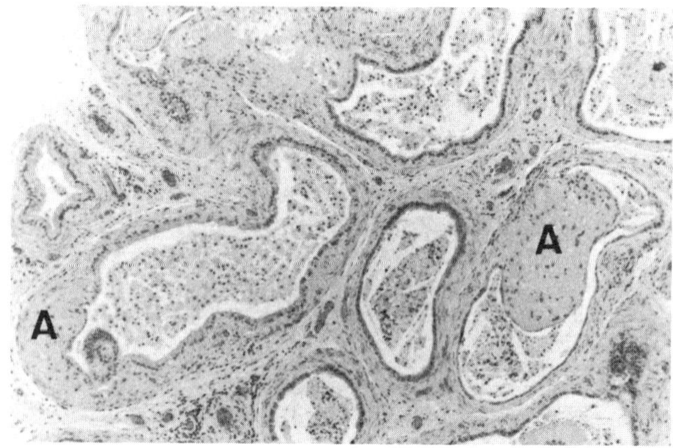

Fig 5–7.—Photomicrograph of the specimen from caput epididymis showing dilated ductuli efferentes, which contain degenerative materials, sperm heads, and prominent cholesterol clefts. Cholesterol granulomas *(A)* are seen. (Reduced from ×40). (Courtesy of Matsuda T, Horii Y, Nishimura K, et al: *Urol Int* 47:53–56, 1991.)

specimen showed normal spermatogenesis, indicating obstructive azoospermia. Results of bilateral vasovesiculography were normal. Microsurgical epididymovasostomy using Silber's specific tubule method was performed in the first patient and the side-to-side method was used in the second, resulting in patency only in the latter patient. Pathologic examination of a specimen from the caput epididymis of the first patient showed dilated ductuli efferentes, which contained acidophilic materials (Fig 5–7); the ductus epididymidis was empty and normal (Fig 5–8).

Conclusion.—The site of seminal tract obstruction in Young's syndrome is the caput epididymis, with obstruction at the most distal region of the ductuli efferentes. Microsurgical epididymovasostomy is the only

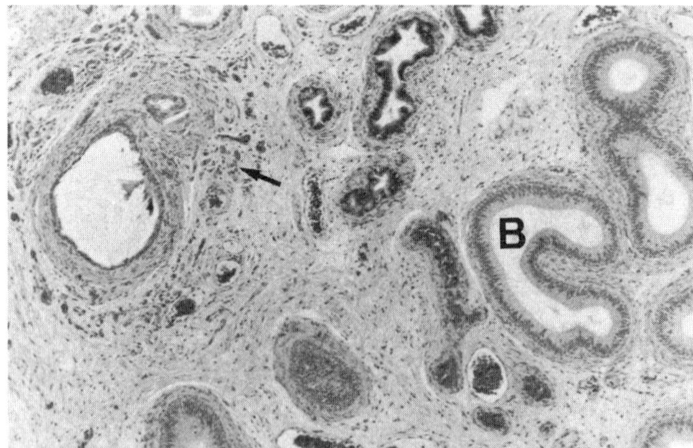

Fig 5–8.—Ductus epididymis *(B)* adjacent to ductus efferentis is empty and normal. In interstitium around ductus efferentis, clusters of cells with lipofuscin are noted *(arrow)*. (Reduced from ×32.) (Courtesy of Matsuda T, Horii Y, Nishimura K, et al: *Urol Int* 47:53–56, 1991.)

treatment, but the patency rate remains low and no incidence of pregnancy has been reported as yet.

▶ These 2 studies (Abstracts 5–19 and 5–20) are placed together in the category of pathophysiology even though the authors of the second report attempted surgical treatment. The basic reason(s) for the epididymal obstruction remain uncertain.—C.A. Paulsen, M.D.

6 Sperm-Cervical Mucus Interaction

Cervical Mucus Score and In Vitro Sperm Mucus Interaction in Spontaneous and Clomiphene Citrate Cycles

Randall JM, Templeton A (Univ of Aberdeen, Scotland)

Fertil Steril 56:465–468, 1991 6–1

Background.—Clomiphene citrate (CC) is commonly used to induce ovulation, but its empirical use in patients with unexplained infertility has been questioned. Clomiphene citrate reportedly has adverse effects on cervical mucus and sperm penetration. In a prospective study, the cervical mucus score and in vitro sperm mucus interaction were evaluated during spontaneous ovulatory cycles and CC-stimulated cycles.

Methods.—The series included 22 women with unexplained infertility lasting for at least 3 years and ovulatory midluteal progesterone level of more than 30 nmol/L for at least 2 cycles. The mean age was 30.4 years, and the mean duration of infertility, 4.4 years. Each woman was studied first during a spontaneous cycle and then in a cycle stimulated by CC, 150 mg on days 5 through 9. Cervical mucus obtained within 12 hours of the luteinizing hormone surge was assessed as to amount, spinnbarkeit, ferning, and viscosity. Sperm-mucus penetration was assessed by a standardized Kremer test.

Results.—The mean cervical mucus score was 9.3 during the spontaneous cycle and 5.6 during the CC-stimulated cycle; all parameters were significantly reduced in the CC cycle (table). The reduction occurred despite a significantly increased mean serum E_2 level in the CC cycle—869 pg/mL vs. 226 pg/mL. The mean sperm penetration scores were 11.4 in the spontaneous cycle and 3.9 in the CC cycle.

Conclusions.—Cervical mucus and sperm-mucus penetration test scores are significantly reduced in CC-stimulated cycles in comparison with spontaneous ovulatory cycles. The components of the cervical mucus score are all relatively reduced. These findings suggest that the empir-

Components of Cervical Mucus Score in Spontaneous and CC Cycles

	Volume	Viscosity	Ferning	Spinnbarkeit	Total score
Spontaneous (n = 22)	2.7 (2.4 to 3.0)	2.6 (2.3 to 2.9)	2.0 (1.7 to 2.3)	1.9 (1.7 to 2.1)	9.3 (8.4 to 10.2)
CC (n = 22)	1.9 (1.5 to 2.3)	1.5 (1.2 to 1.8)	1.4 (1.0 to 1.8)	0.8 (0.6 to 1.0)	5.6 (4.6 to 6.6)
Wilcoxon 1 sample test	$P < 0.01$	$P < 0.0001$	$P < 0.05$	$P < 0.0001$	$P < 0.001$

Note: Values are means with 95% confidence interval in parentheses.
(Courtesy of Randall JM, Templeton A: *Fertil Steril* 56:465–468, 1991.)

ical use of CC in ovulatory women with unexplained infertility should be reassessed.

▶ Although this study shows that a high dose of CC, 150 mg/day for 5 days, when administered from days 5 to 9 in the ovulatory cycle impairs cervical mucus amount and function, it does not indicate that the drug causes impaired sperm transport in preovulatory mucus of women with anovulatory cycles treated with it. Hammond et al. (1) showed that the monthly fecundability rate in women without infertility factors other than anovulation who ovulated with CC did not cause infertility in these women. Furthermore, Frisch et al. (see the 1990 YEAR BOOK OF INFERTILITY, p 175) showed that women with unexplained infertility treated with CC at a dose of 100 mg/day for days 2–6 had a significant increase in their pregnancy rate. The dose of CC used in this study was too high and was given too late in the ovulatory cycle.—D.R. Mishell, Jr., M.D.

Reference

1. Hammond MG, et al: *Obstet Gynecol* 62:196, 1983.

7 Immunologic Factors

Comparison of the Indirect Immunobead, Radiolabeled, and Immunofluorescence Assays for Immunoglobulin G Serum Antibodies to Human Sperm

Haas GG Jr, D'Cruz OJ, DeBault LE (Univ of Oklahoma, Oklahoma City)

Fertil Steril 55:377–388, 1991 7 1

Introduction.—If intact, unfixed, and motile sperm are used as the antigen in different assays with different probes for sperm-associated Ig, it seems logical that the same results would be achieved in all of the assays regardless of the probe used.

Methods.—To investigate this hypothesis, the results of an indirect radiolabeled antiglobulin assay, an indirect immunobead test, and an indirect immunofluorescence assay using unfixed, motile sperm as the antigen source were compared. Eighteen immunobead test positive sera and 18 negative sera served as the standard for the other 2 assays.

Results.—Of the 18 positive sera, 77% were positive in the immunofluorescence assay and 27% were positive in the radiolabeled antiglobulin assay. Of the low-titer immunobead test positive sera, 22% were negative according to the immunofluorescence and radiolabeled antiglobulin assay. The correlations between the results of the immunofluorescence assay and the radiolabeled antiglobulin assay, and between the results of the radiolabeled antiglobulin assay and the titer of the immunobead test, were significant and positive. The use of an unselected sperm population in the radiolabeled antiglobulin assay and the classic indirect immunofluorescence method using methanol-fixed sperm yielded false positive findings in the radiolabeled antiglobulin assay and the immunofluorescence assay.

Conclusion.—These results confirmed the hypothesis in question. Any differences in the results depend on the sensitivity of the assay, not on its specificity. Immunoglobulin G antisperm antibody sera may be reactive to sperm surface and internalized sperm antigens.

▶ The issue of improving testing for clinically significant, sperm associated antibodies is very important for clinicians who send most of their samples to outside labs. The physician should be provided with adequate quality control information.—C.A. Paulsen, M.D.

Effect of Sperm-Associated Antibodies on the Acrosomal Status of Human Sperm

Lansford B, Haas GG Jr, Debault LE, Wolf DP (Univ of Oklahoma, Oklahoma City; Oregon Regional Primate Research Ctr, Beaverton)

J Androl 11:532–538, 1990 7–2

Introduction.—Certain environmental influences are necessary for sperm to become capable of fertilization. This maturational process, called capacitation, encompasses changes that sperm undergo from ejaculation to acrosome reaction initiation. The effect of antisperm antibodies on the acrosomal status of human sperm was studied. The specific binding of *Pisum sativum* lectin to the acrosomal matrix was studied to assess the acrosomal status of sperm.

Results.—The IgG fractions of plasma positive for IgG antisperm antibodies either inhibited, initiated, or had no effect on acrosomal loss. Acrosomal loss before exposure to calcium ionophore was noted in 2 of 5 sperm samples associated in vivo with only IgG and in 6 of 8 samples associated with both IgA and IgG, but not in the 1 sample associated with only sperm-associated IgA. Two samples associated with IgG and/or IgA were inhibited from undergoing acrosome loss after exposure to calcium ionophore. None of the 7 antibody-negative samples had an increased spontaneous acrosomal loss or were inhibited from undergoing acrosomal loss after exposure to calcium ionophore.

Conclusion.—Antisperm antibodies affected acrosomal loss in different ways. Acrosomal loss was either inhibited or initiated prematurely, or was unaffected. Most sperm associated with Ig in vivo had spontaneous acrosomal loss before calcium ionophore was added. A crucial step in human sperm function, the acrosome reaction, can apparently be changed by antisperm antibodies; this change may then result in infertility.

▶ These authors show that antisperm antibodies may exert variable effects on the timing of acrosomal changes. Naturally, this implies poloyclonal composition of such antibodies.—C.A. Paulsen, M.D.

Monoclonal Antibody Recognizing an Apparent Peptide Epitope of Human Seminal Plasma Glycoprotein and Exhibiting Sperm Immobilizing Activity

Batova I, Kameda K, Hasegawa A, Koyama K, Tsuji Y, Isojima S (Hyogo Med College, Nishinomiya, Japan)

J Reprod Immunol 17:1–16, 1990 7–3

Introduction.—Murine and human hybridomes directed to human sperm and human seminal plasma (HSP) secreting monoclonal antibodies (Mabs) with strong sperm immobilizing and agglutinating activities have long been established. A Mab that recognizes a small linear sequential peptide epitope of sperm antigen would be a highly specific, sensitive probe for screening and cloning cDNA libraries obtained from male sexual accessory glands to obtain the DNA producing target antigen. In addition, sperm immobilizing Mabs directed to protein moieties on sperm membrane, including sperm coating antigens, may be a suitable tool for assessing the location of the functional gene products, which would cover the sperm during maturation of sperm cells.

Methods.—A hybridoma, 3B2-F7, was established that secretes a Mab directed against a peptide determinant of human seminal plasma glycoprotein (HSP-gP). The HSP-gP deglycosylation was performed chemically with TFMS hydrolysis and enzymatically with detergent and further treated with periodic acid after fixing deglycosylated HSP on plastic wells.

Results.—The Mab 3B2-F7 showed sperm immobilization activity and inhibited sperm binding to human zona pellucida. Human epididymis, pancreatic islets of Langerhan's, and distal tubulus of kidney were strongly labeled. Other tissues were essentially negative by avidin-biotin complex tissue staining with this Mab. The antigen epitope to the Mab was found in the 36-kDa molecule of human HSP-gP. Six different proteases destroyed the antigenic determinant recognized by Mab 3B2-F7, which was resistant to *N*-glycanase and other carbohydrate-splitting enzymes. Peptide fragments after proteolysis of the HSP molecule with *Staphylococcus aureus* V8 protease and trypsin retained antigenicity.

Conclusion.—The epitope is likely to be composed of a polypeptide chain. The epitope corresponding to the Mab may be a peptide chain and not dependent on the conformational structure of the polypeptide. The possible side effects of Mab 3B2-F7 in vivo are unclear.

▶ These data move us closer to specific peptides. Even though it is stated, that these antibodies are monoclonal, they appear to have different actions.—C.A. Paulsen, M.D.

Role of Testicular Autoantigens and Influence of Lymphokines in Testicular Autoimmune Disease

Yule TD, Mahi-Brown CA, Tung KSK (Washington Univ, St Louis; Univ of California, Davis)

J Reprod Immunol 18:89–103, 1990 7–4

Introduction.—Testicular autoimmune disease, a model of organ-specific autoimmunity, provides a unique opportunity to dissect the afferent and effector mechanisms of the autoimmune response. The role of testicular autoantigens and the influence of lymphokines in testicular autoimmune disease were examined.

Discussion.—The CD4+ helper type T cells appear to be responsible for adoptive transfer of murine experimental autoimmune orchitis (EAO). The earliest lymphoid cell infiltration is confined to terminal segments of seminiferous tubules in passive EAO. Orchitis and vasitis can beoth develop. Any location of the testis is affected in active EAO. The subcapsular seminiferous tubules are often involved. In passive EAO. the location of maximum histopathologic condition coincides with the site that expresses maximal Ia in the normal testis. The demonstration of IgG in the testis after immunization with testicular antigens or after transfer of sera from orchiectomized mice immunized with testis reveals the presence of autoantigens on the germ cells outside the Sertoli cell barrier. This suggests that dynamic protective mechanisms exist against immune responses to the nonsequestered autoimmunogenic germ cells in normal persons.

Conclusion.—A working hypothesis for the pathogenetic basis and target autoantigens in murine EAO was formulated based on these previous findings. Activated CD4+ T cells are pivotal in disease induction and are directly responsible for lesions in the straight tubules and vas deferens. Germ cell autoantigens that leak out of the straight tubules are presented to activated, autoreactive CD4+ T cells. Lesion pathogenesis in the seminiferous tubules requires Ia expression on interstitial macrophages that is up-regulated by adjuvants and antibodies to germ cells outside the Sertoli cell barrier. Antigen-antibody complex shedding may follow binding to the germ cells. After being processed by interstitial macrophages, the antigens in the complexes are presented to activated CD4+ T cells. In addition, germ cells carry antibodies passively across the blood-testis barrier to enter the adluminal compartment where they can disrupt the integrity of the germ cell epithelium.

▶ More evidence that the blood-testis barrier is not complete. Weininger et al. (1) showed that antibodies also pass through the epididymal epithelium into lumen.—C.A. Paulsen, M.D.

Reference

1. Weininger RB, et al: *J Reprod Fertil* 66:251, 1982.

8 Treatment of Male Infertility

A Prospective Trial of Intrauterine Insemination of Motile Spermatozoa Versus Timed Intercourse

Kirby CA, Warnes GM, Flaherty SP, Matthews CD, Godfrey BM (Univ of Adelaide; Queen Elizabeth Hosp, Woodville, South Australia)

Fertil Steril 56:102–107, 1991 8–1

Background.—The use of intrauterine insemination (IUI) as a treatment for male subfertility remains controversial. Prompted by the initial success with luteinizing hormone (LH)-timed IUI using motile sperm, a 5-year trial extended the use of IUI to a larger group of patients with male factor and to couples with cervical mucus hostility or unexplained infertility.

Study Design.—A prospective, randomized sequential trial compared the efficacy of IUI with LH-timed intercourse. The cycles of IUI were alternated with cycles of LH-timed intercourse. A modified swim-up procedure and discontinuous Percoll gradients were used to recover motile sperm, and the inseminations were timed for 40 hours after the start of the endogenous LH rise. A total of 285 couples, including 73 with unexplained fertility, 24 with cervical mucus hostility, 110 with moderate semen defect, and 78 with severe semen defect, underwent 600 IUI cycles and 505 LH-timed intercourse cycles.

Outcome.—Intrauterine insemination was significantly more effective than LH-timed intercourse, with a pregnancy rate of 6.2% vs. 3.4% per cycle. However, the marked improvement was found only in the group with severe semen defects, in which the pregnancy rate was 5.6% vs.

TABLE 1.—The Outcome of LH-Timed Intercourse and IUI Cycles With Respect to Infertility Category

	Timed intercourse			IUI		
Category	No. of couples	No. of cycles	No. of pregnancies	No. of cycles	No. of pregnancies	Logrank test
Mucus hostility	24	52	4 (7.8)*	58	7 (12.1)	$P > 0.05$
Unexplained	73	123	3 (2.4)	145	6 (4.1)	$P > 0.05$
Moderate semen defect	110	177	8 (4.5)	218	14 (6.4)	$P > 0.05$
Severe semen defect	78	154	2 (1.3)	179	10 (5.6)	$P < 0.05$
Overall	285	505	17 (3.4)	600	37 (6.2)	$P = 0.05$

*Values in parentheses are percentages.
(Courtesy of Kirby CA, Warnes GM, Flaherty SP, et al: *Fertil Steril* 56:102–107, 1991.)

TABLE 2.—The Effect of the Number of Cycles of Treatment on the PR for Timed Intercourse and IUI in All the Patient Categories Combined

	Timed intercourse		IUI	
Cycle no.	No. of cycles	No. of pregnancies	No. of cycles	No. of pregnancies
1	226	9 (4.0)*	266	27 (10.2)
2	125	5 (4.0)	141	7 (5.0)
3	79	2 (2.5)	98	2 (2.0)
4	49	1 (2.0)	56	1 (1.8)
5	19	0 (0.0)	27	0 (0)
6	7	0 (0.0)	12	0 (0)

*Values in parentheses are percentages.
(Courtesy of Kirby CA, Warnes GM, Flaherty SP, et al: *Fertil Steril* 56:102–107, 1991.)

1.3% (Table 1). In addition, the first IUI cycle of treatment was more effective when compared with subsequent IUI cycles and the initial LH-timed cycle (Table 2). A total of 74% of the IUI pregnancies occurred in the first cycle, for a pregnancy rate of 10.2% per cycle.

Conclusion.—Intrauterine insemination is more effective than LH-timed intercourse in the treatment of severe male subfertility, but only in the first cycle of treatment. Given the low expectation of pregnancy, however, continued IUI is considered unrewarding, particularly if successful in vitro fertilization/gamete intrafallopian transfer programs are available.

▶ This prospective, randomized, sequential trial provides evidence that IUI is more effective than LH-timed natural intercourse in couples whose male partner has a severe abnormality on semen analysis, including abnormal motility or morphology in addition to sperm concentration. The pregnancy rate of 6% per cycle with IUI is not as high as that occurring with gamete intrafallopian transfer or in vitro fertilization, but the success rate will probably increase if ovarian hyperstimulation is used in addition to IUI.—D.R. Mishell, Jr., M.D.

Intrauterine Insemination With Semen of Oligozoospermic Men: Effectiveness of the Continuous-Step Density Gradient Centrifugation Technique

Kobayashi T, Sato H, Kaneko S, Aoki R, Ohno T, Nozawa S (Keio Univ, Tokyo; Ichikawa Gen Hosp, Chiba, Japan)

Andrologia 23:251–254, 1991 8–2

Background.—In 1987 an improved method of Percoll density gradient centrifugation was described, i.e., the continuous-step density gradient, for selective concentration of progressively motile sperm. The efficacy of intrauterine insemination was assessed quantitatively using the method of life-table analysis.

Methods.—Forty-six infertile couples with oligozoospermia and/or athenozoospermia were studied. Selection criteria included sperm concentration of less than 20×10^6 mL^{-1} and/or motility of less than 40% throughout semen analysis repeated 3 or more times.

Results.—Intrauterine insemination was done in a total of 222 cycles. Seventeen patients had ovulation induction for at least 1 cycle. Pregnancy occurred in 13 patients, 11 of whom had full-term deliveries. By the fifth attempt at insemination, pregnancy had occurred in 9 patients. Nineteen patients decided to drop out of the program. The last conception to occur was in the 11th cycle. The pregnancy rate per insemination cycle was 5.9%, and per patient it was 28.3%. The value of cumulative probability of conception rose as intrauterine insemination was repeated in sequence, reaching 57% after cycle 11. Improvement in sperm quality was seen after processing in all cases. In patients in whom the total motile sperm count was less than 10×10^6, the degree of improvement was significantly higher in pregnant than nonpregnant cases. On the other hand, in those whose total motile sperm count was 10×10^6 or more, there was no difference in the degree of improvement between pregnant and nonpregnant cases.

Conclusions.—Intrauterine insemination is an effective treatment for oligo- and asthenozoospermia. Pregnancy rates exceed 25% if the sperm is processed by continuous-step density gradient centrifugation. Intrauterine insemination deserves to be repeated up to 10 times, as long as spermatogenesis is not severely impaired.

▶ The pregnancy rate per cycle with intrauterine insemination in this study, 5.8%, was nearly identical to the 6.2% reported in abstract 8–1. However, in contrast to the findings of Kirby et al., in whose series no patients conceived after the fourth treatment cycle, in this study 4 of the 13 patients who conceived did so within 6–11 treatment cycles. Some of the female partners in this study received ovulation-inducing drugs, but the results indicate that it is contraindicated to continue intrauterine insemination as treatment of oligo-asthenozoospermia for at least 6 months and possibly longer.—D.R. Mishell, Jr., M.D.

Direct Intraperitoneal Insemination: Clinical Results and Comparison Between Two Methods of Sperm Preparation

Karlström P-O, Bergh T, Bakos O, Lundkvist O, Palmstierna M (Uppsala Univ, Uppsala, Sweden)

Fertil Steril 56:939–945, 1991 8–3

Background.—Direct intraperitoneal (IP) insemination is another treatment of unexplained infertility, mild endometriosis, cervical factor, and male subfertility. Sperm preparation with a self-migration method in sodium hyaluronate was compared with a centrifugation/swim-up method, and the efficacy of IP insemination was investigated.

Methods.—Fifty-three couples with unexplained infertility, 17 with endometriosis, and 9 with cervical factor were enrolled. Sodium hyaluronate and centrifugation/swim-up were used randomly in alternating cycles for direct IP insemination. There was an interval of at least 1 untreated cycle in each treatment. If ovulation occurred on a weekend, natural insemination by coitus was used instead of IP. Controlled ovarian hyperstimulation was done with clomiphene citrate and gonadotropins.

Results.—Similar conception rates were achieved with sodium hyaluronate and centrifugation/swim-up techniques. However, sodium hyaluronate recovered more motile spermatozoa than the centrifugation/swim-up method. The percentage of patients becoming pregnant after direct IP insemination or controlled ovarian hyperstimulation only was significantly greater than that after untreated cycles.

Conclusions.—Preparing sperm with sodium hyaluronate is an alternative to centrifugation/swim-up. Direct IP insemination seems to increase the cycle fecundity. Whether direct IP insemination/controlled ovarian hyperstimulation is more effective than controlled ovarian hyperstimulation alone has yet to be established.

▶ This study indicates that both techniques of sperm concentration are equally effective for achieving pregnancy after IP insemination but that the self-migration method in sodium hyaluronate recovers more motile spermatozoa than the centrifugation swim-up method. Therefore, the former technique may be more successful when treating couples with male factor infertility by hyperstimulation and intrauterine insemination.—D.R. Mishell, Jr., M.D.

Transvaginal Intratubal Embryo Transfer: A New Treatment of Male Infertility

Diedrich K, Bauer O, Werner A, van der Ven H, Al-Hasani S, Krebs D (Univ of Bonn, Germany)

Hum Reprod 6:672–675, 1991 8–4

Purpose.—Transvaginal intratubal embryo transfer is a recently developed treatment approach in male infertility. The results of intratubal em-

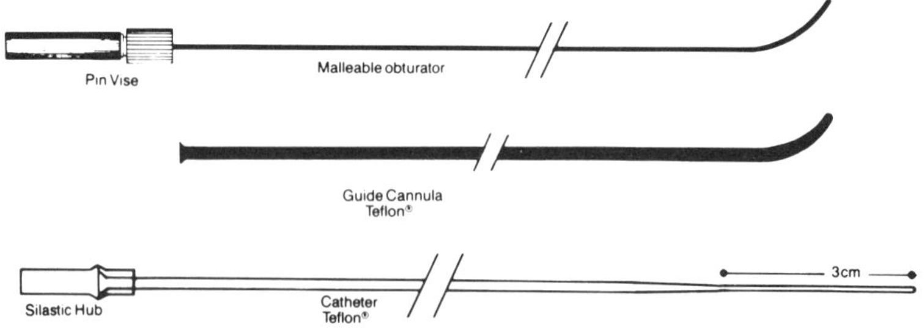

Fig 8–1.—Instrument set for transvaginal intratubal embryo transfer. (Courtesy of Diedrich K, Bauer O, Werner A, et al: *Hum Reprod* 6:672–675, 1991.)

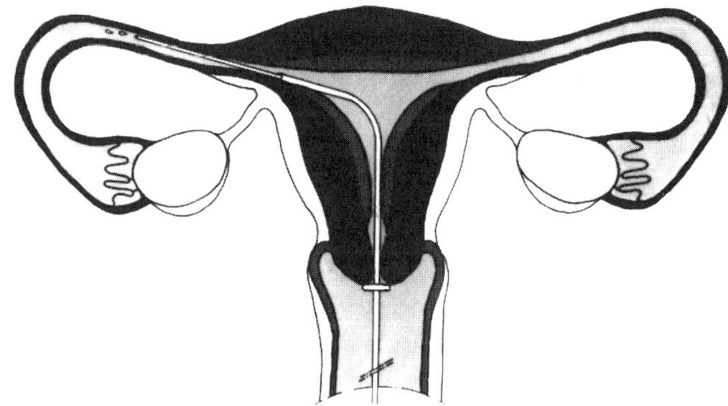

Fig 8–2.—The transvaginal intratubal embryo transfer. (Courtesy of Diedrich K, Bauer O, Werner A, et al: *Hum Reprod* 6:672–675, 1991.)

bryo transfer were assessed in 113 couples with male infertility factor.

Procedure.—Intratubal embryo transfer was undertaken when patients had proven patency of at least 1 fallopian tube, when there was at least 1 good embryo, and when male factor was the only cause of infertility. The transfer was performed 48 hours after transvaginal sonographic oocyte retrieval and successful in vitro fertilization (IVF). The Hansen and Anderson intratubal transfer catheter (Fig 8–1) was introduced transvaginally to the internal os using a metallic guiding rod. The guiding rod was then removed and the Teflon catheter was introduced carefully into the tubal angle. After resistance was reached, the catheter was advanced further by 1 mm–2 mm. The embryo was aspirated into the internal catheter, which was pushed through the Teflon catheter until it reached the cornual part of the tube and a slight resistance was noted (Fig 8–2).

Results.—Transvaginal intratubal embryo transfer was performed in 95 of 113 patients with male factor infertility, with an average of 2.3 embryos transferred per patient. There were 29 pregnancies, for a pregnancy rate of 31% per transfer, or 23% per attempt. In addition, there was 1 abortion and no ectopic pregnancies. No complications occurred. In the remaining 18 patients the catheter could not be introduced into the tube, producing a failure rate of 16%.

Discussion.—Transvaginal intratubal embryo transfer offers the advantages of IVF and gamete intrafallopian transfer. The sperm/oocyte contact can be established favorably under in vitro conditions, and embryonic development occurs in the physiologic milieu of the oviduct. The transvaginal intratubal embryo transfer may improve IVF success rates, particularly in couples with male infertility.

▶ For women with normal oviducts, transferring a fertilized embryo directly into the patent tube may result in a higher pregnancy rate than following in vitro fertilization with embryo transfer (IVF-ET) into the endometrial cavity, because initial embryoma development would occur under more physiologic conditions. In contrast to gamete intrafallopian transfer (GIFT), transvaginal intratubal embryo transfer provides evidence that fertilization and embryo formulation has actually occurred. Thus this technique may be more advantageous than either GIFT or IVF-ET in the treatment of male infertility. In this study, pregnancy occurred in nearly one fourth of the couples so treated.—D.R. Mishell, Jr., M.D.

In-Vitro Fertilization, Gamete- or Zygote Intra-Fallopian Transfer for the Treatment of Male Infertility

Tournaye H, Camus M, Khan I, Staessen C, Van Steirteghem AC, Devroey P (Vrije Universiteit Brussel, Brussels, Belgium)

Hum Reprod 6:263–266, 1991 8–5

Background.—In vitro fertilization and embryo transfer (IVF-ET) had been proposed as a means of treating male infertility, although alternate methods exist. A review was made of the results of a retrospective study comparing IVT-ET, gamete intrafallopian transfer (GIFT), and zygote intrafallopian transfer (ZIFT, by laparoscopy) techniques among 266 couples with male infertility.

Methods.—A total of 318 consecutive cycles in 266 couples with male infertility were reviewed retrospectively between January 1987 and April 1989. The treatment groups consisted of 163 cycles (133 couples) with IVF-ET, 45 cycles (43 couples) with GIFT, and 110 cycles (90 couples) with ZIFT. Ovarian stimulation, oocyte retrieval and incubation and sperm preparation were similar in each procedure.

Results.—The mean age of the couples and the duration of infertility were similar among the 3 treatment groups. Sperm values for insemination were poor in all 3 groups. Embryo transfer could be performed in 48.5% of the IVF-ET procedures, and zygotes were replaced in 62.7% of the ZIFT attempts. Oocyte transfer resulted in an average of embryo replaced in IVF-ET, 2.9 oocytes in GIFT, and 1.6 zygotes in ZIFT, a significant intertreatment difference. Conception occurred in 23 women treated by IVF-ET (14.1% per cycle), in 8 undergoing GIFT (17.8% per cycle), and in 23 patients having ZIFT (20.9% per cycle). Although the number of conceptions with ZIFT tended to be higher than the number after IVF-ET, the outcome did not reach statistical significance. The take-home infant rate per couple was 20% after ZIFT, 13.5% after IVF-ET, and 7% after GIFT.

Implications.—In the treatment of male infertility, these findings have led to the authors' policy of not using GIFT because of lack of confirmation of fertilization and of preferring the use of ZIFT because of the good take-home infant rate when no tubal factor complicates the patient's status. As an alternative method, IVF-ET is used when a tubal factor is present or if repeated treatments may be required.

▶ Although this was a retrospective study, the results confirm the findings observed in Abstract 8–4. In this study the zygotes were transferred to the oviduct under laparoscopic visualization, whereas in the Diedrich et al.'s study they were transferred transvaginally. The similar pregnancy rates indicate that in couples with patent tubes and male factor infertility, ZIFT may be the treatment of choice if ovarian hyperstimulation and IVF are unsuccessful.—D.R. Mishell, Jr., M.D.

Subzonal Insemination for the Alleviation of Infertility

Fishel S, Johnson J, Jackson P, Grossi S, Antinori S, Versaci C (Queen's Med Ctr, Nottingham, England; Casa Di Cura Nomentana, Rome)

Fertil Steril 54:828 835, 1990 8–6

Background.—A significant number of women are unable to conceive by in vitro fertilization (IVF) because of lack of fertilization. In some cases the spermatozoa bind with apparently normal affinity to the zona pellucida, whereas in others binding does not take place. In still other instances the male is subfertile.

Study Design.—In patients with severe male factor subfertility, half of the oocytes were assigned to subzonal insemination and the rest to in vivo insemination. Spermatozoa were prepared by standard methods including double centrifugation and swim-up. Micropipettes and microneedles prepared from borosilicate glass capillary tubes were fitted to a micromanipulator. Subzonal insemination was carried out using an inverted microscope. A mean of 3.4 spermatozoa were injected into the perivitelline space of each oocyte.

Results.—Oocytes were recovered from 85 patients. Fertilization was achieved when there were 2% to 10% motile sperm, but not when there were 5% to 30% motile sperm. On attempted subzonal insemination, 15% of oocytes were fertilized and an equal proportion were damaged by the procedure. In 38% of patients, at least 1 oocyte was fertilized by the subzonal technique. There were 1 twin and 2 singleton pregnancies in 31 replacements. Sixteen percent of subzonally inseminated oocytes were fertilized. as were 11% of those used for in vitro insemination.

Discussion.—Seven more pregnancies occurred in later trials. At present, subzonal insemination offers some, but not much hope to infertile patients.

Routine Application of Partial Zona Dissection for Male Factor Infertility

Tucker MJ, Bishop FM, Cohen J, Wiker SR, Wright G (Reproductive Biology Associates, Atlanta; Cornell Univ Med College, New York)

Hum Reprod 6:676–681, 1991 8–7

Background.—Male factor infertility remains a problematic occurrence, and its causes are imprecisely understood. Partial zona dissection (PZD) attempts to increase the chance of fertilization by improving the access of spermatozoa to the perivitelline space, thereby aiding those spermatozoa that cannot penetrate the zona pellucida (and possibly those that do not penetrate the oolemma well). In bypassing the zona pellucida, PZD may also increase the rate of polyspermy.

Study Design.—Partial zona dissection was used to treat male infertility in 70 in vitro fertilization cycles attempted in 67 patients. In 61 couples, male factor infertility was the principal finding. Oocytes were aspirated by transvaginal ultrasound. Those not fertilized after conventional insemination were micromanipulated to open the zona pellucida before reinsemination. Partial zona dissection was done without hyaluronidase pretreatment or shrinkage in sucrose. Up to 4 embryos were replaced in the uterus.

Outcome.—In the first 35 cycles, fertilization occurred at a rate of 23% with initial PZD and 33% with PZD reinsemination. There were 4 pregnancies. In 19 other cycles, fertilization failed to occur with either PZD or conventional insemination. In 16 cycles the fertilization rates were similar with PZD and conventional insemination, but polyspermy occurred at a rate of 48% in those having PZD. Ten pregnancies occurred in this group. No broad correlations were found between patient or seminal parameters and the outcome of PZD, although normal morphology was least frequent when no fertilization occurred.

Conclusions.—The chance of fertilization can improve with PZD when the spermatozoa are unable to normally penetrate the zona pellucida or fuse with the oolemma.

Partial Zona Dissection or Subzonal Sperm Insertion: Microsurgical Fertilization Alternatives Based on Evaluation of Sperm and Embryo Morphology

Cohen J, Adler A, Alikani M, Talansky BE, Malter HE, Rosenwaks Z (New York Hosp-Cornell Med Ctr, New York)

Fertil Steril 56:696–706, 1991 8–8

Introduction.—The 3 main types of microsurgical fertilization methods available for promoting sperm-egg fusion for human in vitro fertilization (IVF) are injecting a single spermatozoon directly into ooplasm, placing spermatozoa into the perivitelline space (i.e., subzonal sperm insertion), and breaching the zona pellucida to facilitate sperm access to the egg, i.e., partial zona pellucida dissection. Sperm parameters, embryo morphology, and fertilization and implantation rates were compared after partial zona dissection and subzonal sperm insertion in 104 couples with severe male factor infertility.

Patients.—During the first part of the study, 57 couples were treated with partial zona dissection. Most were considered to have little chance of spontaneous fertilization after standard IVF. Partially zona-dissected oocytes were inseminated with low numbers of motile spermatozoa to avoid polyspermy. A maximum of 4 embryos were replaced. In the second part of the study, subzonal sperm insertion was performed on all or some of the oocytes in 47 couples.

Results.—Embryo replacement was successful in 21 of the 104 women

(20%), 9 of whom (19%) became clinically pregnant—4 after partial zona dissection and 5 after subzonal sperm insertion. Couples in whom standard IVF had failed had a chance of pregnancy after the use of micromanipulation similar to that of first-time patients. In a subgroup of 15 patients in whom IVF had failed because of insufficient numbers of motile sperm, the rate of fertilization in subzonally inserted eggs was significantly higher than that with partially zona-dissected eggs, indicating that the latter require a higher concentration of motile sperm than needed for subzonal sperm insertion. Partially zona-dissected embryos from couples with severe teratozoospermia, defined as 5% or less normal forms, had significantly more morphological abnormalities than embryos from couples with moderate teratozoospermia, defined as 6% to 10% normal forms. In couples with severe teratozoospermia significantly fewer partially zona-dissected than subzonally inserted embryos were implanted.

Conclusion.—Choosing the best microsurgical fertilization method for a given couple could possibly be based on careful examination of sperm morphology.

▶ Micromanipulation of the ovary to partially dissect the zona pellucida, as well as to insert the sperm directly beneath the zona into the perivitelline space (subzonal insemination), are experimental techniques to treat the failure of routine IVF in couples with male factor infertility. These methods require a great amount of technical expertise. Therefore, the conception rates after the use of these procedures varies among centers for many reasons, primary among them being the technicians' experience. It remains to be determined which of these techniques is preferable to use in certain cases of male factor infertility.—D.R. Mishell, Jr., M.D.

Comparison of Gonadotropin-Releasing Hormone and Gonadotropin Therapy in Male Patients With Idiopathic Hypothalamic Hypogonadism

Schopohl J, Eversmann T, Mehltretter G, von Werder K, von Zumbusch R (Klinikum Innenstadt, München, Germany)

Fertil Steril 56:1143–1150, 1991 8–9

Objective.—The efficacy of treatment with pulsatile gonadotropin-releasing hormone (GnRH) was compared with that of gonadotropin therapy in a prospective series of 36 men who had hypogonadotropic hypogonadism. Puberty had not occurred by age 18 years in 34 of the 36 men.

Treatment.—Eighteen patients, 10 with idiopathic hypothalamic hypogonadism and 8 with Kallmann's syndrome, received pulsatile GnRH treatment. Eighteen age-matched patients, 9 with idiopathic hypothalamic hypogonadism and 9 with Kallmann's syndrome, received gonadotropins (human chorionic gonadotropin and human menopausal gonadotropin).

Results.—Levels of testosterone and estradiol rose significantly more in gonadotropin-treated patients than in those given GnRH therapy. Gynecomastia developed in 5 of the former patients. The increase in testicular volume was more marked with GnRH therapy. Ten patients given GnRH and 8 given gonadotropins had positive sperm counts, which were achieved more rapidly in the GnRH recipients. Pregnancies were achieved by both patients for whom this was a goal.

Conclusions.—Gonadotropin-releasing hormone treatment of patients with hypogonadotropic hypogonadism leads more rapidly to spermatogenesis than does gonadotropin therapy and does not cause gynecomastia. The treatment, however, requires good patient compliance. Gonadotropin therapy remains an effective alternative for those patients who are not able or willing to carry an infusion pump for a year or longer.

▶ Treatment of men whose infertility results from lack of adequate endogenous GnRH is the most predictable and successful management of male infertility. The above study compares 2 methods designed to produce sufficient gonadotropin levels to stimulate testicular function.—C.A. Paulsen, M.D.

Possible Role of Pure Human Follicle-Stimulating Hormone in the Treatment of Severe Male-Factor Infertility by Assisted Reproduction: Preliminary Report

Acosta AA, Oehninger S, Ertunc H, Philput C (Eastern Virginia Med School, Norfolk)

Fertil Steril 55:1150–1156, 1991 8–10

Introduction.—Patients with male-factor infertility and severe impairment of sperm parameters often do not achieve fertilization in the in vitro fertilization (IVF) system. The potential of systemic follicle-stimulating hormone (FSH) to improve sperm fertilizing capacity in IVF was assessed in 14 patients (41 cycles) in whom IVF failed and in 22 (32 cycles) with severe quantitative and qualitative semen abnormalities indicating poor fertilization.

Methods.—The patients were treated with FSH, 150 units intramuscularly 3 times a week for 3 months. Endocrine profiles, basic semen analysis, and fertilization and pregnancy rates were recorded before and after treatment.

Results.—There were no significant changes in endocrine profiles or semen parameters. In some individuals the sperm concentration and motility improved. There was a significant increase in the fertilization rate of preovulatory oocytes, with 7 term pregnancies achieved.

Conclusion.—Some infertile men whose sperm are unable to fertilize oocytes in the human in vitro system can be helped by systemic treatment with pure FSH before IVF/embryo transfer. These men are characterized mainly by severe abnormal morphology or a combination of abnormal parameters. A multicenter, randomized, double-blind trial with crossover is warranted to explore the possibilities of this treatment.

▶ An interesting observation that requires confirmation. Furthermore, a placebo-treated population should be used as controls. Previous studies using human menopausal gonadotropin failed to provide conclusive evidence of efficacy; however, IVF was not used in those studies (1).—C.A. Paulsen, M.D.

Reference

1. Paulsen CA, et al: Current Concepts in the Management of Male Infertility, Troen P, Nankin HR (eds): *The Testis in Normal and Infertile Men.* New York, Raven Press, 1977, pp 549-559.

Placebo-Controlled Trial of High-Dose Mesterolone Treatment of Idiopathic Male Infertility

Gerris J, Peeters K, Comhaire F, Schoonjans F, Hellemans P (Antwerp Univ, Antwerp, Belgium; State Univ Hosp, Ghent, Belgium)

Fertil Steril 55:603–607, 1991 8–11

Introduction.—Male infertility is often the result of idiopathic oligoasthenospermia or teratozoospermia. In a double-blind trial, mesterolone or placebo was administered to men with idiopathic infertility to assess the drug's potential benefit for semen improvement.

Methods.—Mesterolone (150 mg/day daily) or placebo was administered for 12 months to 52 men with idiopathic infertility. Gynecologic causes of infertility were ruled out. Two semen samples were examined before initiation of treatment, and semen analyses were repeated at 3, 6, 9, and 12 months during drug intake.

Results.—The pregnancy rates in the mesterolone-treated group and the placebo-treated group were similar (26% vs. 48%, respectively). During treatment, a significant increase in motility and proportion of spermatozoa with normal morphology was seen in the patients given mesterolone. Increases in motility were also found in patients taking placebo after 3 months and 12 months, but only borderline improvement in spermatozoa with normal morphology was observed.

Discussion.—The improvement of sperm after treatment with mesterolone did not increase the pregnancy rate to any higher degree than that in the group given placebo. Regardless of treatment, men with better initial sperm morphology had a greater chance of initiating pregnancy. High-dose mesterolone did not have a significant effect on male fertility in patients with idiopathic testicular failure.

▶ A not too surprising, but important study, because placebo controls were included.—C.A. Paulsen, M.D.

Clinical Experience and Successful Impregnation Using an Artificial Spermatocele

Miura K, Matsuhashi M, Takanami M, Ishii N, Shirai M (Toho Univ, Tokyo)

Urol Int 47:149–152, 1991 8–12

Background.—No successful therapy has been developed for male infertility caused by bilateral congenital vas deferens deficiency, sperm passage disorders (e.g., insufficiency or obstruction), or extensive damage of the bilateral vas deferens. Artificial insemination of the husband (AIH) with semen collected from an artificial spermatocele installed in the epididymis was successful in 2 patients.

Technique.—A brimlike eave of Teflon mesh is attached to an artificial silicone spermatocele for easy adhesion and is sutured to the epididymis. Semen collection is accomplished by piercing the spermatocele percutaneously and suctioning the fluid into a syringe containing a medium for culturing sperm. After the fluid is subjected to fertility tests, it is used for AIH.

Results.—The artificial spermatocele was installed in 33 men, and sperm specimens with good fertility were collected and used for AIH in 11 cases. Artificial insemination could be performed only 1–9 times. Subsequent histologic tests on the region where the spermatocele was installed showed that the incised epididymal surface had become obstructed with fibrous tissue. Because lower levels of sperm activity are found in the head and body of the epididymis, implantation of the artificial spermatocele in the tail region of the epididymis is preferred.

Conclusions.—In 11 of 33 patients in whom an artificial spermatocele was installed, sperm with good fertility was collected. Pregnancy was achieved after the second AIH in 1 case and after the first AIH in another. Artificial insemination of husband is possible only for several months because natural blocking of the incised site in the epididymal duct occurs. A key point for inducing pregnancy is to attempt AIH as quickly as possible upon collecting semen. These 2 cases are part of a very small number of reported successful pregnancies achieved through the use of artificial spermatoceles.

▶ Another suggestion about a surgical approach to solving the vexing problem of ductile obstruction, either congenital or acquired.—C.A. Paulsen, M.D.

Semen Retrieval in Spinal Cord Injured Men

Rawicki HB, Hill S (Caulfield Gen Med Ctr, Caulfield, Vic, Australia; Hampton Rehabilitation Hosp, Hampton, Vic, Australia)

Paraplegia 29:443–446, 1991 8–13

Background.—Infertility is a usual sequel to cord injury in men; only 1% of untreated men with a complete cord lesion are fertile. Semen quality, particularly sperm motility, usually is poor whether or not ejaculation is aided.

Management.—Various methods were used to enhance fertility in 39 cord-injured men. They first were asked to try masturbating if they had not already done so. Electroejaculation, using a rectal probe to deliver a 30-volt, 10-Hz current to the nerves of the seminal vesicles and vas deferens, remains an effective method. Vibration ejaculation is a method of stimulating the glans, frenulum, or penile base. Another method is to inject physostigmine subcutaneously in conjunction with an anticholinergic agent.

Experience.—Thirty-five men were treated with various combinations of these methods. Semen was obtained as an external ejaculate from 18 of 24 men with lesions at T-8 or above and in a retrograde manner in 3 others. Semen was obtained from only 3 of 10 men with lesions at T-10 to T-12. Among 15 couples treated for 6 months or longer, 6 have had 8 pregnancies.

Conclusions.—It is feasible to obtain semen from many cord-injured men with lesions above T-10. In these cases the major goal is to improve the quality of the obtained sperm to maximize the chance of fertility.

▶ Additional experience in dealing with a difficult problem. Reasonable results were obtained by these authors even in men with lesions at T-8 or above.—C.A. Paulsen, M.D.

The Application of Pentoxifylline in the Stimulation of Sperm Motion in Men Undergoing Electroejaculation

Sikka SC, Hellstrom WJG (Tulane Univ, New Orleans)

J Androl 12:165–170, 1991 8–14

Introduction.—Electroejaculation can cause production of a semen sample for use in artificial insemination in most men with spinal cord injury, but low pregnancy rates usually result. This may be because the mo-

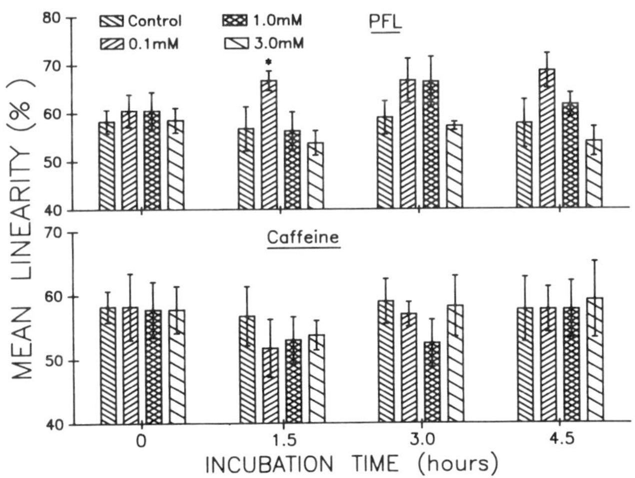

Fig 8–3.—Comparison of the effect of pentoxifylline *(PFL)* and caffeine on mean linearity of electroejaculated human sperm. Incubations were performed with various doses as shown, and the results are presented as the mean ± SEM from 5 patients. *Asterisk* indicates $P < .05$ compared with the control at the same time period. (Courtesy of Sikka SC, Hellstrom WJG: *J Androl* 12:165–179, 1991.)

Summary of Semen Evaluations of Electroejaculation (EE) Program Patients

Patient no.	Etiology	Number of EE attempts	Antegrade sample: Volume (ml)	Antegrade sample: Count (10^6/ml)	Antegrade sample: Motility (%)	Retrograde sample: Volume (ml)	Retrograde sample: Count (10^6/ml)	Retrograde sample: Motility (%)	Normal morphology (%)
1	RPLND	4†	1.2 ± 0.5	352 ± 132	6 ± 3	45 ± 15	144 ± 54	9 ± 5	65 ± 2
2	Spinal	2	0.6 ± 0.1	81 ± 14	1 ± 1	65 ± 5	106 ± 86	1 ± 1	48 ± 6
3	RPLND	5	3.0 ± 0.2	217 ± 41	23 ± 6	33 ± 2	64 ± 21	18 ± 3	49 ± 4
4	Spinal	3	0.4 ± 0.1	68 ± 8	7 ± 4	36 ± 9	47 ± 22	13 ± 6	64 ± 3
5	Psychogenic	6	2.7 ± 0.5	84 ± 7	11 ± 1	70 ± 6	23 ± 11	13 ± 3	56 ± 2
6	Spinal	4	1.0 ± 0.5	18 ± 12	6 ± 3	170 ± 30	5 ± 3	1 ± 1	49 ± 4
Mean ± SEM		4 ± 0.6	1.5 ± 0.4	137 ± 50	9 ± 3	70 ± 20	65 ± 21	9 ± 2	55 ± 3

*Represents prestimulated values (mean ± SEM) of different EE attempts for each patient.
†Denotes birth of a normal, healthy infant using GIFT after sperm stimulation.
(Courtesy of Sikka SC, Hellstrom WJG: *J Androl* 12:165–179, 1991.)

tility of sperm obtained from these patients is usually low. There is evidence that pentoxifylline, a trisubstituted methylxanthine derivative, can enhance sperm activity.

Methods.—The movement characteristics of sperm obtained from electroejaculated samples after stimulation by pentoxifylline were studied in 6 neurologically impaired men who underwent multiple electroejaculation procedures. Washed sperm were incubated with 0, .1, 1, or 3 mmol of either pentoxifylline or caffeine per liter. Sperm motility was evaluated using videomicrography and computer-assisted sperm analysis.

Results.—The mean sperm concentration of antegrade samples was $137 \pm 50 \times 10^6$/mL for antegrade samples and $65 \pm 21 \times 10^6$/mL for retrograde samples. The mean motility was only 9% (table). After 3-hour incubation with pentoxifylline, the sperm showed dose-dependent increases in percent motility. Pentoxifylline and caffeine significantly increased both the curvilinear and straight line velocity of sperm. Incubation of sperm for 1.5 hours with pentoxifylline, .1 mmol/L, but not with caffeine, resulted in significant stimulation of mean linearity, a measure of swimming straightness (Fig 8–3). Neither drug affected lateral head displacement of electroejaculated sperm. The pentoxifylline-stimulated samples were used for gamete intrafallopian transfer or intrauterine insemination in 4 couples, resulting in 1 normal pregnancy.

Conclusion.—Pentoxifylline is a greater stimulus than similar doses of caffeine to the motility characteristics of asthenospermic sperm obtained by electroejaculation. Treatment of sperm with pentoxifylline does not impair fertilization and may be useful in improving the fertility of neurologically impaired young men.

Transcatheter Embolization of Testicular Vein for Varicocele Testis

Kuroiwa T, Hasuo K, Yasumori K, Mizushima A, Yoshida K, Hirakata R, Komatsu K, Yamaguchi A, Masuda K (Kyushu Univ; Sanshinkai Hara Hosp, Fukuoka, Japan)

Acta Radiol 32:311–314, 1991 8–15

Introduction.—High ligation of the testicular vein has been performed to treat varicocele testis; however, varicocele recurrence and surgical complications have been reported. Data were reviewed on 28 men with clinically palpable varicoceles who underwent percutaneous transcatheter embolization with stainless steel coils.

Methods.—All of the patients had oligospermia or infertility of more than 3 years' duration. Embolization was performed using Seldinger's technique. The left vein in 26 patients and bilateral veins in 2 were embolized using 3-, 5-, or 8-mm stainless steel coils. The volume of sperm, sperm motility, and sperm density were analyzed about 1 month before and 3–6 months after the procedure.

Results.—Varicocele grade improved after embolization in 82% of the men. The effective sperm count significantly increased from 34.5 to 65.1 after embolization. However, pregnancy was achieved in only 1 case. The basilic vein approach was believed to be superior to the femoral vein or jugular vein approach.

Conclusion.—Testicular venography and transcatheter embolization for varicoceles using the basilic approach are fairly simple procedures. There is no significant risk of complications. These procedures may be indicated in virtually all infertile men with a clinical diagnosis of varicoceles for both confirmation of the diagnosis and possible cure.

▶ This and various other studies using chemicals, coils, and the like to induce embolization are of interest, but based on my experience, it is not certain that all centers report their adverse reactions. Perhaps more importantly, comparisons of various surgical techniques are rarely studied in the same clinic and then published.—C.A. Paulsen, M.D.

Study of Bilateral Histology and Meiotic Analysis in Men Undergoing Varicocele Ligation

Wang Y-X, Chandley AC, Lei C, MacIntyre M, Dong S-G, Hargreave TB (Western Gen Hosp, Edinburgh)

Fertil Steril 55:152–155, 1991 8–16

Background.—Scrotal varicoceles are a major cause of primary testicular failure and infertility. Whether conventional histopathology or the findings from meiosis could predict who would benefit from varicocele ligation was determined.

Methods.—Fifty men aged 19–40 years underwent testicular biopsy at the time of varicocele ligation. All had involuntary infertility of 2 or more years' duration. The biopsy specimens were scored, and part of each specimen was analyzed meiotically. The men were then followed for a mean of 19.3 months.

Findings.—No consistent histologic or meiotic abnormalities were found. Nor was there any evidence that the varicocele side was more defective than the contralateral side. Thirteen pregnancies occurred, but only when the mean Johnsen score from 1 or the other testis was more than 6.

Conclusions.—Pregnancies are not likely to occur after varicocele ligation unless 1 or the other testicle has a biopsy Johnsen score of at least 6. The benefit of having this information must be weighed against the risks of the invasive procedure of biopsy. When biopsy is done, it must be bilateral. In this study, the physicians were not able to identify specific meiotic findings associated with the presence of a varicocele, although such findings were abnormal even when the Johnsen score was toward the high end of the scale.

▶ Interesting study, but the data do not provide convincing evidence that testicular biopsy is useful in this setting.—C.A. Paulsen, M.D.

Results of 1,469 Microsurgical Vasectomy Reversals by the Vasovasostomy Study Group

Belker AM, Thomas AJ Jr, Fuchs EF, Konnak JW, Sharlip ID (Univ of Louisville; Cleveland Clinic Found; Oregon Health Sciences Univ, Portland; Univ of Michigan; Univ of California, San Francisco)

J Urol 145:505–511, 1991 8–17

Introduction.—Data were reviewed on 1247 first-time and 222 repeated microsurgical vasectomy reversals performed by 5 surgeons from 1976 to 1985 to examine the relationships of various preoperative and intraoperative factors to postoperative results.

Methods.—Patient characteristics are shown in Table 1. Surgeons recorded intraoperative observations on the gross appearance and sperm content of the fluid from the testicular end of the vas deferens, the presence or absence of a sperm granuloma at the vasectomy site, and the type of anesthesia used. Either microsurgical 2-layer or modified 1-layer vasovasostomy was performed. Periodic postoperative semen analyses and information about postoperative pregnancies were continued for 2 years (Table 2). Postoperative rates of patency and pregnancy were recorded according to yearly obstructive intervals (Fig 8–4).

Results.—If the obstructive interval had been for less than 3 years, the patency rate was 97% and the pregnancy rate, 76%. After 15 years the

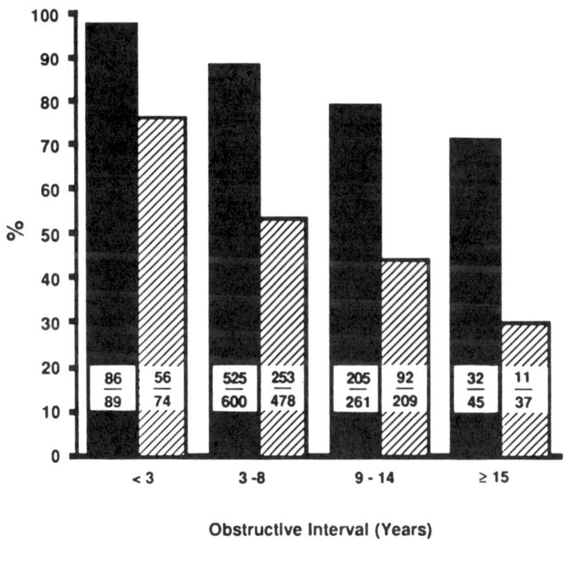

Fig 8–4.—New obstructive interval guidelines may be useful to predict postoperative patency and pregnancy rates. *Numerator* equals number of patients achieving patency or pregnancy, *denominator* equals total number of patients in each group. (Courtesy of Belker AM, Thomas AJ Jr, Fuchs EF, et al: *J Urol* 145:505–511, 1991.)

TABLE 1.—Characteristics of 1,247 Patients Undergoing a First Microsurgical Vasectomy Reversal Procedure

Demographics:	Range	Mean
Pt. age (yrs.)	20.3–67.4	36.9
Wife's age (yrs.)	17.0–46.0	29.6
Prior No. children/pt.	0.0–9.0	1.8
Obstructive interval (yrs.)	<1.0–33.0	7.0
No. wives previously pregnant/total No. wives (%)	391/1,011	(39)
Reasons for reversal in 1,213 pts.:	**No.**	**%**
Divorce and remarriage	897	73.9
Religion	7	0.6
Scrotal pain	19	1.6
Child died	31	2.6
Divorced, not remarried	20	1.6
Other	239	19.7
Procedures performed in 1,247 pts.:	**No.**	**%**
Unilat. vasovasostomy	28	2.3
Bilat. vasovasostomy	1,166	93.5
Vasovasostomy 1 side, vasoepididymostomy other side	36	2.9
Unilat. vasoepididymostomy	2	0.2
Bilat. vasoepididymostomy	12	1.0
Unspecified	3	0.2

Note: Percentage may total greater than 100 because of rounding.
(Courtesy of Belker AM, Thomas AJ Jr, Fuchs EF, et al: *J Urol* 145:505–511, 1991.)

TABLE 2.—Postoperative Follow-up Information for First Reversals

No. lost to or excluded from postop. followup (% of 1,247 first reversals):	
No postop. semen analysis	235 (18.9)
Pregnancy information:	
Excluded	192 (15.4)
<2-yr. followup	245 (19.6)
Had semen analysis	155 (12.4)
No semen analysis	90 (7.2)
No. reasons for exclusion from pregnancy rate calculations:	
Reversal reasons:	
Religion	3
Scrotal pain	12
Divorced, not remarried	24
Never married	7
Total	46
Postop. reasons:	
Divorced postop.	13
Used contraception postop.	19
Wife found to have fertility problem	70
Total	102
Combined reasons	
2 of above reasons	37
3 of above reasons	6
4 of above reasons	1
Total	44

(Courtesy of Belker AM, Thomas AJ Jr, Fuchs EF, et al: *J Urol* 145:505–511, 1991.)

patency rate was 71% and the pregnancy rate, 30%. These rates were not significantly better with 2-layer than with 1-layer procedures. When sperm was absent from the intraoperative vas fluid bilaterally and the patient underwent bilateral vasovasostomy rather than vasoepididymostomy, patency occurred in 60% of patients and pregnancy in 31% of couples. Of the 222 repeat reversal procedures, 75% produced patency, and pregnancy was reported in 43% of couples.

Conclusion.—The pregnancy rate after vasectomy reversal is inversely related to the duration of the obstructive interval. When comparing the success of microsurgical vasectomy reversals to nonmicrosurgical reversals, the obstructive interval guidelines must be considered. The results of microsurgical reversals are sufficiently superior to justify the increased expense and operating time.

▶ The authors of this multicenter study are providing solid clinical data with respect to vasectomy reversals. The time between the vasectomy and the attempt at reversal is an important point when counseling patients.—C.A. Paulsen, M.D.

The Appropriate Upper Age Limit for Semen Donors: A Review of the Genetic Effects of Paternal Age

Bordson BL, Leonardo VS (Reproductive Resources, Inc, Metairie, La; Univ of Nebraska, Omaha)

Fertil Steril 56:397–400, 1991 8–18

Background.—The American Association of Tissue Banks has set an upper age limit of 35 years for semen donors to minimize the chances of age-related genetic abnormalities occurring. The literature on the incidence of genetic anomalies associated with increased paternal age was reviewed, with particular attention to the paternal age contribution to genetic disorders in liveborn infants.

Discussion.—Nondisjunction during a meiotic division is the primary cause of aneuploidy. Nondisjunction during spermatogenesis is not rare. In 1 study of sperm from 30 normal men, a mean 4.7% of the sperm had abnormal chromosome numbers. Other research done on normal men has shown similar high proportions of aneuploid sperm. Although there is little evidence that advanced paternal age is associated with the incidence of chromosome anomalies, the incidence of serious nonchromosomal birth defects increases with paternal age. This is especially true for those arising from new autosomal mutations. Risk estimates have been reported for advanced paternal age and contribution to new dominant mutations.

Conclusions.—The association between increased paternal age and new autosomal mutations, and the fact that most disorders from such mutations cannot be diagnosed prenatally, may be important in setting the upper age limit for semen donors. The literature suggests that men should be advised to have their children before age 40 years. This advice would not only benefit immediate offspring, but possibly successive generations as well.

▶ Sperm banks should notice. The American Fertility Society (1) has suggested 40 years as the upper age limit for donors.—C.A. Paulsen, M.D.

Reference

1. American Fertility Society: *Fertil Steril* 56:396, 1991.

Therapeutic Donor Insemination: A Prospective Randomized Study of Scheduling Methods

Odem RR, Pineda JA, Durso NM, Strickler RC, Long CA, Gast MJ (Washington Univ, St Louis)

Fertil Steril 55:976–982, 1991 8–19

Introduction.—Accurate appointment scheduling is crucial to the successful outcome of therapeutic donor insemination treatment. The therapeutic efficacy and economic benefit of 2 commonly used methods for scheduling therapeutic donor insemination appointments were compared.

Patients.—During a 16-month period, 113 women attending an infertility clinic were enrolled in the study. Of these, 57 (mean age, 33 years) were randomly allocated to urinary luteinizing hormone (LH) monitoring for scheduling their 6 monthly therapeutic donor insemination appointments; 56 (mean age, 34 years) had their appointments scheduled on the basis of daily basal body temperature (BBT) graphs. Inclusion criteria were devised to insure a population with pure male factor infertility. Only

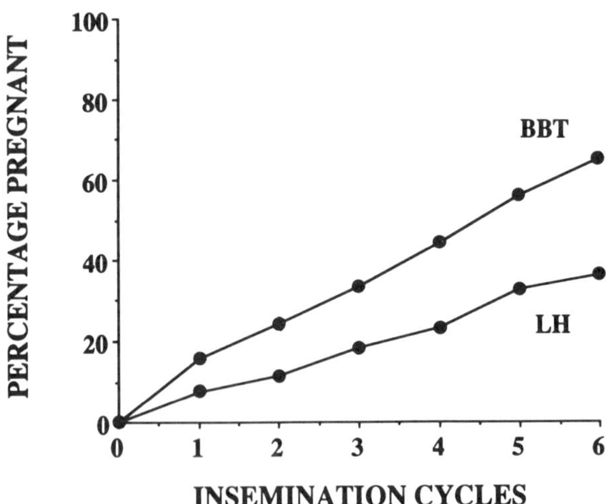

Fig 8–5.—The 6-cycle cumulative probability of pregnancy calculated by life table analysis in the BBT and urinary LH groups was significantly different ($P < .025$). (Courtesy of Odem RR, Pineda JA, Durso NM, et al: *Fertil Steril* 55:976–982, 1991.)

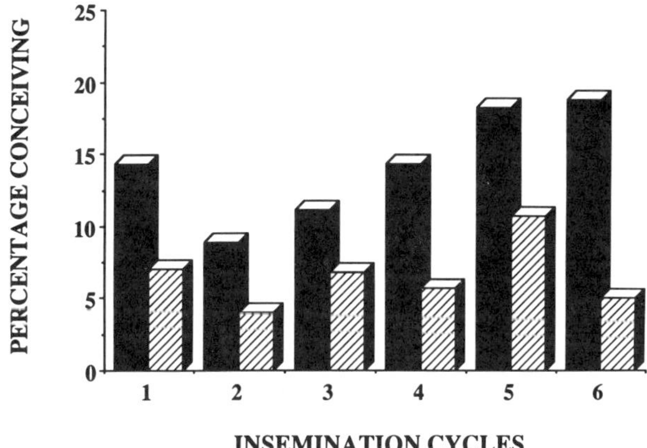

Fig 8–6.—Cycle fecundity rates for each cycle are shown. The fecundity rates for patients in the BBT group *(filled bars)* and for patients using urinary LH monitoring *(striped bars)* are significantly different ($P = .033$). (Courtesy of Odem RR, Pineda JA, Durso NM, et al: *Fertil Steril* 55:976–982, 1991.)

cryopreserved sperm that had been quarantined in liquid nitrogen for at least 6 months was used for insemination.

Results.—Of the 113 women enrolled in the study, 74 completed it by either receiving 6 insemination cycles or attaining pregnancy; 18 had ongoing treatment at the end of the study, and 21 withdrew for various reasons. By life-table analysis, the 6-month probability of pregnancy was 65% for women whose appointments were scheduled by the BBT method and 36% for those assigned to urinary LH monitoring (Fig 8–5). The difference was statistically significant. In women whose appointments were scheduled on the basis of urinary LH monitoring, fecundity rates remained constant throughout the 6 cycles. In women who used BBT graphs, fecundity rates increased with each successive cycle, with the highest individual fecundity rates achieved in cycle 6 (Fig 8–6). The total

Cost Analysis of Treatment

Category	LH group	BBT group
All study patients (n = 113)		
Initial cost	$424	$391
Insemination cost	$1,211	$1,536 *
Total cost	$1,635	$1,927
Total cost/pregnancy	$6,212	$3,997 †
Study patients who conceived (n = 42)		
Initial cost	$452	$377
Insemination cost	$905	$1,259
Total cost/pregnancy	$1,357	$1,637

Note: Values are means, rounded to the nearest whole dollar.
*$P < .02$ for the comparison between groups.
†$P < .001$ for the comparison between groups.
(Courtesy of Odem RR, Pineda JA, Durso NM, et al: *Fertil Steril* 55:976–982, 1991.)

cost per pregnancy was $6,212 for women assigned to LH monitoring and $3,997 per pregnancy for women who maintained daily BBT graphs (table).

Conclusions.—The use of daily BBT graphs to schedule therapeutic donor insemination appointments has significant therapeutic and economic advantages over daily urinary LH monitoring.

▶ This is an interesting comparison. Perhaps the results using the BBT method indicate this clinic's experience and ability to advise their patients—for example, their criteria for cancelling insemination appointments based on temperature readings. Perhaps judgment as to the timing of the LH surge was associated with less satisfactory results.—C.A. Paulsen, M.D.

Motile Sperm Recovery From Fresh and Frozen-Thawed Ejaculates Using a Swim-Up Procedure

Graczykowski JW, Siegel MS (Univ of Southern California, Los Angeles)
Fertil Steril 55:841–843, 1991 8–20

Background and Methods.—Frozen-thawed semen has recently replaced freshly ejaculated semen in artificial insemination by donor (AID) programs. The recovery of motile sperm and the quality of sperm movement after centrifugation and swim-up were compared in freshly ejaculated and frozen-thawed specimens of fertile semen provided by 8 healthy donors of proved fertility. Each specimen was divided into 4 aliquots, 2 of which were processed immediately. The other 2 were frozen first, then thawed and processed.

Results.—The recovery of motile sperm in swim-ups from fresh semen washed and centrifuged once was 33%. For semen washed and centrifuged twice, the recovery rate was 22%. For frozen-thawed semen, the recovery rates were only 7% and 5%, respectively. Straight-line velocity of sperm was increased after sperm swim-up. Changes in the lateral sperm head movement were not as evident.

Conclusions.—A significant loss of motile sperm occurred in the swim-up from freshly ejaculated semen specimens. In AID programs in which frozen-thawed semen is used, several factors reduce the number of motile sperm available for insemination. They include the number of semen vials used for insemination, dilution of semen with equal volumes of freezing medium, loss of motile sperm from freezing and thawing, and poor recovery of post-thaw motile sperm in swim-ups.

▶ Same story. The technique of freezing and thawing impairs human sperm. The National Institute of Child Health and Development is sponsoring a multicenter effort to improve present methods of cryopreserving sperm. We shall watch for results.—C.A. Paulsen, M.D.

Psychological Factors Related to Donor Insemination
Klock SC, Maier D (Univ of Connecticut, Farmington)
Fertil Steril 56:489–495, 1991 8–21

Background and Methods.—Therapeutic donor insemination (TDI) is commonly used to treat male factor infertility. There have been many studies regarding the medical aspects of TDI, but little is known about its psychological effects. To investigate these ramifications of TDI, survey questionnaires were mailed to 70 married couples who conceived as a result of TDI. Thirty-five couples returned completed questionnaires.

Results.—Fifty-six percent of couples waited 6 months or less after the diagnosis of male factor infertility before initiating TDI, but 20% waited for more than 2 years. Most respondents were indifferent to the gender of the inseminator, but of the 31% who had a preference, all preferred a female inseminator. Sixty percent of respondents told someone about the TDI, but in retrospect, 87% reported that they would tell no one. When asked if they planned to tell the child, 86.5% said they did not, most frequently citing unnecessary complications in the child's life as the reason. For the overall sample, marriage adjustment was rated average. Both men and women indicated that their biggest concern was the genetic and medical history of the donor. Although 88% of the patients had no psychological counseling after TDI, 39% believed that it should be mandatory.

Conclusions.—Most patients initiated TDI relatively soon after receiving the diagnosis of male factor infertility. In retrospect, most couples regretted having told others about the TDI, and most did not plan to tell the child. The major concern for couples was the genetic and medical history of the donor. Psychological counseling should be available to couples undertaking TDI.

▶ Fortunately, there is increasing interest in critical evaluation of the psychological aspects involved in donor insemination. This study and that reviewed in Abstract 8–22 provide important information in this area.—C.A. Paulsen, M.D.

Sperm Donors: Their Attitudes Toward Providing Medical and Pyschosocial Information for Recipient Couples and Donor Offspring
Mahlstedt PP, Probasco KA (Baylor College of Medicine, Houston)
Fertil Steril 56:747–753, 1991 8–22

Introduction.—Physicians in the United States long have recommended donor insemination as a means of achieving pregnancy when a husband is infertile or there is concern over transmitting genetic disease. Sperm donors have allowed thousands of such couples to achieve parenthood, but they remain without any personal, social, or medical identity to these couples.

Objective.—Seventy-nine sperm donors in 2 donor programs, 36 of whom were new donors, were asked about their willingness to provide medical and psychosocial information when applying and to share the information with recipient families.

Findings.—All but 10% of the donors were willing to complete a lengthy form providing medical and psychosocial information, and 96% were willing to share this information with recipient families as long as they were not identified. Sixty percent of the donors were willing to meet the child at age 18 years or to provide identifying information at that time. More than two thirds of the donors left personal messages for their potential offspring.

Recommendations.—Detailed medical and psychosocial information should be acquired from sperm donors and given to recipients as a means of personalizing this very important process. In addition, knowledge of family history can help to anticipate and prevent potential intergenerational health problems.

▶ Perhaps these authors' suggestions will improve the total picture in therapeutic donor insemination, but care must be exercised in this area. More data are needed with respect to the psychological profiles of the infertile husband, the recipient wife, and the donor. What type of information is important to each participant? This whole process of donor insemination has been in the investigational closet long enough.—C.A. Paulsen, M.D.

9 Ovulation Induction

Luteal Insufficiency: Correlation Between Endometrial Dating and Integrated Progesterone Output in Clomiphene Citrate-Induced Cycles

Hecht BR, Bardawil WA, Khan-Dawood FS, Dawood MY (Northwestern Univ, Chicago; Univ of Texas, Houston; Univ of Illinois, Chicago)

Am J Obstet Gynecol 163:1986–1991, 1990 9–1

Introduction.—When clomiphene citrate is given to induce or augment ovulation, a luteal phase defect and failure to conceive may occur in some cycles. The histologic diagnosis of luteal phase defect may be imprecise because the true postovulatory luteal age is unknown. In a controlled study in normal ovulatory women, luteal histologic findings were compared with the midcycle luteinizing hormone (LH) surge and integrated progesterone output. Also the effects of clomiphene citrate on luteal phase endometrial development were assessed.

Methods.—Ten normal, fertile women with regular ovulatory menstrual cycles were studied. The first cycle was untreated and served as a control. Clomiphene was given at a dose of 50 mg/day from day 5 to day 9 of the second cycle and at a dose of 150 mg/day from day 5 to day 9 of the third cycle. Eight to 12 days after the LH surge was observed, endometrial biopsy specimens were taken.

Findings.—All 3 cycles were ovulatory. Control and low-dose clomiphene citrate cycles showed endometrial maturation within 48 hours of the expected date. One high-dose clomiphene citrate cycle produced endometrium out of phase by 4 days. The mean integrated progesterone level was 6.6 ng/mL in control cycles, 117.5 ng/mL in low-dose clomiphene citrate cycles, and 152.1 ng/mL in high-dose clomiphene citrate cycles. The high-dose cycle with out-of-phase endometrium showed an integrated progesterone level of only 28 ng/mL.

Conclusions.—The incidence of luteal phase defects or inadequacy resulting from clomiphene citrate induction of ovulation appears to be low in ovulatory women—5% in the present study. When it occurs, it probably indicates inadequate progesterone production during the luteal phase.

▶ There is a common misconception that clomiphene citrate produces luteal insufficiency and may therefore cause infertility. As Hammond (1) has shown, the monthly fecundability rate in anovulatory women successfully treated with clomiphene citrate is .22, similar to the .20 rate in normal fertile couples. Thus the discrepancy between ovulation rates and pregnancy rates in anovulatory women treated with clomiphene citrate is not because the drug leads to infertility by causing thick cervical mucus or luteal insufficiency, but because the woman has not been treated for a sufficient number of ovulatory cycles. With a monthly fecundability of 0.20, only half of normal fertile couples conceive within 3 months and only 75% in 6 cycles. The rate is no different when ovulation is induced with clomiphene citrate. There is no evidence that clomiphene citrate produces luteal insufficiency. As a matter of fact, clomiphene citrate increases serum progesterone levels, as shown in this study, by causing more than 1 follicle to become luteinized.—D.R. Mishell, Jr., M.D.

Reference

1. Hammond CB, Halme JK, Talbert LM: *Obstet Gynecol* 62:196–202, 1983.

Endocrinology of Gonadotropin-Releasing Hormone Induced Cycles in Hypothalamic Amenorrhea: The Role of the Pulse Dose

Braat DDM, Schoemaker J (Academic Hosp Vrije Universiteit, Amsterdam)
Fertil Steril 56:1054–1059, 1991 9–2

Background.—Pulsatile gonadotropin-releasing hormone (GnRH) has been administered in pulse intervals ranging from 60 minutes to 120 minutes with equally good results in restoring ovulation in patients with hypothalamic amenorrhea. There is a higher multiple pregnancy rate in GnRH-induced pregnancies, however, if higher pulses are used. The treatment regimen that gives the maximum chance of ovulation with a minimal risk of multiple follicular development was determined.

Methods.—Fifteen women with amenorrhea of suprapituitary origin received randomly assigned pulse doses of GnRH at 5, 10, and 20 μg. Patients were treated intravenously for 1–3 cycles, with different pulse doses, at pulse intervals of 120 minutes. The endocrine parameters of the induced cycles were compared with those of spontaneous menstrual cycles in 14 women. The number of ovulations per pulse dose, luteinizing hormone (LH), follicle-stimulating hormone (FSH), total urinary estrogens (Es), and pregnanediol excretion were measured per cycle day and per stimulation day.

Results.—The endocrine values of cycles induced with intravenous GnRH were normal at 5-, 10-, or 20-μg pulse doses. There was a significantly higher percentage of anovulation in the 5-μg dose group. A low LH level in the first 10 days of an anovulatory cycle suggests that anovulation might have been prevented by a higher pulse dose. Significantly higher estrogen levels were found during the luteal phase of treated cycles compared with normal cycles; pregnanediol excretion did not change.

Conclusions.—Ovulatory cycles were within the normal range with the production of large follicles at pulse doses of 5-, 10-, and 20-μg. A pulse dose of 5 μg is recommended for the first treatment cycle because the first cycle has a higher ovulation rate. If no conception occurs, the dose should be raised to 10 μg per pulse. After ovulation the pulse interval should be changed to 240 minutes.

▶ The use of intravenous GnRH for induction of ovulation is becoming popular again, although this has been around for some time. This paper shows clearly that doses larger than 5 μg per pulse may be needed to induce ovulation, even in patients with hypothalamic amenorrhea. It was surprising that, in this study, body weight was taken into account. Several years ago, Crowley's group showed that the optimum dose of GnRH is 75 ng/kg for a single pulse. Whereas the physiologic amounts of GnRH within the portal system are no more than about 25 ng/kg, it requires larger doses such as the 75 ng/kg per pulse dose to effectively induce ovulation. A key clinical point is the misconception that, to induce ovulation in patients who do not respond, an increased pulse frequency is required. Here the authors used a pulse frequency of approximately every 120 minutes, and all that was necessary was an increase in the pulse amount keeping the pulse frequency constant. Another important point is that, if luteal support is not afforded by human chorionic gonadotropin, the pulse frequency should be decreased to the physiologic time of once every 240 minutes, as suggested here; otherwise, a perturbed estrogen/progestin status may ensue.—R.A. Lobo, M.D.

Adjusting the Dose to the Individual Response of the Patient During the Induction of Ovulation With Pulsatile Gonadotropin-Releasing Hormone

Mais V, Antinori D, Melis GB, de Ruggiero A, Strigini F, Fioretti P (Univ of Cagliari, Cagliari; Univ of Pisa, Pisa, Italy)

Fertil Steril 55:80–85, 1991 9–3

Introduction.—A systematic study to identify the effective dose of gonadotropin-releasing hormone (GnRH) necessary to induce ovulation in patients with chronic anovulation of various causes has not been conducted. The results of pulse GnRH studies in which the GnRH level was the only factor progressively adjusted were reviewed.

Methods.—Forty patients with chronic anovulation were divided into 4 treatment groups and underwent 90 treatment cycles for anovulation with GnRH. Nine patients had idiopathic hypogonadotropic hypogonadism (IHH), 13 had secondary hypoestrogenic amenorrhea, 6 had normoandrogenic oligomenorrhea, and 12 had polycystic ovarian syndrome (PCOS). The GnRH pulses were given intravenously for 90 minutes at about 5 μg per pulse. The dose was increased progressively by 2.5 μg per pulse if no follicular development occurred within 16–20 days. The effectiveness of GnRH was assessed by plasma estradiol radioimmunoassay and ultrasonography of the follicular growth.

Results.—The 9 patients with IHH underwent 16 GnRH treatment cycles, with the pulse dose of 5 μg sufficient in 11 cycles. During the treatment phase, 62.5% of patients with IHH who wanted to become pregnant did so. The 5 μg per pulse dose of GnRH was 100% effective in the 13 patients with functional hypothalamic amenorrhea and in the 6 patients with normoandrogenic oligomenorrhea, with 25% achieving pregnancy in the former group and 33% in the latter group. Administration of 5 μg per pulse induced ovulation only in 4 consecutive cycles in 2 of the 12 patients with PCOS; but with increasing dosage, two thirds of these patients ovulated. Nevertheless, conception occurred in only 12%

of those who wanted to become pregnant. The side effects of intravenous GnRH administration was minimal, and only 1 patient had mild hyperstimulation over 2 cycles.

Conclusion.—These findings allowed the adjustment of GnRH dosage so that 100% efficacy was achieved for patients with IHH, functional hypothalamic amenorrhea, and normoandrogenic oligomenorrhea. Dose adjustment of GnRH also improved results for patients with PCOS.

▶ The pulsatile administration of GnRH is infrequently used in the United States to treat anovulatory women who fail to ovulate with clomiphene citrate therapy and/or have low endogenous estrogen levels because of hypothalamic-pituitary insufficiency. This study confirms that pulsatile GnRH therapy is effective in inducing ovulation in thse women and can be offered as an alternative to treatment with hMG. A progressive increase in the dosage of GnRH resulted in an increased rate of presumptive ovulation in women with PCOS, but not in pregnancy, so these women may not have actually ovulated.—D.R. Mishell, Jr., M.D.

Life Table Analysis of Fecundity in Intravenously Gonadotropin-Releasing Hormone-Treated Patients With Normogonadotropic and Hypogonadotropic Amenorrhea

Braat DDM, Schoemaker R, Schoemaker J (Academic Hosp, Vrije Universiteit, Amsterdam)

Fertil Steril 55:266–271, 1991 9–4

Study Design.—The success of pulsatile gonadotropin-releasing hormone (GnRH) therapy administered intravenously to patients with normogonadotropic and hypogonadotropic amenorrhea was evaluated using life-table analysis. Forty-nine patients received GnRH for 272 cycles, with pulses given at either 60-, 90-, or 120-minute intervals. A total of 244 cycles in 48 patients were studied retrospectively.

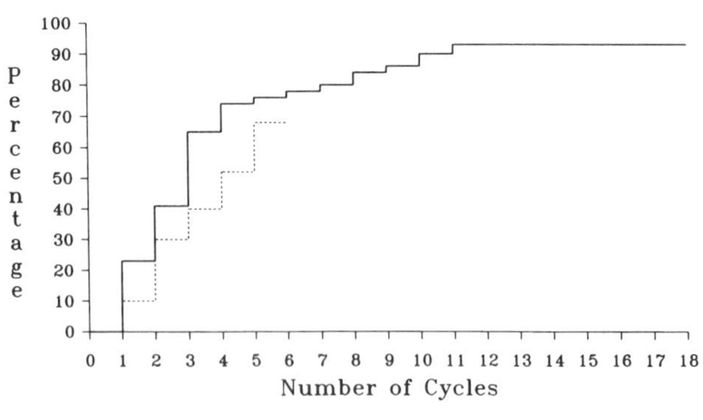

Fig 9–1.—Cumulative conception rates of all ovulatory cycles (n = 244) and of cycles 7 to 12 (n = 36). (Courtesy of Braat DDM, Schoemaker R, Schoemaker J: *Fertil Steril* 55:266–271, 1991.)

Findings.—One patient had only anovulatory cycles. The cumulative conception rate after 12 cycles was 93%, with a mean conception rate of 22.5% per cycle (Fig 9–1). Cumulative conception rates did not differ significantly between cycles 1 and 6 and cycles 7 and 8. The estrogenic status, weight history, actual weight, and whether amenorrhea was primary or secondary did not affect the outcome of GnRH therapy. The life-table curves of patients with and without additional infertility factors, however, were significantly different. In patients without additional infertility factors, the cumulative pregnancy rate was 84% after 6 cycles and 100% after 8 cycles, with a mean conception rate of 29.6% per cycle. In contrast, in patients with additional infertility factors, the cumulative pregnancy rate was 60% after 6 cycles and 100% after 11 cycles, with a mean conception rate of 15.8% per cycle.

Conclusion.—These data show that GnRH given intravenously is successful in patients with normogonadotropic and hypogonadotropic amenorrhea.

▶ As reported in this abstract, pulsatile GnRH therapy is extremely effective for the treatment of anovulation in amenorrheic women with low gonadotropin levels. These women usually do not ovulate after treatment with clomiphene. Despite the fact that pulsatile GnRH treatment requires less monitoring than treatment with human menopausal gonadotropin (hMG) and is associated with a lower rate of hyperstimulation and multiple pregnancies, GnRH is used much less frequently than hMG in the United States. Perhaps American women would rather be monitored more frequently than wear an intrauterine pump for several weeks. Nevertheless, they should be offered the option of GnRH therapy because it is just as effective as hMG—23% pregnancy rate per cycle—and is associated with fewer complications.—D.R. Mishell, Jr., M.D.

Ovarian Hyporesponsiveness in Combined Gonadotropin-Releasing Hormone Agonist and Menotropin Therapy Is Associated With Low Serum Follicle-Stimulating Hormone Levels

Ben-Rafael Z, Lipitz S, Bider D, Mashiach S (The Chaim Sheba Med Ctr; Sackler School of Medicine, Tel Hashomer, Israel)

Fertil Steril 55:272–275, 1991 9–5

Background.—The combination of gonadotropin-releasing hormone analogues (GnRH-a) before and during ovulation induction and human menopausal gonadotropin (hMG) is used to synchronize follicular development, minimize the premature luteinization, and increase the overall success rate. Findings have suggested that the analogue induces ovarian hyporesponsiveness. The serum level of follicle-stimulating hormone (FSH) during hMG stimulation in patients treated with GnRH-a and hMG and in a control group not treated with the analogue was evaluated to determine whether ovarian hyporesponsiveness is related to suboptimal serum levels of FSH.

Methods.—Thirty-four patients undergoing in vitro fertilization-embryo transfer were divided into 3 groups. Two groups of 12 patients each were suppressed with GnRH-a; stimulation was with a fixed dose of hMG. A control group of 10 patients received equal doses of hMG only.

Results.—The follicular phase and the number of hMG ampules required were significantly higher in the study group than in the controls. The patients treated with GnRH-a had significantly lower basal FSH levels and lower FSH levels during hMG treatment. The 2 study groups and the controls had similar peak levels of estradiol and similar outcomes after in vitro fertilization.

Conclusions.—The delay in ovarian response in patients treated with a combination of GnRH-a and hMG may be attributable to lack of an endogenous contribution of FSH, which results in low circulating levels of that hormone. Administering higher doses of hMG can increase serum levels of FSH and reverse the ovarian desensitization that is encountered after use of the analogue.

▶ It has been known for some time that use of the GnRH agonist before gonadotropin therapy increases the length of time of stimulation and also the number of ampules required. A raging debate has continued as to whether or not ovarian insensitivity to gonadotropins is induced by the analogue (a direct ovarian effect), or whether it is related to changes in the endogenous gonadotropin. Most of the data would suggest the latter, which this paper confirms. In humans, direct GnRH agonist ovarian effects have not been demonstrated, nor have specific receptors been found. Most of the data suggest that profound suppression of endogenous gonadotropins for some period of time before stimulation results in hyporesponsiveness to exogenous gonadotropins.

In this paper, measurements of serum FSH were carried out in 2 groups receiving Decapeptyl and in patients receiving hMG alone. The assays for immunoreactivity of FSH are difficult to assess and often do not accurately predict suppression with agonist. Bioassay of FSH on immunofluorometric assays is probably a better way to detect profound suppression of FSH. The findings here, although significant, would seemingly be enhanced further with this type of approach.

Nevertheless, the data are clear in that the predominant reason for the large gonadotropin requirement is that endogenous FSH is decreased, and it takes a longer time for FSH in larger doses to overcome this barrier for follicular recruitment. This adds weight to the rationale for protocols that start stimulation with a high dose of FSH or hMG and continue until follicular recruitment begins.—R.A. Lobo, M.D.

Results of Ovulation Induction Using Human Menopausal Gonadotropin or Purified Follicle-Stimulating Hormone in Hypogonadotropic Hypogonadism Patients

Shoham Z, Balen A, Patel A, Jacobs HS (Middlesex Hosp, London)

Fertil Steril 56:1048–1053, 1991 9–6

Background.—Follicle-stimulating hormone (FSH) stimulates gonadal differentiation and maturation via its regulatory action on the granulosa cell in the ovary. Luteinizing hormone (LH) also has a role in the follicular phase and in stimulation of the follicle, but the optimal amount of LH or the ratio of FSH:LH in gonadotropin therapy has not been determined. Ovarian performance and hormonal levels in patients with isolated hypogonadotropic hypogonadism were compared after ovulation induction using 2 different gonadotropin drugs.

Method.—Nine patients with isolated hypogonadotropic hypogonadism were treated during consecutive cycles with human menopausal gonadotropin (hMG) in the first treatment cycle and purified FSH in the second cycle. Human menopausal gonadotropin has an equal amount of FSH and LH, and the purified form of FSH used in the second cycle has <1.0 IU of LH per ampule. Measurements included duration of stimulation, number of leading follicles, serum estradiol (E_2) concentration, and endometrial thickness at the time of human chorionic gonadotropin (hCG) administration, as well as the occurrence of ovulation.

Findings.—Significantly more ampules of purified FSH were used per cycle compared with hMG, but the serum level of E_2 was significantly higher after the hMG cycle. In the hMG cycle, the endometrium was significantly thicker, there were more follicles with a diameter >16 mm, and there was a higher incidence of ovulation.

Conclusions.—Patients treated with FSH had a significantly reduced serum E_2 concentration, less endometrial thickness, and a lower ovulation rate than patients treated with hMG. The use of FSH is not recommended for induction of ovulation in hypogonadotropic patients. The superior efficacy of hMG, which had an equal amount of FSH and LH, supports the 2-cell, 2-gonadotropin hypothesis. Luteinizing hormone supports and augments the regulatory function of FSH during ovarian steroidogenesis.

▶ The controversy rages on as to whether or not there is a difference in the efficacy of hMG vs. FSH for induction of ovulation. Whereas most studies do not find a benefit of FSH over hMG or vice versa, this paper suggests that in this category of patients—those with hypothalamic amenorrhea and those who do not have adequate quantities of endogenous gonadotropins—the use of hMG with LH and FSH is preferable to the use of FSH alone. This is somewhat at odds with data in the monkey. Hodgen used an antagonist to block endogenous gonadotropins in the macaque and showed that FSH was very efficient in recruiting follicles. Nevertheless, this was not compared directly with the use of hMG.

The other issue that comes to mind is that with urinary gonadotropins there are batch to batch differences, and it could be that the bio FSH used in the urinary FSH preparation was less active than that of hMG. Even so, these data imply that a small quantity of LH is extremely important in recruiting follicles, which, as suggested by the authors, is presumably because of the 2-cell theory in which androgen production by the theca is important for granulosa estrogen production.—R.A. Lobo, M.D.

A Comparative, Randomized Study of Low-Dose Human Menopausal Gonadotropin and Follicle-Stimulating Hormone in Women With Polycystic Ovarian Syndrome

Sagle MA, Hamilton-Fairley D, Kiddy DS, Franks S (St Mary's Hosp Med School, London)

Fertil Steril 55:56–60, 1991 9–7

Background and Methods.—In the treatment of clomiphene-citrate-resistant anovulation in women with polycystic ovary syndrome (PCOS), low-dose follicle-stimulating hormone (FSH) results in a high rate of ovulation and pregnancy, but it is not clear whether the success of the treatment is because of the use of pure FSH or low doses of gonadotropin. In a randomized controlled study, 30 women with anovulatory infertility associated with PCOS were treated with either FSH or human menopausal gonadotropin (hMG) given in low doses for a maximum of 3 cycles. Of the 30 patients, 25 had oligomenorrhea, and 20 had hirsutism and/or acne.

Results.—Ovulation occurred in 75% of women and in 77% of cycles induced with FSH; the mean total dose of FSH was 19.3 ampules per cycle. Ovulation occurred in 94% of women and in 85% of cycles treated with hMG; the mean total dose of hMG was 14.4 ampules per cycle. Overall, 70% of FSH- and 65% of hMG-induced cycles were single follicle ovulations. Five pregnancies occurred in each treatment group, but 4 pregnancies ended in early spontaneous miscarriage in 3 of the FSH-treated and 1 of the hMG-treated patients. All other pregnancies resulted in single live births. The overall pregnancy rate was 30% in both groups, and the cumulative conception rate was 36.5% at 3 months.

Conclusion.—Low doses of FSH and hMG are equally successful in inducing ovulation, suggesting that the success of treatment depends on the low dose of gonadotropin used rather than the presence or absence of luteinizing hormone in the preparation.

▶ The results of this randomized study of prolonged treatment with low doses of gonadotropins, either FSH or hMG, replicate the findings of randomized trials with standard dose regimens of these 2 agents. There is no advantage in treating anovulatory women with PCOS who do not respond to clomiphene with pure FSH instead of hMG.—D.R. Mishell, Jr., M.D.

Ovulation Induction by Step-Down Administration of Purified Urinary Follicle-Stimulating Hormone in Patients With Polycystic Ovarian Syndrome

Mizunuma H, Andoh K, Takagi T, Ibuki Y, Yamada K, Igarashi M (Gunma Univ, Maebashi, Gunma, Japan)

Fertil Steril 55:1195–1196, 1991 9–8

Background.—Purified urinary follicle-stimulating hormone (FSH) would appear to be an ideal treatment for anovulatory women with elevated levels of endogenous luteinizing hormone (LH). Clinical attempts have been made using fixed doses, but results have not always been promising. Step-down administration might be effective because it mimics the physiologic secretion of endogenous FSH release.

Methods.—All 23 infertile women with polycystic ovarian syndrome were amenorrheic and had an LH/FSH ratio greater than 2; LH levels were more than 25 mIU/mL. All patients received a daily intramuscular injection of urinary FSH. Fourteen received a fixed dose, starting with a daily dose of 150 IU for 7 days; this could be increased as high as 225 IU. In 3 cycles the starting dose of 75 IU was used; 1 was treated with a starting dosc of 225 IU. Nine patients were treated by the step-down regimen, consisting of 225 IU/day for the first 2 days and 75 IU/day thereafter, with the daily dose increased to 150 IU after 7 days if follicular diameter did not increase. In 2 cycles, 75 IU or 150 IU were given on the second day.

Results.—The urinary FSH dose had to be increased in 3 of 17 cycles in the step-down group. Women in the step-down group required 11.8 75-IU ampules of urinary FSH, significantly less than the 16.5 ampules required by the fixed-dose group. The step-down group also had fewer intermediate-sized follicles and less excessive ovarian enlargement. The pregnancy rate per cycle was 17.6% in the step-down group and 7.7% in the fixed-dose group, although this difference did not reach significance. Excessive ovarian enlargement occurred in 23 cycles, but it did not require medication.

Conclusions.—In women with polycystic ovarian syndrome, the step-down administration of urinary FSH can be a useful way of inducing ovulation. Compared to the fixed-dose method, it requires less FSH and results in a lower incidence of excessive ovarian enlargement.

Polycystic Ovarian Syndrome: Safety and Effectiveness of Stepwise and Low-Dose Administration of Purified Follicle-Stimulating Hormone

Shoham Z, Patel A, Jacobs HS (Middlesex Hosp, London)

Fertil Steril 55:1051–1056, 1991 9–9

Background.—Ovulation induction in patients with polycystic ovarian syndrome (PCOS) remains difficult. No single method has emerged as the treatment of choice. An attempt was made to induce ovulation with 1 dominant follicle in patients with PCOS.

Methods.—Of the 8 patients studied, 6 had not responded adequately to the conventional protocol. Ultrasound appearances and estradiol (E_2) measurements during treatment with a low-dose protocol using purified follicle-stimulating hormone, starting at 75 IU/day and escalating by 37.5 IU/day every 7 days, were compared with those obtained after conventional treatment with the same drug. Rate of cancellation of cycles, number of leading follicles, and serum E_2 levels at ovulation were the main outcome measures.

Results.—Treatment with the low-dose protocol significantly reduced the number of leading follicles. Serum E_2 levels also were significantly decreased with low-dose treatment. The patients in the low-dose group had a higher rate of ovulation; 5 of these women became pregnant, all with singletons. One woman miscarried at 22 weeks of gestation because of premature contractions and cervical incompetence; the remaining 4 delivered healthy infants.

Conclusions.—This low-dose protocol permitted safe, successful ovulation induction in selected patients with PCOS. These patients had been difficult to treat with the conventional ovulation induction protocol. A double-blind controlled study is currently underway to verify these findings.

▶ There is no ideal way to induce ovulation in patients with PCOS who are clomiphene resistant. There tend to be very individual responses. Some women do well with conventional gonadotropin therapy and others have aberrant responses. The studies reviewed in Abstracts 9–8 and 9–9 were not randomized trials, and both groups of authors suggest that this is clearly necessary. Primary because of the heterogeneity of the patient population and the different types of responses encountered, there is no way that a blanket endorsement of either one of these regimens can be made.

Presented here are 2 different approaches to the induction of ovulation in the "difficult-to-manage patient" with polycystic ovaries. Others have tried down-regulation first with a gonadotropin-releasing hormone (GnRH) agonist followed either by human menopausal gonadotropin (hMG) or pure follicle-stimulating hormone (FSH), and this has clearly been shown not to be of any greater advantage. Indeed, there is often a higher risk of hyperstimulation when this is tried. Ovarian cautery has become more popular in resistant patients. Also, the pulsatile administration of GnRH, either alone or in conjunction with the GnRH agonist, is be efficacious. In terms of using hMG or pure FSH, most data suggest that one is not superior to the other, as suggested by one of the groups here.

Nevertheless, although both reports focused on FSH, divergent approaches were taken. The paper from Japan (Abstract 9–8) suggests that what is necessary is FSH, starting with a high bolus of 3 ampules a day and then tapering the dose. It was noted in this paper, however, that some patients required changes in the regimen; this was not really a fixed protocol, and variations in dose requirements occurred. The data are encouraging, however, as the authors point out that the physiologic bolus effect of FSH early in the cycle, which is often the strategy used for controlled hyperstimulation in in vitro fertilization cycles, might be the preferred technique.

In the paper from Jacobs' group (Abstract 9–9), the authors showed that using a low fixed-dose regimen with increments of only half an ampule after 7 days was beneficial. They compared this regimen in only 6 patients who had previously failed to respond to conventional therapy and in 2 others, a total of 8. Of interest, the regimen of conventional therapy was not very different: an increase of 1 ampule after 7 days as opposed to half an ampule. The slower protocol was not very different from the method Jacobs et al. advocate. Indeed, somewhat of a surprise was that the length of treatment, means of 12 days and 13 days, was not different between the 2 groups. Use of this regimen decreased the rate of complications. The authors point out that this approach requires a randomized trial for confirmation, and one is now being run. We anxiously await the results of these studies.

The purpose of this comment is to suggest that because there is heterogeneity in responses, it is unlikely that one single definitive regimen will be found to suit all patients with polycystic ovaries, and it is important for the reader to know that there are 2 different gonadotropin stimulation regimens advocated. Perhaps these could be tried alternatively in patients who prove to be difficult to manage.—R.A. Lobo, M.D.

Low-Dose Gonadotrophin Therapy for Induction of Ovulation in 100 Women With Polycystic Ovary Syndrome

Hamilton-Fairley D, Kiddy D, Watson H, Sagle M, Franks S (St Mary's Hosp Med School, London)

Hum Reprod 6:1095–1099, 1991 9–10

Background.—In women with anovulation caused by polycystic ovary syndrome (PCOS), multiple follicles are likely to develop during treatment with gonadotropin. Their risk of multiple pregnancy is therefore high. A low-dose regimen was assessed in such patients.

Methods.—One hundred women with clomiphene-resistant PCOS were treated. A low dose of gonadotropin was injected intramuscularly every day. Eighty-three received human menopausal gonadotropin and 17 received follicle-stimulating hormone. Initial doses were maintained for up to 14 days in the first cycle and for up to 7 days in later cycles. The dose was increased from 1 to 1.5 ampules per day if no response was seen on ultrasound. This dose was then maintained for another 7 days before it was raised by .5 ampules a day. This stepwise increase was continued to a maximum of 3 ampules daily; if no ovarian response occurred at this dose, the patient was considered unresponsive and treatment was stopped. Once ovarian activity was seen ultrasonically, the same dose was continued until complete follicular maturation. Human chorionic gonadotropin, 5000 IU, was administered to induce ovulation.

Results.—Ninety-five women ovulated at least once. Of the 401 cycles induced, 72% were ovulatory and 73% of these were uniovulatory. The overall 6-month cumulative conception rate was 55%. Only 2 multiple pregnancies occurred. The rate of early pregnancy loss was 32%. The prevalence of complications was low. There were no cases of severe hyperstimulation, and less than 5% of cycles were abandoned because multiple follicles developed. An increased baseline or midfollicular level of luteinizing hormone, or both, was associated with a poor response to treatment, anovulation, ovulation without conception, or early pregnancy loss. None of the women whose levels of luteinizing hormone were persistently raised during ovulatory cycles had good pregnancy outcomes.

Conclusions.—Low-dose gonadotropin treatment is a safe, effective way to induce ovulation. It is associated with a high incidence of single follicular development and a low multiple pregnancy rate.

▶ Overall pregnancy rates after attempts at ovulation induction with human menopausal gonadotropin (hMG) in women with polycystic ovaries who fail to ovulate with clomiphene citrate therapy are not very high. The results of this regimen of a low dose of hMG administered for a prolonged period of time to such women are encouraging, with ovulation occurring in 95 of 100 women so treated and a 55% cumulative pregnancy rate after 6 cycles of therapy. Although some centers have reported that the use of gonadotropin-releasing hormone agonists enhances the success of hMG in these women, others have not been able to confirm these findings (see Abstract 9–12). Thus the regimen reported here should be tried by other investigators to determine whether these good results can be confirmed.—D.R. Mishell, Jr., M.D.

Transvaginal Ultrasound-Guided Follicular Aspiration in the Management of Anovulatory Infertility Associated With Polycystic Ovaries
Mio Y, Terado H, Toda T, Harada T, Tanikawa M, Terakawa N (Tottori Univ, Yonago, Japan)
Fertil Steril 56:1060–1065, 1991 9–11

Background.—Polycystic ovarian disease (PCOD) is associated with anovulation and hormonal abnormalities. Polycystic ovaries (PCO) without hormonal abnormalities have also been reported in patients with menstrual irregularity and inability to conceive. Whether transvaginal ultrasound-guided follicular aspiration can effectively induce ovulation and facilitate pregnancy in anovulatory women with PCO was investigated.

Methods.—Eight patients with PCOD and 10 with PCO who failed to ovulate with medical therapies were studied. Most persistent follicles were punctured and their contents aspirated thoroughly during the midluteal phase. The ovarian stimulation regimen used in previous cycles were used in the cycles after aspiration. Evidence of ovulation and subsequent pregnancy was monitored ultrasonically after aspiration. The responsiveness of pituitary gonadotropins to gonadotropin-releasing hormone was assessed.

Results.—Patients with PCOD had ovulation rates of 87.5% per person and 52.6% per cycle. Patients with PCO had rates of 100% per person and 63.3% per cycle. Half of the patients with PCOD and PCO became pregnant after the aspiration. There was a significant drop in basal and peak serum levels of luteinizing hormone after aspiration.

Conclusions.—Transvaginal ultrasonically guided follicular aspiration is a much less invasive and simpler technique for oocyte pick-up in an in vitro fertilization-embryo transfer program. This method seems preferable for treating anovulatory patients with PCOD or PCO without hormonal abnormalities. It is also helpful for clarifying the pathophysiology of anovulation such as PCOD and luteinized unruptured follicles.

▶ As mentioned in the discussion of Abstract 9–10, attempts to induce ovulation with human menopausal gonadotropin in women with PCOS who fail to ovulate with clomiphene citrate are not highly successful. In efforts to replicate the success achieved decades ago with the surgical procedures of ovarian wedge resection, various investigators have destroyed portions of ovarian tissue by electrocautery or laser vaporization under laparoscopic visualization. Good success has been reported with these procedures, but they require general anesthesia and use of an operating room facility. The minor operative procedure described in this study did not require general anesthesia or use of an operating room, and the patients were ambulatory and discharged within 30 minutes after the procedure was completed. Further studies of this innovative technique should be undertaken.—D.R. Mishell, Jr., M.D.

Combined Growth Hormone and Gonadotropin Treatment for Ovulation Induction in Patients With Non-Responsive Ovaries

Homburg R, West C, Ostergaard H, Jacobs HS (Middlesex Hosp, London; Novo-Nordisk A/S, Gentofte, Denmark)

Gynecol Endocrinol 5:33–36, 1991 9–12

Introduction.—The ovarian response to stimulation by human menopausal gonadotropin (hMG) can be markedly enhanced by coadministering growth hormone (GH). This approach was tried in 4 women who exhibited no ovarian response to hMG alone.

Results.—A woman aged 28 with idiopathic hypogonadotropic hypogonadism and undetectable serum gonadotropin had failed to respond to pulsatile luteinizing hormone-releasing hormone or to hMG alone. When GH was given with the same daily dose of hMG, the serum estradiol level rose markedly within a week and ovulation occurred after administration of human chorionic gonadotropin. A woman aged 30 with autoimmune Addison's disease had a similar response to combined treatment with hMG and GH after failing to respond to hMG alone. The other 2 patients failed to respond to combined hormonal treatment.

Conclusions.—The combined administration of hMG and GH initiates an ovarian response in some women who fail to respond to hMG alone. Those with clear evidence of primary ovarian failure, however, cannot be expected to respond to this treatment.

▶ Other investigators have reported in nonrandomized studies that treatment with gonadotropin-releasing hormone (GnRH) analogs, combined with hMG, successfully induces ovulation in women with polycystic ovarian syndrome (PCOS) who do not ovulate after treatment with hMG alone. This randomized study of women with PCOS who failed to ovulate with clomiphene indicates that it is not beneficial to treat them all with a combination of a GnRH analog and hMG as this expensive regimen may be unnecessary. This combination therapy should be reserved for those women who fail to ovulate with hMG alone because it requires greater amounts of hMG and a longer duration of therapy.—D.R. Mishell, Jr., M.D.

Follicular Size at the Time of Human Chorionic Gonadotropin Administration Predicts Ovulation Outcome in Human Menopausal Gonadotropin-Stimulated Cycles

Silverberg KM, Johnson JV, Olive DL, Groff TR, Burns WN, Schenken RS (Univ of Texas, San Antonio)

Fertil Steril 56:296–300, 1991 9–13

Background.—Certain data from in vitro fertilization-embryo transfer programs correlate follicle size with oocyte maturity. An attempt was made to correlate follicle size with ovulation outcomes in cycles of controlled ovarian hyperstimulation with human menopausal gonadotropins, to learn whether follicular size on the day of human chorionic gonadotropin (hCG) treatment predicts ovulation incidence, and, if so, to develop a mathematical model to predict the number of expected ovulations in any given cycle of controlled ovarian hyperstimulation.

Methods and Results.—Data were analyzed retrospectively on 49 consecutive patients undergoing 122 cycles of controlled ovarian hyperstimulation in a tertiary care setting. Sonography was used to determine follicular size and evidence of ovulation. The rate of ovulation per follicle size was the main outcome measure. The percentages of patients who subsequently ovulated on the day of hCG administration were .5% of those with follicles measuring 14 mm or less, 37.4% of those with follicles of 15–16 mm, 72.5% of those with follicles of 17–18 mm, 81.2% of those with follicles of 19–20 mm, and 95.5% of those with follicles greater than 20 mm. Thus follicular size on the day of hCG administration did correlate with ovulation incidence. Using the equation developed, the expected number of ovulations in any given controlled ovarian hyperstimulation cycle may be predicted with 95% confidence.

Conclusions.—Ovulation rates depend on follicle size at the time of hCG administration. Serum estradiol (E_2) levels can be predicted on the basis of follicle size and number. The ovulation prediction equation developed in this study provides the first objective criterion correlating ovulation with follicle size on the day of hCG administration in cycles stimulated by human menopausal gonadotropin. The regression equation to predict E_2 values may be useful clinically by obviating the need for expensive daily serum E_2 determinations.

▶ This interesting report correlates follicle size with ovulation efficiency. Conventional wisdom has suggested that in Pergonal cycles, follicles mature at around 15 or 16 mm, and traditionally that is believed to be the size at which triggering of ovulation with hCG occurs. This retrospective study offers us some more refined measurements for clinical use. The authors suggest that ovulation efficiency is closely correlated with follicle size, and 95% of those whose follicles were greater than 20 mm ovulated, whereas with follicles 15–16 mm in size the ovulation rate was only 37%.

The authors provide 2 equations that they believe are useful for determining the number of ovulations as well as what the E_2 levels would be. For the expected number of ovulations, the equations they provide is 0.96 (A) + 0.81 (B)

+ 0.73 (C) + 0.37 (D) + .005 (E) in which A, B, C, D, and E refer to mean follicular diameters of more than 20 mm, 19–20 mm, 17–18 mm, 15–16 mm, and 14 mm or less, respectively. This gives a rough idea of the number of ovulations with multiple follicles that one would expect.

Of interest in this study, the number of ovulations did not correlate with fecundity. Extrapolating from these data, one would suggest that increasing the number of follicles in any given cycle does not necessarily increase fecundity. This concept goes against our superovulation strategies for unexplained infertility and other surgical situations in infertility. The authors admit, however, that their statistical power for truly evaluating this is not great and that more data are needed to confirm or refute these findings. Nevertheless, another point the authors make is that for clinical induction of ovulation, the E_2 level often can be predicted and although they provide a formula, it may not be necessary.

The bottom line message for me in this report is that often a follicle is not mature, even when Pergonal is administered, until it is close to 20 mm or even larger in size. Although a considerable variation exists among patients, the clinician should be alert to the possibility the follicles may not be mature at a lower follicle size, particularly when there are only 1 or 2 present.—R.A. Lobo, M.D.

Is It Possible to Run a Successful Ovulation Induction Program Based Solely on Ultrasound Monitoring? The Importance of Endometrial Measurements

Shoham Z, Conway GS, Di Carlo C, Jacobs HS, Patel A (Middlesex Hosp, London)

Fertil Steril 56:836–841, 1991 9–14

Background.—Ovarian ultrasonography is a standard way to monitor ovulation induction. The results of an ovulation induction program monitored solely by ultrasound were studied prospectively. The ease and accuracy of uterine measurements compared with serum estradiol (E_2) measurements also was assessed.

Methods.—Twenty patients with hypogonadotropism and 29 patients with polycystic ovaries that were ultrasonically diagnosed were enrolled. Serial ultrasound measures were used to monitor ovulation induction with human menopausal gonadotropin and human chorionic gonadotropin (hCG) or E_2 levels at the end of each cycle. The main outcome measures were follicular growth, uterine measures, endometrial thickness, and serum E_2 levels.

Results.—Estradiol levels were highly correlated with follicular growth, uterine measures, and endometrial thickness. Endometrium on the day of hCG administration was significantly thicker in the conception than in the nonconception cycles. There were no significant differences in serum E_2 levels. No pregnancy occurred when hCG was administered if the endometrial thickness was 7 mm or less. Midluteal endometrial thickness of 11 mm or greater was a good prognostic indicator for detecting early pregnancy.

Conclusions.—Ultrasound used alone for the monitoring of ovulation induction is safe, accurate, and cost effective. Ultrasound examinations can also be used in the midluteal phase to help to predict pregnancy.

▶ Monitoring for induction of ovulation has gone through quite a revolution with time. Fifteen years ago, estrogen monitoring by urinary or serum determinations was the sole mechanism for determining follicular development and triggering ovulation. Since that time, with the advent of ultrasound, we now rely far more heavily on that technique and use estrogen determinations as fine tuning or as a check on the system.

The use of ultrasound has not only revolutionized the concepts of induction of ovulation, but it has, in my view, greater success. Shoham et al. purport that ultrasound alone is all that is necessary to determine induction of ovulation. Whereas I would agree in general, I think the purists among us would still like to have a few, albeit not daily, estradiol determinations to assure maturation of the follicles. This is particularly true when selection of a follicle is difficult to determine; it is perhaps more important in monitoring in vitro fertilization, in which the number of mature follicles are best determined by estradiol levels and high estrogen levels are to be avoided because of concerns about the endometrium.

In this study, ultrasound criteria were used to assess follicular maturation with the triggering of ovulation at approximate 16 mm of follicular diameter. In recent years, based on knowledge of estradiol levels, we have tended to push follicle size beyond this point with the expectation of a greater pregnancy rate. A concept that is expanded in this paper and that recently has received much attention is endometrial thickness and its correlation with estrogen status. In general terms, endometrium of a certain thickness has been associated with a good outcome; as shown in this paper, endometrial thickness of less than 7 mm at the time of hCG administration suggested a poor prognosis. These more subtle findings with vaginal ultrasound provide some means of fine tuning the art of induction of ovulation.—R.A. Lobo, M.D.

Increased Circulating Levels of Bromocriptine After Vaginal Compared With Oral Administration

Katz E, Schran HF, Weiss BE, Adashi EY, Hassell A (Univ of Maryland, Baltimore; Sandoz Research Inst, East Hanover, NJ)

Fertil Steril 55:882–884, 1991 9–15

Background.—Bromocriptine mesylate is the treatment of choice for prolactin (PRL)-producing pituitary tumors. Intravaginal administration has been used successfully to overcome the side effects of nausea and vomiting. The circulating levels of bromocriptine after oral and vaginal administration were compared.

Methods.—Seven ovulatory women were randomly allocated to receive 2.5 mg of bromocriptine either orally or vaginally. In a second session the subjects received the drug by the alternate route. One patient with hyperprolactinemia received bromocriptine only, vaginally. Serum

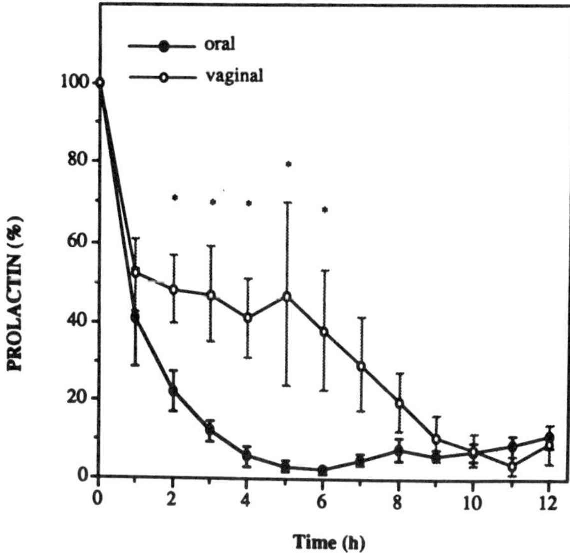

Fig 9–2.—Circulating levels of PRL (±SEM) expressed as percent from baseline after oral (n = 7) and vaginal (n = 8) administration of bromocriptine mesylate (2.5 mg). (Courtesy of Katz E, Schran HF, Weiss BE: *Fertil Steril* 55:882–884, 1991.)

levels of bromocriptine and prolactin were measured hourly for 12 hours in the normal volunteers and for 10 hours in the patient with hyperprolactinemia.

Results.—Serum PRL levels decreased dramatically in both groups, but the reduction was significantly greater between 2 hours and 6 hours in the group given the drug orally (Fig 9–2). Circulating levels of bromocriptine peaked at 1 hour in the orally treated group, but they were significantly higher after 7 hours in the group treated vaginally. Only 1 patient in each group complained of nausea and dizziness.

Conclusions.—Vaginal administration of bromocriptine resulted in significantly higher and longer-lasting levels of circulating bromocriptine compared with oral administration. Prolactin levels after oral administration were lower during the first 6 hours, but vaginal administration may allow an overall dose reduction without sacrificing therapeutic efficacy.

▶ This paper extends the work of Vermesh et al. (1) who showed that vaginal bromocriptine is efficacious, particularly in those patients with elevated levels of PRL who have nausea and vomiting associated with bromocriptine use. The interesting aspect of this report is the pharmacokinetics of oral vs. vaginal bromocriptine. Whereas oral administration results in a very early rise, with vaginal administration levels peak only after about 10 hours and are higher than with those achieved by the oral route by this time. Because of the early absorption of bromocriptine when given orally, PRL levels fall earlier and are much lower in the first 2–6 hours than when the vaginal route is used (see Fig 9–3). Perhaps this bolus effect with the oral route is the very reason why patients experience nausea. Although oral therapy is very effective, the levels on the graphs extend only to 12 hours and we do not know whether they start creeping up beyond that point in time; I suspect they do. Bromocriptine is usually given in twice-a-day dosage for patients who require larger doses. With vaginal administration, the PRL level is lowered as well as with oral after 8–10 hours; perhaps because of these pharmacokinetics the 24-hour profile will be valuable. In patients who are relatively intolerant to oral bromocriptine, the vaginal route is clearly worth a try.—R.A. Lobo, M.D.

Reference

1. Vermesh M, et al: *Obstet Gynecol* 72:693, 1988.

Clinical Use of Growth Hormone-Releasing Factor for Induction of Superovulation

Volpe A, Coukos G, Barreca A, Giordano G, Artini PG, Genazzani AR (Univ of Cagliari; Univ of Modena; Univ of Genoa, Italy)

Hum Reprod 6:1228–1232, 1991 9–16

Background and Methods.—The ovarian follicular cycle appears to be regulated not only by gonadotropins but also by growth factors such as the insulin-like growth factor I (IGF-I) and possibly growth hormone (GH). Positive results have been reported in the use of exogenous GH combined with gonadotropins in inducing ovulation or superovulation. In vitro fertilization/embryo transfer-gamete intrafallopian transfer (IVF/ET–GIFT), combined with GH-releasing factors (GRF) and gonadotropins, was attempted in 10 women with a previously normal response to gonadotropins. The effects of GRF supplementation on follicular fluid GH, IGF-I, epidermal growth factor (EGF), and steroids were studied.

Findings.—After administration of GRF combined with gonadotropins, the stimulatory cycle was shortened and there was a reduced number of gonadotropin ampules used per patient relative to a previous stimulatory cycle with gonadotropins alone. The number of follicles recruited was significantly higher in the GRF-supplemented cycle, but the number of oocytes retrieved per patient was similar with both treatments. There was a significant increase of both follicular fluid IGF-I levels and plasma GH levels immediately after administration of GRF and throughout the GRF cycle.

Conclusions.—Consistent with previous reports, GRF combined with gonadotropins induced faster follicular growth and a significant increase in follicular fluid IGF-I and progesterone levels compared to a cycle in which superovulation was induced by gonadotropins alone. Potentiation of the ovarian response to gonadotropins by GRF may be attributable to direct action of the peptide on the ovary or to activation of the GH-IGF-I axis.

▶ This is clearly a very important trend in induction of ovulation, and much has been written, and more will be written, on the use of GH and analogs to stimulate the GH/IGF axis in facilitating ovulation induction. It is important to note that, in this series, normal patients were compared. Although the approach used shortened the time required for induction of ovulation and more follicles resulted, a similar number of eggs were retrieved, perhaps because these were normal patients who did not necessarily have a deficiency or an abnormal requirement for GH. This is probably not the case for patients who have poor gonadotropin responses; these are the real targets for various strategies of GH treatment.

In this study the strategy was to use GH-releasing hormone (RH) to release endogenous growth hormone. The IGF-I levels in follicular fluid increased. A test dose of 1 mg/kg, used intravenously, showed a normal response in all of the patients. The standard dose used was 5 mg/kg subcutaneously daily during each of day of induction of ovulation with gonadotropin. Several regimens have been described, including alternate-day therapy and different doses, as well as intravenous and subcutaneous administration. More of these refinements will be forthcoming.

The authors suggest that the data may imply direct GH-RH action on the ovary. Although this is possible, I do not believe it to be the primary mechanism, because GH itself results in similar findings with co-gonadotropin therapy. Of some use to the reader, perhaps, other recent papers concerning this aspect of the treatment of infertility are listed below (1–3).—R.A. Lobo, M.D.

References

1. Burger HG, et al: *Clin Endocrinol* 35:119–122, 1991.
2. Blumenfeld Z: *J In Vitro Fertil Embryo Transf* 8:127–136, 1991.
3. Katz E, Adashi EY: *Contemp OB/Gyn* 37:12–28, 1991.

Interest of Growth Hormone-Releasing Administration for Improvement of Ovarian Responsiveness to Gonadotropins in Poor Responder Women

Hugues J-N, Martin-Pont B, Torresani T, Tamboise A, Herve F, Santarelli J (Hôpital Jean Verdier, Bondy, France; Univ of Zurich)

Fertil Steril 55:945–951, 1991 9–17

Background.—Growth hormone (GH) has been used to initiate ovarian activity, to improve folliculogenesis in humans, to correct the delay in puberty usually observed in GH-deficient children, and to improve the ovarian response to human menopausal gonadotropin (hMG) in chronic anovulating women. Whether growth hormone-releasing hormone (GH-RH) administration would improve the ovarian response to gonadotropins of women undergoing an in vitro fertilization (IVF) protocol was investigated.

Methods.—Twelve women who had responded poorly to previous stimulation with gonadotropin-releasing hormone analogue (GnRH-a) and human menopausal gonadotropins (hMG) were selected. In an IVF protocol, 500 μg of GH-RH$^{1\text{-}29}$ was administered twice daily concomitantly with GnRH-a and hMG from day 2 of the cycle to the time of ovulation. The overnight urinary GH output, plasma GH, insulin-like growth factor I (IGF-I), and follicular fluid (FF) IGF-I values were measured. Plasma estradiol levels were determined and follicular data were collected.

Findings.—The use of GH-RH was associated with significant improvement of urinary and plasma concentrations and of the hormonal response to hMG. Plasma IGF-I concentrations had a biphasic plasma variation. There was a slight increase in recruited follicles, retrieved oocytes, and FF IGF-I content.

Conclusions.—Prolonged stimulation of the somatotroph axis by repetitive daily administration of GH-RH[1-29] improves the hormonal ovarian response to hMG in poor responders, as shown by a sustained increase in plasma and urinary GH levels and a slight increase in the number of both mature follicles and retrieved oocytes. The IGF-I plasma levels have a biphasic variation, with a slight increase during the first part of the follicular phase and a decrease thereafter. In this study, the fertilization rate was not improved and no pregnancy resulted. However, GH-RH may be a useful adjunctive therapy to improve follicular maturation.

▶ This paper was selected because of its point of view that GH therapy may not be an absolute panacea. In this paper, GH-RH hormone was used as in the previous report. Very much larger doses were used, 500 μg twice a day. Yet, although hormonal increases were evident (e.g., an increase in GH, which was anticipated), the clinical results were not really improved, although the authors suggest a trend in this direction. It is clear that we do not have all the answers as yet, and there are many that need to be done, e.g., assessing what constitutes normal or abnormal endogenous GH responses initially and the ideal ways of co-administering gonadotropins and GHs or GH-RH.—R.A. Lobo, M.D.

Gonadotropin-Releasing Hormone Agonist (Leuprolide Acetate) Induced Ovarian Hyperstimulation Syndrome in a Woman Undergoing Intermittent Hemodialysis

Hampton HL, Whitworth NS, Cowan BD (Univ of Mississippi, Jackson)
Fertil Steril 55:429–431, 1991 9–18

Background.—Gonadotropin-releasing hormone agonists (GnRH-a) have been used to induce therapeutic hypogonadism. Ovarian hyperstimulation developed in a woman treated with leuprolide acetate for a menstrual disorder.

Case Report.—Woman, 21, with hypertension and renal failure secondary to glomerulonephritis, was evaluated for severe menorrhagia. Renal transplantation had failed, and the patient required dialysis 3 times weekly. After administration of leuprolide acetate to establish gonadotropic amenorrhea, the patient was hospitalized with crescendo pelvic pain. Ultrasound examination revealed a 9-cm right ovary and a 5-cm left ovary with multiple cystic structures. Her pain was alleviated after she received 7.5 mg of depot leuprolide acetate. Fifteen days after a second dose of leuprolide acetate, the pain, ovarian enlargement, and hyperestrogenemia were resolved. Amenorrhea was maintained for 6 months, during which time the hematocrit increased to 28%.

Discussion.—Leuprolide acetate administered to a patient with severe menorrhagia stopped the bleeding but produced moderate ovarian hyperstimulation syndrome with painfully enlarged ovaries and hyperestrogenemia. Ovarian hyperstimulation may have developed because renal dialysis affected circulating concentrations of leuprolide acetate. Sustained secretion of gonadotropins occurred because the pituitary receptors for GnRH were incompletely down-regulated, and ovarian hyperstimulation occurred secondary to endogenous gonadotropins. When a second dose of leuprolide acetate was administered 15 days after the first dose, gonadotropin concentrations increased minimally. The pituitary ultimately was desensitized to further GnRH-a stimulation by the initial dose of agonist.

Conclusion.—Women with renal failure who undergo hemodialysis may have increased "ovarian responsiveness" to endogenous gonadotropins. The development of ovarian hyperstimulation in this patient suggests that long-acting GnRH-a could be used for endogenous follicular stimulation.

▶ This is an interesting case of hyperstimulation induced by the agonist. Whereas we know that the GnRH-a causes hyperstimulation and results in ovarian stimulation before down-regulation, patients receiving hemodialysis may constitute a high-risk group because of the metabolism of the agonist. What is suggested in this report is that initial administration of the GnRH-a may have resulted in exaggerated stimulation for the first week to 10 days. Therefore, it may be prudent to use something to block the pituitary response (e.g., a progestin) before down-regulation actually occurs. We have found 10 mg of norethindrone daily to be of benefit; if started 2 days before administration of the agonist, it may block the pituitary from the agonistic effects of the GnRH analog.—R.A. Lobo, M.D.

10 Disorders of the Fallopian Tube

Salpingitis Isthmica Nodosa in Female Infertility and Tubal Diseases

Skibsted L, Sperling L, Hansen U, Hertz J (Gentofte Hosp, Copenhagen)

Hum Reprod 6:828–831, 1991 10–1

Background.—Salpingitis isthmica nodosa (SIN), or nodular thickening of the proximal fallopian tube, is characterized by small diverticula in an irregularly hypertrophied myosalpinx. The occurrence, distribution, and frequency of SIN were examined in Danish women who underwent salpingectomy because of tubal pregnancy or salpingitis. An attempt was made to correlate SIN with infertility, pregnancies, outcome of pregnancies, births, pelvic inflammatory disease, and salpingitis.

Methods.—Sections from the isthmus of 223 fallopian tubes obtained from 193 patients were analyzed by the same pathologist. The results were compared among patients with and without SIN.

Findings.—Twenty-four women had SIN; only 1 had SIN in both tubes. The disease was located in the isthmus only in 72% and in both the isthmus and ampulla in 28%; it never involved the ampulla alone. The median age of women with SIN was 32.5 years and of those without SIN, 31 years. The incidence of SIN was 12.3% (19 of 155) in tubal pregnancies and 19.4% (12 of 62 in infertile women. Of 15 women with both SIN and tubal pregnancy, 40% had more than 1 tubal pregnancy. Women with SIN had a greater risk of 2 or more tubal pregnancies than women without SIN (17.3%). Primary infertility was more common in the group with SIN. The frequency of births before salpingectomy did not differ significantly among women with or without SIN. After SIN was diagnosed, no children were born to the women with SIN, but this finding did not differ significantly from that in women without SIN. Although women with SIN more often had histologic signs of salpingitis, this did not influence the number of children or tubal pregnancies.

Conclusion.—Salpingectomized women have reduced fertility. Women with SIN give birth to as many children as women without SIN, but they have a greater risk of 2 or more tubal pregnancies. The frequency of salpingitis is increased in women with SIN and tubal pregnancy.

▶ The cause of SIN has not been clarified completely. Some believe that the condition occurs after tubal infection, and others that it occurs in the absence of salpingitis, similar to the development of adenomyosis. Its cause most likely is not congenital, because SIN is not found in the oviducts of children and is rarely found in the second decade of life. A causal relationship of SIN with infertility has not been established, as both entities increase with age and SIN has been demonstrated in about 10% of oviducts removed at the time of postpartum sterilizations. In this study, 11 of the 243 women with SIN had given birth previously, compared with 100 of 169 without SIN, an insignificant difference.—D.R. Mishell, Jr., M.D.

Fallopian Tube Catheterization and Recanalization Under Ultrasonic Observation: A Simplified Technique to Evaluate Tubal Patency and Open Proximally Obstructed Tubes

Lisse K, Sydow P (Humboldt Univ, Berlin)

Fertil Steril 56:198–201, 1991 10–2

Introduction.—A sonoscopic technique was developed for transvaginal catheterization and recanalization. The use of this technique, diagnostically and therapeutically, was evaluated in 19 patients with bilateral proximal tubal obstruction. Transvaginal tubal catheterization was performed with ultrasonographic observation.

Results.—Proximal fallopian tube recanalization was successful in 1 tube in 16 of 19 patients (87.2%); 21 of 38 tubes (55.3%) were successfully cannulated (table). Within a 6-month period, 5 of the 16 successfully cannulated patients (31.6%) were found to have an intrauterine pregnancy. Reocclusion occurred in 6 of 14 treated tubes (42.9%).

Discussion.—The patients had an average of 4 years of infertility. This technique appeared to be effective in recanalizing obstructed fallopian tubes. Its success questions the application of microsurgery in many patients with proximal tubal obstruction who are infertile. Further studies are needed to confirm the diagnostic and therapeutic effectiveness of this method.

▶ Several nonsurgical methods to treat proximal tubal obstruction using fluoroscopic or hysteroscopic visualization have been described previously by Kumpe, Thurmond, and Confino (see the 1991 YEAR BOOK OF INFERTILITY, pp

Results of Sonoscopic Fallopian Tube Recanalization for Proximal Obstruction

Patients successfully recanalized*/patients with bilateral obstruction	16/19 (84.2)†
Tubes recanalized/tubes attempted	21/38 (55.3)
IUPs at a 6-month follow-up interval/patients recanalized*	5/16 (31.6)
Patients with reoccluded tubes* 6 months following the procedure/patients recanalized	5/11 (45.5)
Tubes reoccluded/tubes recanalized	6/14 (42.9)

*One or both tubes.
†Values in parentheses are percents.
(Courtesy of Lisse K, Sydow P: *Fertil Steril* 56:198–201, 1991.)

182–183). The technique of ultrasonographic visualization described here should be less costly than the techniques using fluoroscopy or hysteroscopy, but it probably requires greater technical experience. Because of the convenience and good results with these transcervical methods of treating proximal tubal obstruction, their use should precede and/or replace microsurgical reanastomosis.—D.R. Mishell, Jr., M.D.

Handling of Tubal Infertility After Introduction of In Vitro Fertilization: Changes and Consequences

Holst N, Maltau JM, Forsdahl F, Hansen LJ (Univ of Tromsø, Norway)

Fertil Steril 55:140–143, 1991 10–3

Introduction.—In vitro fertilization (IVF) is replacing surgery as the main treatment of tubal infertility. The changes in management of tubal infertility at one clinic were investigated, along with the quantifiable consequences of these changes, their economic impact, and the pregnancy and birth rates associated with tubal surgery and IVF.

Study Groups.—Two groups of patients who had tubal surgery were studied. Group 1 comprised 206 patients who had a tubal operation between 1980 and 1982, and group 2 comprised 104 patients who had surgery between 1986 and 1988.

Findings.—The number of operations decreased by nearly half between these 2 periods as indications for surgery became more limited. The proportion of salpingostomies decreased, and the proportion of operations carried out solely for adhesions increased correspondingly, but these changes were not significant. The decreased number of operations increased the available operating room time by about 3 weeks and reduced the need for hospitalization by almost 250 days yearly because IVF was always done on an outpatient basis. Sick leave was reduced by 3.5 man-years per year. The birth rate for all tubal surgery patients was 23.7%, and that for all patients who entered the IVF program after 1986 was 24.8% (Fig 10–1). However, birth rate for patients who had complete IVF treatment was 72.3%. The rate of ectopic pregnancies was 9.2% in tubal surgery group 1 and 1.3% among those who had IVF.

Conclusion.—In vitro fertilization has narrowed the indications for tubal surgery, reducing the number of operations by almost 50%. Based on a cost of $4,000, this corresponds to a cost savings of about $140,000 per year, which is about half the yearly budget of one IVF unit. Also, IVF improves pregnancy rates and increases the availability of hospital resources.

▶ This longitudinal study in one center shows the effect that the introduction of the IVF technique has had in the treatment of infertility caused by tubal disease. An argument can be made that if the extent of tubal disease is so severe that it cannot be treated by laparoscopic surgery on an outpatient basis, as reported by Dubuisson et al. (see the 1991 YEAR BOOK OF INFERTILITY, p 181), the patient should not have a laparotomy but be treated by 1 or more cycles of IVF.—D.R. Mishell, Jr., M.D.

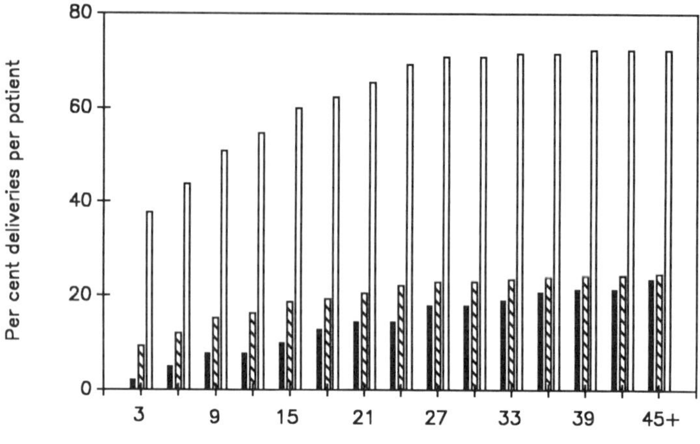

Fig 10–1.—Life table analyzing the cumulative rate of deliveries comparing 177 patients having tubal surgery *(filled in area)*; all 389 patients entering the IVF program *(stippled area)*; and 128 patients having a complete IVF treatment *(open area)*. (Courtesy of Holst N, Maltau JM, Forsdahl F, et al: *Fertil Steril* 55:140–143, 1991.)

Neosalpingostomy for Distal Tubal Obstruction: Prognostic Factors and Impact of Surgical Technique

Schlaff WD, Hassiakos DK, Damewood MD, Rock JA (Johns Hopkins Med School, Baltimore)

Fertil Steril 54:984–990, 1990 10–4

Introduction.—Microsurgical technique appears to have improved the results of neosalpingostomy for occlusion of the fallopian tubes. A retrospective study was done to analyze prognostic factors for pregnancy outcome and evaluate the success of conventional vs. microsurgical neosalpingostomy in comparable patients.

Study Design.—Records of all patients who underwent microsurgical neosalpingostomy during a 5.5-year period were reviewed. The procedure was defined as creation of an opening in the distal end of an occluded fallopian tube regardless of the presence or absence of fibriae. The size of the hydrosalpinx, condition of the fimbriae, degree of adhesion, and rugal pattern on hysterosalpingogram were used to classify patients as having mild, moderate, or severe disease. The disease was severe in 37 patients.

Results.—Of the 64 patients who had bilateral surgery, 18 conceived; 5 of these were tubal ectopic pregnancies. Of 31 patients who had unilateral surgery, 8 conceived; there were 2 tubal ectopic conceptions. The rates of gestation were similar in these groups. Only 2 of 18 patients whose contralateral tube was irreparable conceived, compared to 6 of 13 whose contralateral tube required only salpingolysis. The mean time to

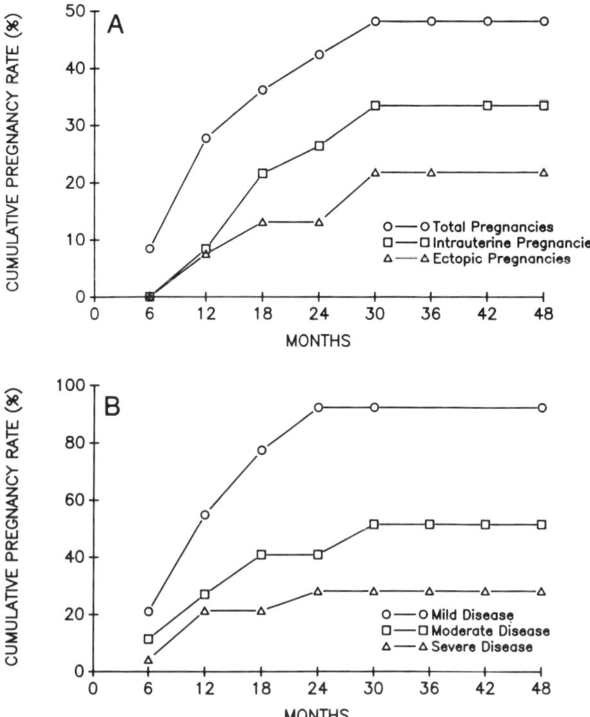

Fig 10–2.—Life table analysis of pregnancy outcome after neosalpingostomy by (**A**) pregnancy location and (**B**) extent of disease. (Courtesy of Schlaff WD, Hassiakos DK, Damewood MD, et al: *Fertil Steril* 54:984–990, 1990.)

pregnancy was 9 months for intrauterine and 12.6 months for ectopic gestations (Fig 10–2). Among patients who conceived, 73% did so within 1 year and 96% within 2 years. Rates of pregnancy were 80% of patients with mild disease, 31% of those with moderate disease, and 16% of those with severe disease; however, the rates of intrauterine pregnancy—17% of patients with mild disease and 12.7% of those with moderate disease—were not significantly different.

Conclusion.—The severity of tubal disease and the extent of adnexal adhesions appear to be the main prognostic factors in neosalpingostomy. Microsurgical technique may improve the pregnancy rate in patients with severe disease, but the difference does not reach significance. Pregnancy rates are no different whether mild or moderate disease is present.

▶ This study confirms what has been reported by others, namely, that the prognosis for pregnancy after distal tubal surgery is directly proportional to the extent of the preexisting tubal disease. This finding supports the contention made in the comments of Abstract 10–3. If the tubal disease cannot be corrected with laparoscopic surgery, it may be better to perform in vitro fertiliza tion. Correcting patent tubes surgically does not insure pregnancy. If the endosalpinx is sufficiently damaged, secretion of necessary nutrients to support metabolic activity of the dividing blastocyst for 3 days will not occur. In this study, even with excellent microsurgical techniques, the intrauterine pregnancy rate in those individuals with severe tubal disease was only 12%. One must remember that the goal of treatment of the infertile couple is to obtain a live infant, not to fertilize an egg.—D.R. Mishell, Jr., M.D.

Treatment of Tubal Ectopic Pregnancy by Salpingotomy With or Without Tubal Suturing and Salpingectomy

Tulandi T, Guralnick M (Sir Mortimer B Davis Jewish Gen Hosp; Royal Victoria Hosp; McGill Univ, Montreal, PQ, Canada)

Fertil Steril 55:53–55, 1991 10–5

Introduction.—Serial measurements of serum β-human chorionic gonadotropin and early ultrasound examination have allowed early detection of unruptured tubal ectopic pregnancy (EP), thus enabling its conservative surgical treatment. Thirty-four women with unruptured tubal EP were randomly assigned to undergo salpingotomy with or without tubal suturing. The reproductive outcome of these patients were compared with that of 24 patients who underwent salpingectomy for unruptured ampullary EP (historical control).

Results.—Life-table analysis showed that the cumulative probability of an intrauterine pregnancy (IUP) was significantly higher after conservative surgical treatment than after salpingectomy. The cumulative probability of IUP was significantly higher after salpingotomy without than after with tubal suturing. At 12 months the cumulative probability of IUP was 45% after salpingotomy without and 21% with tubal suturing. The cumulative probability of recurrent EP did not differ significantly after salpingotomy with or without tubal suturing, but was significantly higher than after salpingectomy.

Conclusions.—These findings suggest that IUP after conservative surgical treatment of tubal EP is higher than after salpingectomy, but recurrent EP also is higher. Intrauterine pregnancy occurs earlier after salpingotomy without tubal suturing than after salpingotomy with tubal suturing, possibly because healing by secondary intention in the former facilitates rapid return of tubal function.

▶ In the United States, the technique of salpingostomy without tubal closure is used for conservative treatment of unruptured tubal gestation, whereas in Europe the incision in the oviduct is usually closed. This randomized study shows that the subsequent IUP rates are relatively similar with either technique, but that conception occurs more rapidly if the incision is left open and allowed to heal by secondary intention. The group of patients treated by salpingectomy had a lower rate of subsequent EP. This group was not randomized, however, and was a historical control. Most studies in the literature indicate that the overall subsequent EP rate is similar whether treatment is radical or conservative.—D.R. Mishell, Jr., M.D.

Laparoscopic Distal Tuboplasty: Report of 87 Cases and a 4-Year Experience

Canis M, Manhes H, Mage G, Wattiez A, Pouly JL, Bruhat MA (Centre Hospitalier Régional et Universitaire, Clermont-Ferrand, France)

Fertil Steril 56:616–621, 1991 10–6

Objective.—Although there have been several reports of the value of laparoscopic distal tuboplasty in the treatment of tubal infertility, the procedure remains controversial. A retrospective study was undertaken to evaluate the fertility results after laparoscopic distal tuboplasty and to compare these results with those obtained previously with laser microsurgery.

Patients.—Between October 1985 and June 1989, a total of 87 patients (mean age, 29 years) underwent laparoscopic surgery for distal tubal occlusion. Forty-two patients were treated for primary infertility and 45 for secondary infertility. The mean duration of infertility was 33 months. Tubal damage was evaluated at laparoscopy by using a classification in which the disease severity was staged I, II, III, or IV, with IV being the worst.

Results.—Twenty-nine patients (33.3%) achieved intrauterine pregnancies (IUPs) and 6 (6.9%) had extrauterine pregnancies (EUPs). Twenty-six of the 29 IUPs occurred during the first year after laparoscopic surgery and 93% of conceptions occurred within 14 months (Fig 10–3). The monthly fecundity rate was 3.3% during the first postoperative year, but only .6% during the following years. The overall monthly fecundity rate was 2.3%. None of the patients with stage IV disease became pregnant. The pregnancy rate was 5.6% among patients with stages

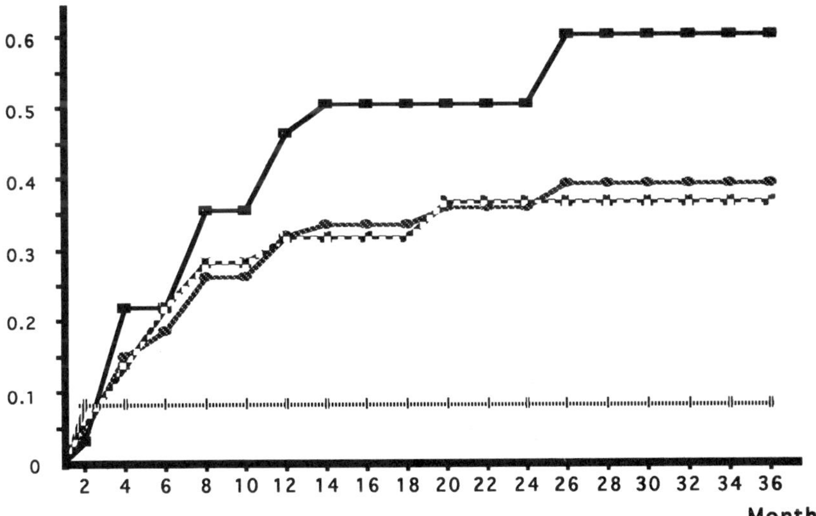

Fig 10–3.—Cumulative pregnancy rates. (Courtesy of Canis M, Manhes H, Mage G, et al: *Fertil Steril* 56:616–621, 1991.)

III and IV tubal disease, compared with 40.6% among patients with stages I and II disease. The difference was statistically significant. The EUP rates were 11.8% of those with stage I disease; 3.3%, stage II; 6.7%, stage III; and 10%, stage IV. Comparison of the pregnancy rates obtained after laparoscopic surgery with those obtained after laser microsurgical distal tuboplasty revealed no statistical difference between the 2 treatment modalities.

Conclusion.—In experienced hands, laparoscopic surgery represents a safe and effective alternative to laser microsurgery in the treatment of distal tubal occlusion.

▶ Although the use of laparoscopic salpingostomy was not prospectively compared with the microsurgical technique performed by laparotomy in this study, the retrospective comparison that was performed indicates that the pregnancy rates were comparable with the 2 techniques. It was recently reported by Schlaff (1) that the results with microsurgery were comparable with those achieved by conventional surgery in management of tubal infertility. It appears that the prognoses for fertility after salpingostomy by any operative technique are correlated more with extent of disease than with type of surgical procedure. Because laparoscopic salpingostomy results in less morbidity, length of hospitalization, and cost than does laparotomy, the former technique should become the procedure of choice to treat distal tubal disease when performed by experienced laparoscopic surgeons.—D.R. Mishell, Jr., M.D.

Reference

1. Schlaff WD: Fertil Steril 54:984, 1991.

Risk Factors for Ectopic Pregnancy in 556 Pregnancies After In Vitro Fertilization: Implications for Preventive Management

Dubuisson JB, Foulot H, Aubriot FX, Mandelbrot L, Mathieu L, de Jolinière JB (Clinique Universitaire Port-Royal, Paris; Clinique Cherest, Neuilly, France)

Fertil Steril 56:686–690, 1991 10–7

Objective.—The proportion of ectopic pregnancies (EPs) after in vitro fertilization (IVF) reported ranges from 4% to 11%. A retrospective analysis was designed to examine the incidence of EP after IVF and to determine the impact of specific risk factors on the rate of EP. The risk factors examined included tubal status, type of ovarian stimulation and luteal phase support, and number of embryos transferred.

Patients.—During a 6-year period 48 EPs occurred among a total of 556 pregnancies after 3103 IVF cycles. The records of these 48 patients and those of the 508 patients who had intrauterine pregnancies (IUPs) after IVF during the same period were analyzed.

Results.—Thirty-seven of the 48 EPs were ampullar, 8 were interstitial, and 3 were isthmic. Forty-six patients underwent salpingectomy, and pathologic examination revealed tubal lesions in all 46 cases. Among the

Rate of EP According to Indication for IVF

Indication	Pregnancies	EP	IUP
Tubal	387[a]	43 (11.1)[b]	344
Endometriosis	48[c]	1 (2.1)[d]	47
Unexplained	89	3 (3.4)[e]	86
Other[f]	32	1[g]	31
Total	556	48	508

[a] Including 11 with male factor.
[b] Values in parentheses are percents of EP.
[c] Including 3 cases with male factor.
[d] $P < .05$ when compared with EP in tubal indications.
[e] $P < .02$ when compared with EP in tubal indications.
[f] Including 13 cases with male factor, 5 with cervical factor, 12 with anovulation, and 2 with immunologic factor.
[g] Male factor.
(Courtesy of Dubuisson JB, Foulot H, Aubriot FX, et al: *Fertil Steril* 56:686–690, 1991.)

508 IUPs 125 ended in miscarriage and 383 in delivery. When the incidence of EP was analyzed according to the indications for IVF, 43 EPs were found to have occurred in women with tubal sterility, 1 in a woman with endometriosis, and 3 in women with unexplained infertility. Thus the ratios of EPs to total pregnancies was significantly greater for tubal sterility than it was for either endometriosis or unexplained infertility (table). The incidence of EP was not related to the protocol of ovarian stimulation, treatment given for luteal phase support, level of estradiol at the time of ovulation induction, or to number of embryos transferred. Nor was the difference in EP rates significant according to whether 1 or both tubes were patent. All 4 heterotopic pregnancies were treated by salpingectomy.

Discussion.—Preexisting tubal pathology is the major risk factor for EP. An extreme approach to reducing the risk of EP after IVF would be systematic bilateral salpingectomy in patients with tubal infertility. Because the incidence of EP among women with tubal infertility was 11%, however, such a policy would lead to unnecessary salpingectomies in almost 89% of patients who did achieve IUPs after IVF and would not eliminate the risk of interstitial pregnancy. The problem of EP after IVF should be managed carefully without overtreatment.

Tubal Ectopic Pregnancy After In Vitro Fertilization and Embryo Transfer: A Role for Proximal Occlusion or Salpingectomy After Failed Distal Tubal Surgery?

Zouves C, Erenus M, Gomel V (Univ of British Columbia, Vancouver; Univ Hosp, Vancouver, BC, Canada)

Fertil Steril 56:691–695, 1991 10–8

Objective.—Ectopic pregnancy (EP) is a well-reported complication of reconstructive surgery for sequelae of pelvic inflammatory disease, but the potential of tubal gestation as a result of in vitro fertilization-embryo

Outcome of 640 Embryo Transfer Cycles in Patients With Tubal Factor Infertility

Prior surgery	No. of cycles	No. of clinical pregnancies	No. of tubal pregnancies
Reconstructive tubal surgery	359 (56)*	64 (17.8)	10 (15.6)†
None	183 (29)	22 (12)	2 (9)†
Sterilization/salpingectomy	98 (16)	14 (13)	0
Total	640 (100)	100 (15)	12 (12)

*Values in parentheses are percents.
†$P < .05$.
(Courtesy of Zouves C, Erenus M, Gomel V: *Fertil Steril* 56:691–695, 1991.)

transfer (IVF-ET) has received less scrutiny. A retrospective analysis was undertaken to identify predisposing factors to tubal pregnancy after IVF-ET.

Patients.—During a 5-year period, 891 ET cycles were performed in the IVF program at the University of British Columbia. Indications for IVF were tubal factor in 640 cycles (72%) and nontubal factors in 251 cycles (28%). The 3 basic protocols used in the IVF program were clomiphene citrate followed by human menopausal gonadotropin, human menopausal gonadotropin alone, and gonadotropin-releasing hormone analogue plus human menopausal gonadotropin.

Results.—Of 1067 cycles initiated, 891 resulted in embryo replacement, 138 (15.5%) resulted in clinical pregnancies, and 13 (9.4%) of these were EPs. Of 640 ET cycles performed in patients with tubal factor infertility, 100 (15.6%) resulted in clinical pregnancies, and 12 of these (12%) were EPs. Of 251 ET cycles performed in patients with nontubal factor infertility, only 38 (15.1%) resulted in clinical pregnancies, and only 1 of these (2.6%) was a tubal gestation. Ten of the 12 patients with tubal factor infertility and an EP had undergone reconstructive tubal surgery (table). Furthermore, the tube that ultimately housed the pregnancy had been a hydrosalpinx in 10 of the 13 patients. There was no statistically significant difference in tubal pregnancy rates for the 3 basic treatment protocols.

Conclusion.—Women who previously had reconstructive tubal surgery for distal tubal disease are at the highest risk of having a tubal pregnancy after IVF. Although prophylactic proximal tubal occlusion may be too radical an approach, such a procedure may be considered in those patients with tubal factor infertility in whom an attempt at tubal reconstruction has failed.

▶ Ectopic pregnancy after IVF is not uncommon, rates varying from 2% to 12%. In these 2 studies (Abstracts 10–7 and 10–8), about 10% of the clinical pregnancies after IVF were ectopic. Because 10 of the 13 ectopic pregnancies in the second study occurred after previous tubal reconstruction surgery, and there were 64 clinical pregnancies in women who had such surgery, about a sixth of pregnancies occurring after IVF in this group of women were ectopic. The authors of the study reviewed in Abstract 10–7 believe that performing salpingectomy in all women with tubal factor infertility before performing IVF is probably unjustified. However, as Zouves et al. note, a persuasive argument can be made for performing salpingectomy before IVF in women who have had unsuccessful tubal reconstructive surgery.—D.R. Mishell, Jr., M.D.

11 Endometriosis

Bone Mineral Density of the Lumbar Spine in Endometriosis Subjects Compared to an Age-Similar Control Population

Lane N, Baptista J, Snow-Harter C (Univ of California, San Francisco; Syntex Labs, Palo Alto, Calif; VA Med Ctr, Palo Alto)

J Clin Endocrinol Metab 72:510–514, 1991 11–1

Background.—Low estrogen levels may be associated with bone loss in healthy women. Bone mineral density (BMD) in patients with endometriosis was compared with that in healthy women of similar age.

Methods.—The series included 85 women with laparoscopically confirmed endometriosis whose mean age was 30.7 years. These patients were enrolled in a clinical trial of the gonadotropin-releasing hormone agonist nafarelin. Each patient completed a questionnaire about her gynecologic and endometriosis history and health habits. The BMD of the lumbar spine was determined by dual-energy radiographic absorptiometry and hormonal values. A group of 52 normal women (mean age, 32 years) with regular menstrual cycles and no major medical problems, also were studied as controls. Both groups consisted of mainly white women.

Results.—Both groups had a mean BMD value of 1.1 g/cm^2, which was 104.8% of normal for their age group. There was no correlation between BMD and the severity or time since the diagnosis of endometriosis. Positive correlations existed between BMD and weight in both groups, BMD and height in the group with endometriosis, and, marginally, between BMD and height in the control group.

Conclusions.—Women with endometriosis have normal BMD of the lumbar spine for their age and no increased risk of vertebral osteoporotic fractures with aging. Bone mineral density is correlated with height and weight but not duration of endometriosis. Interleukin-1 activity may increase peritoneal inflammation and fibrosis in endometriosis without affecting bone turnover systemically.

▶ This is an important paper only because it is provocative and challenges a previous report on the relationship between endometriosis and bone mass. What is the answer here? Is or is not bone mass decreased in patients with endometriosis? Clearly, this is extremely important. If there is a decrease in bone mass or vulnerability for a reduction in bone mass in patients with endometriosis, then gonadotropin-releasing hormone agonist therapy, which decreases estrogen secretion, would have to be used very carefully; otherwise, acceleration of the decline in bone mass could occur.

The report by Comite et al. (1) is what is challenged here. Those investigators used the QCT of the distal radius to demonstrate a reduction in bone mass. Here, the Dexa technique was used, which appears to be state of the art. Also, in this study, the vertebrae were the targets of Dexa imaging, whereas the forearm was used in Comite et al.'s study. Clearly, there could be a difference depending on the site of bone mass measurement. What this concept challenges, however, is that the cytokine abnormalities of endometriosis (e.g., the release of compounds such as interleukin-1) may not necessarily be related to increased bone resorption, at least at the vertebrae.

It is extremely difficult to evaluate these studies because of the heterogeneous nature of the patient populations; more studies are needed to provide a definitive answer on this topic. However, the clinical significance is the mere suspicion that there may be alterations in patients with endometriosis. A difference between the status of the patients in the 2 studies, and specifically their estrogen status, may help to explain these opposing conclusions. In terms of clinical management, because of this concern we must evaluate our endometriotic patients very carefully, particularly before initiating agonist treatment. Specifically, patients who are thin, immobile, and who smoke, and those who do not take in adequate amounts of calcium, should be counseled very carefully and followed for bone loss and osteopenia.—R.A. Lobo, M.D.

Reference

1. Comite F, et al: *J Clin Endocrinol Metab* 69:837, 1989.

Menstrual Symptoms in Women With Pelvic Endometriosis

Mahmood TA, Templeton AA, Thomson L, Fraser C (Aberdeen Maternity Hosp, Aberdeen, Scotland)

Br J Obstet Gynaecol 98:558–563, 1991 11–2

Purpose.—The symptomatology of endometriosis is not clear. A prospective, questionnaire-based study examined menstrual symptoms in women with pelvic endometriosis.

Setting.—Of the 1250 questionnaires sent to women before planned admission for laparotomy or hysterectomy, 1200 (96%) were completed. The frequencies of dysmenorrhea, menorrhagia, menstrual regularity, premenstrual spotting, deep dyspareunia, and pelvic pain were evaluated in 598 women undergoing laparoscopic sterilization, 312 undergoing laparoscopy for infertility, 156 having laproscopy because of chronic pelvic pain, and 134 undergoing abdominal hysterectomy for dysfunctional uterine bleeding.

Findings.—Of the 201 women (17%) with endometriosis, 73% had mild disease. The remaining patients had either postinfective pelvic adhesions (23%) or normal pelvic organs (60%). Dysmenorrhea occurred more frequently in women with endometriosis than in those with a normal pelvis or postinfective pelvic adhesions (table). Deep dyspareunia, pain after intercourse, and recurrent pain unrelated to menstruation or coitus occurred more often in women with endometriosis or postinfective pelvic adhesions than in women with a normal pelvis. Menorrhagia, menstrual irregularity, and premenstrual spotting were noted with equal

A Comparison of Menstrual Symptoms in Women With and Without Endometriosis (n = 1,200)

Variables	Endometriosis (n = 201)		Pelvic adhesions (n = 278)		Normal pelvis (n = 721)		Significance with 2 df	
	n	(%)	n	(%)	n	(%)	χ^2	P
Dysmenorrhoea	137	(68)	140	(50)	358	(50)	24·48	<0·001
Present periods regular	154	(77)	206	(74)	632	(88)	9·92	<0·02
Menorrhagia	110	(55)	125	(45)	365	(51)	4·89	>0·05
Premenstrual spotting	56	(30)	79	(28)	190	(26)	2·28	>0·05
Deep dyspareunia	75	(37)	93	(33)	168	(23)	25·64	<0·001
Pain after intercourse	29	(14)	42	(15)	72	(10)	6·41	<0·05
Pelvic pain	118	(59)	165	(59)	346	(48)	17·95	<0·001

(Courtesy of Mahmood TA, Templeton AA, Thomson L, et al: *Br J Obstet Gynaecol* 98:558–563, 1991.)

frequency in all groups. There was no relationship between symptomatology and the severity of endometriosis.

Conclusion.—Menstrual symptoms are not reliable indices of disease in women with pelvic endometriosis. Although dysmenorrhea is the most common symptom reported by women with endometriosis, other menstrual symptoms are also frequent in women with pelvic pathology.

▶ Other retrospective studies have suggested that women with endometriosis have a higher frequency of abnormal bleeding than those without this disease, and that therefore endometriosis may be a cause of abnormal uterine bleeding. However, as shown in this nonrandomized, prospective study, women with endometriosis undergoing laparoscopy for a variety of reasons, including tubal sterilization, do not have a greater frequency of abnormal uterine bleeding than women without endometriosis. Dysmenorrhea, as expected, occurred significantly more frequently in women with endometriosis. Endometriosis does not appear to cause abnormal uterine bleeding, as it most likely does not cause infertility, unless the disease causes tubal pathology.—D.R. Mishell, Jr., M.D.

12 Uncommon Causes and Unexplained Infertility

Ultrasound-Guided Transcervical Metroplasty

Querleu D, Brasme TL, Parmentier D (Clinique Universitaire de Gynécologie Obstétrique et Pathologie de la Reproduction, Roubaix, France)

Fertil Steril 54:995–998, 1990 12–1

Introduction.—Transcervical metroplasty under ultrasonic guidance is a means of sectioning the uterine septa without hysteroscopy or laparoscopy. Twenty-four patients underwent this procedure.

Patients.—Twelve patients had had 2 or more spontaneous first- or second-trimester losses. Nine others were seen with primary infertility of at least 18 months' duration. Three women had asymptomatic uterine septa.

Technique.—Under general anesthesia or neuroleptanalgesia, the bladder is filled with saline and sonography is carried out using a real-time scanner to measure the septum. Endoscopic scissors are used to divide the septum at a point equidistant from the anterior and posterior uterine surfaces. No intrauterine device is inserted. Cyclical hormone therapy was given for 5 months in this series.

Results.—No patient had significant bleeding or uterine perforation. Eleven of 18 evaluable patients had an excellent outcome with no significant indentation of the uterine fundus. Two patients had a residual septum divided under hysteroscopic control. Eighteen women conceived; 1 had a first-trimester abortion. Two of the 6 women who did not conceive did not wish to do so, and 2 others had another cause of infertility.

Conclusions.—Ultrasound-guided transcervical metroplasty leaves no myometrial scar or pelvic adhesions and is an expeditious procedure. The obstetric outcome has been satisfactory.

▶ It is established that a septate uterus can be the cause of recurrent abortion, but a causal relationship between the presence of a uterine septum and primary infertility has not been established. In this study, 6 of the 9 patients with infertility conceived after the septum was divided, but this result does not demonstrate that the septum was the cause of their infertility. The technique described appears easy to learn and may be tried if an individual with hysteroscopic surgical training is not available to perform the metroplasty.—D.R. Mishell, Jr., M.D.

Lectin Binding of Endometrium in Women With Unexplained Infertility

Klentzeris LD, Morrison L, Bulmer JN, Warren A, Li T-C, Cooke ID (Univ of Sheffield, Sheffield, England; Univ of Leeds, Leeds, England)

Fertil Steril 56:660–667, 1991 12–2

Background.—Lectins have a specific affinity for nonimmunologic binding with the terminal oligosaccharides of complex glycoconjugates; this binding can be inhibited by sugars of low molecular weight. Endometrial glycoconjugates probably take part in endometrial events occurring during the "implantation window" and they may affect the outcome of blastocyst implantation. Endometrial biopsy specimens and lectin histochemistry were used to assess endometrial function during the peri-implantation phase in women with unexplained infertility and those with normal fertility.

Methods.—Eighteen normal fertile women, seen for sterilization or reversal of sterilization, and 18 women with unexplained infertility were studied. The mean age was 32 years in the former group and 33 years in the latter group; in those patients the mean duration of infertility was almost 6 years. Endometrial biopsy specimens were obtained from each woman 5, 7, and 9 days after the luteinizing hormone surge. In addition, lectin histochemistry studies were performed using 5 biotinylated lectins as analytic probes: concanavalin A (ConA); wheat germ, soybean, and peanut agglutinins; and *Ulex europaeus I*. The avidin-biotin peroxidase method was used to assess lectin binding by endometrial glands, surface epithelium, stromal cells, and vessels.

Results.—The fertile women had staining of the subnuclear glandular cytoplasm, glandular lumen, stromal cells, and surface epithelium with ConA. In contrast, the infertile women had no or only equivocal conA binding to the glandular or surface epithelium. With wheat germ agglutinin, the glandular cytoplasm and stromal cells stained on days 5 and 7 in the fertile women, whereas in the infertile women the stroma stained but the glands did not.

Conclusions.—Women with unexplained infertility may have defective biosynthesis and distribution of glycoconjugates in the glandular and surface epithelium of the endometrium. This may negatively affect the endometrial environment during the peri-implantatin phase. One possible mechanism is suboptimal expression of certain oligosaccharides on the cellular surface, resulting in failure of recognition between the blastocyst and endometrium.

▶ This is an interesting paper on a potentially important finding in unexplained infertility. It is difficult to know what really constitutes unexplained infertility. In some patients, clearly, there is no infertility, and it merely requires a longer time for pregnancy to occur. Others truly have defects, albeit subtle, that interfere with the process of fertilization and/or successful implantation. This paper focuses on lectins. Lectins are glycoproteins that are apparently important for intercellular adhesion, allowing cell processes to adhere, and for antigenic recognition, cellular differentiation, growth, transformation, and perhaps also for endometrial implantation.

In this study the immunoperoxidase technique was used and biopsy material was stained for the presence of lectins, specifically concanavalin A and wheat germ agglutinin. Both were noted to be decreased in patients with unexplained infertility. The problems with immunoperoxidase staining include the possibility of nonspecific binding and the potential for difficulties in the quantification of binding to specific compounds. It is not clear whether those patients who had decreased binding of these lectins would be considered to have an inadequate luteal phase, which may be a cause of unexplained infertility. Yet, we are told that these patients all had normal, in-phase endometria, as determined in previous biopsy specimens.

If these data prove to be true, they would suggest that the major problem of patients with unexplained infertility is blastocyst implantation. How often this occurs is not clear. It would be interesting to confirm these data by other techniques, e.g., measurement of the production of these compounds in endometria rather than by binding techniques using immunoperoxidase. It would then also be important to know whether these defects can be altered by, for example, superovulation, which is efficacious in patients with unexplained infertility.—R.A. Lobo, M.D.

The Effects of Clomiphene Citrate Upon Ovulation and Endocrinology When Administered to Patients With Unexplained Infertility

Randall JM, Templeton A (Univ of Aberdeen, Scotland)

Hum Reprod 6:659–664, 1991 12–3

Background.—Clomiphene citrate enhances follicular development in ovulatory women and has been used therapeutically in patients with unexplained infertility. However, numerous reports of adverse effects have included luteinized unruptured follicle (LUF) syndrome, reduction of cervical mucus score, reduced endometrial thickness, and effects on embryonic development. Increased follicular size, weakening of the follicle wall, and actions of prostaglandins may be implicated in follicular rupture. The incidence of LUF when clomiphene citrate is administered to ovulatory women was assessed in 24 women with unexplained infertility.

Methods.—All 24 patients had spontaneous ovulatory cycles as documented by follicular collapse viewed by transvaginal sonography. The women then received 150 mg of clomiphene citrate on days 5–9. Ultrasonography was performed on a daily basis for at least 2 days after the day of the luteinizing hormone (LH) peak and luteinization.

Findings.—In 25% of the cycles stimulated by clomiphene citrate, LUF occurred, and in 2 of the 6 LUF cycles there was no apparent LH surge. In the LUF cycles significantly elevated LH levels were noted in the follicular phase, but there was no apparent difference in the serum estradiol level compared with those in ovulatory clomiphene-citrate-treated cycles. Multifollicular development occurred in 87.5% of cycles in which clomiphene citrate was given, with significantly elevated serum levels of estradiol. Levels of LH and follicle-stimulating hormone (FSH) were elevated in the follicular phase of the clomiphene-citrate-treated cycles compared with the spontaneous cycles.

Conclusions.—In clomiphene-citrate-stimulated cycles in ovulatory patients with unexplained infertility, the incidence of LUF was 25%; also, gonadotropin levels were increased, follicular development was enhanced, and levels of LH and FSH were elevated in the follicular phase compared with levels in spontaneous cycles. The high incidence of LUF when clomiphene citrate is administered does not support the use of this drug in patients with ovulatory infertility.

▶ This is potentially a problem. Clomiphene is often used in patients with unexplained infertility to enhance follicular development. A note of caution is suggested by this report in which a high incidence (25%) of the LUF syndrome was encountered. In general, patients who do not really need clomiphene (ovulatory) are the ones who end up with problems associated with clomiphene therapy. In these normally ovulatory women, 150 mg of clomiphene induced approximately 3 follicles. However, LH levels were high throughout the cycle; high LH levels may be associated with problems such as premature luteinization, as evidenced by earlier progesterone rises in these same patients. These data may not be relevant if human chorionic gonadotropin is used with clomiphene instead of depending on the spontaneous LH surge, but this remains to be determined.

There is a lot that we do not as yet understand. Most other reports have suggested beginning clomiphene earlier, such as on day 3 of the cycle rather than on days 5 through 9, as was done in this study. This paper merely brings to our attention the potential concern we should have when we administer clomiphene to otherwise ovulatory patients with unexplained infertility.—R.A. Lobo, M.D.

A Randomized, Controlled Trial of Clomiphene Citrate and Intrauterine Insemination in Couples With Unexplained Infertility or Surgically Corrected Endometriosis

Deaton JL, Nakajima ST, Gibson M, Badger GJ, Blackmer KM, Brumsted JR (Univ of Vermont, Burlington)

Fertil Steril 54:1083–1088, 1990 12–4

Purpose.—Because few randomized, controlled studies have compared treatments of unexplained infertility or infertility associated with endometriosis, such a study of 4 treatment and 4 control groups was undertaken in which ovulation was enhanced by clomiphene citrate therapy. Timed intrauterine insemination (IUI) was then performed in couples with unexplained infertility or surgically corrected endometriosis.

Findings.—In 67 couples there were 14 pregnancies in 148 treated cycles compared with 5 pregnancies in 150 untreated cycles. In the 2 groups the fecundity rate of .095 compared to .033 was statistically significant, but comparison of pregnancy outcome was not. Comparison of cycles of conception and nonconception during treatment detected no differences between the size of the lead follicle or number of dominant follicles. The only complication was the tubal pregnancy rate of 11% in 19 conceptions.

Conclusions.—The resulting 14 pregnancies during treatment cycles and 5 pregnancies during control cycles show that treatment with clomiphene citrate and IUI improves fecundity over periovulatory intercourse in couples with unexplained fertility or surgically corrected endometriosis. The prospective, randomized trials and life-table analysis are valuable methods for treatment evaluation.

▶ Infertile couples should be divided into 2 categories: (1) those who are sterile and therefore cannot conceive without treatment (e.g., women with complete distal tubal occlusion), and (2) those who are subfertile, whose fecundibility rate (pregnancy rate per cycle) is significantly less than the normal population. The couples enrolled in this study belong to the latter group. Therefore, over time a certain percentage will conceive without any treatment. To determine whether any therapeutic regimen is truly superior to no treatment in such couples, it is essential that prospective, randomized trials such as this be performed and the results analyzed by life-table analysis to learn whether the monthly fecundity rate is significantly better in the treated group compared with the untreated group. In this study, the use of clomiphene citrate and washed IUI was more effective than withholding treatment. Therefore, it should be offered to couples with unexplained infertility or treated endometriosis before the more expensive and complicated in vitro fertilization or gamete intrafallopian transfer procedures are undertaken.—D.R. Mishell, Jr., M.D.

The Effect of Treatment on Pregnancy Among Couples With Unexplained Infertility

Collins JA, Milner RA, Rowe TC (McMaster Univ, Hamilton, Ont; Univ of British Columbia, Vancouver, BC, Canada)

Int J Fertil 36:140–152, 1991 12–5

Background.—The effectiveness of treatment for couples with unexplained infertility is not known, although treatment is offered such couples in the hope of augmenting the normal mechanisms of conception. A prospective cohort study used proportional-hazards analysis to evaluate the occurrence of pregnancy, adjusting for covariates such as the duration of infertility.

Methods.—Findings in 130 couples with unexplained infertility who were treated were compared with those in 470 couples with unexplained infertility who were not treated. Overall, 117 couples had secondary infertility. The patients were registered at 11 Canadian infertility clinics and had a mean duration of infertility of 40 months. The duration of observation was a mean of 14.5 months; 9.4% of couples were lost to follow-up after 1 year and 22.1% were lost after 2 years. Treatments included clomiphene, gonadotropins, intrauterine inseminations, in vitro fertilizations, gamete intrafallopian transfer (GIFT), and bromocriptine. Advice, reassurance, counseling and other subjective therapy were not defined as treatment in this analysis.

Results.—Untreated couples were observed for a mean of 13 months, compared with 19 months for treated couples (8 months before and 11 months after treatment). The likelihood of couples receiving treatment increased with longer duration of infertility and longer observation at a clinic. Couples who received treatment also differed from those who did not by being more likely to have had a laparoscopy. The pregnancy rate was 34% among untreated couples and 25% among treated couples. This difference was largely the result of early pregnancies among untreated couples. Among couples who conceived, the mean time to pregnancy was 6 months in untreated and 10 months in treated couples. The cumulative probability of pregnancy during treatment, stratifying for laparoscopy status, was twice as high among treated as among untreated couples. The adjusted relative likelihood of pregnancy for couples treated with clomiphene was 1.9; with IVF or GIFT, 3; with gonadotropins, 1.1; with intrauterine insemination, 1.1; and with bromocriptine, .4. Longer

Duration of Infertility ≤ 36 Months

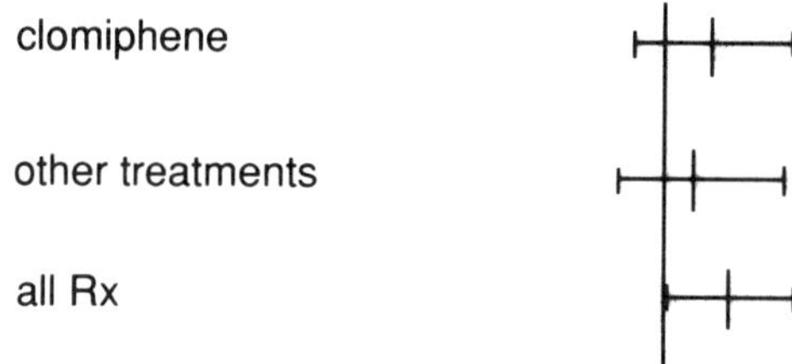

Duration of Infertility > 36 Months

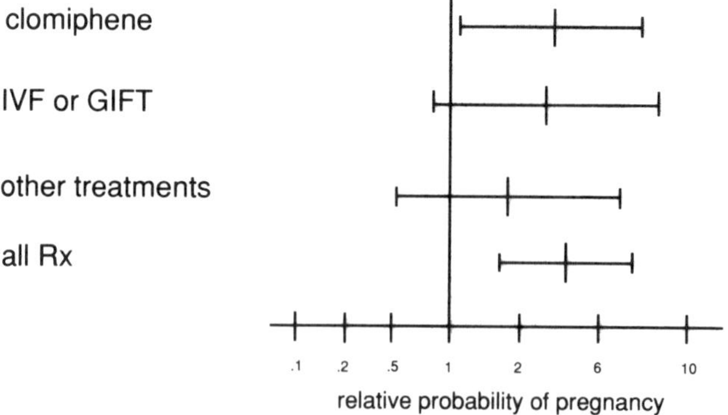

Fig 12–1.—Relative likelihood of pregnancy with clomiphene and other treatments stratified by duration of infertility. *Horizontal bars,* 95% confidence interval. (Courtesy of Collins JA, Milner RA, Rowe TC: *Int J Fertil* 36:140–152, 1991.)

durations of infertility were associated with significantly increased effects of treatment (Fig 12–1).

Conclusions.—As in other studies the treated group comprised a biased selection of couples: those with infertility of longer duration. Statistical correction for this bias resulted in the conclusion that the probability of pregnancy was doubled compared to that in the untreated group. The subgroup most likely to achieve pregnancy included women who had undergone laparoscopy, couples with infertility of more than 3 years' duration, and women receiving their first treatment.

▶ The results of this study are in agreement with the prospective randomized study by Glazener et al. (see the 1991 YEAR BOOK OF INFERTILITY, p 199). Couples with more than 3 years of unexplained infertility have a significantly higher pregnancy rate when treated with clomiphene citrate or other therapy than those not treated. However, it does not appear beneficial to treat women with less than 3 years of unexplained infertility with clomiphene, because pregnancy rates in this series were not significantly different with and without such therapy.—D.R. Mishell, Jr., M.D.

A Controlled Study of Human Chorionic Gonadotrophin Induced Ovulation Versus Urinary Luteinizing Hormone Surge for Timing of Intrauterine Insemination

Martinez AR, Bernadus RE, Voorhorst FJ, Vermeiden JPW, Schoemaker J (Free Univ Hosp, Amsterdam)

Hum Reprod 6:1247–1251, 1991 12–6

Background.—It is not known whether permitting the natural process of maturation to occur, as in luteinizing hormone (LH)-monitored ovulation, improves pregnancy rates compared with insemination after human chorionic gonadotropin (hCG)-induced rupture of the dominant follicle. The results of a controlled study of hCG-induced ovulation vs. urinary LH surge for timing of intrauterine insemination were evaluated.

Methods.—Forty-eight patients, most with unexplained infertility, in intrauterine insemination program were enrolled. All underwent stimulation with clomiphene citrate and were inseminated by random assignment after follicular rupture induced by hCG or after a spontaneous LH surge. Human chorionic gonadotropin was administered when follicles of 18–22 mm in diameter were seen on ultrasound. Intrauterine insemination was done within 37–40 hours afterward. Urinary LH peaks were monitored using a rapid urinary LH test. Intrauterine insemination was done about 22 hours after LH surges were detected.

Results.—The overall pregnancy rates were 9.3% after hCG-induced ovulation and 20.5% after spontaneous ovulation. Midcycle event analysis showed that, based on sonographic criteria, the hCG injection was done significantly earlier in the cycle when compared with the LH surge. Also, the mean diameter of the preovulatory follicles was significantly smaller and insemination was markedly earlier in the hCG-induced cycles.

Conclusions.—A beneficial effect seems to be associated with permitting the natural process of final follicular maturation to occur. Because of the sample size, the 20% overall conception rate resulting from insemination timed after detection of a spontaneous LH surge was not significantly different from 9% rate associated with hCG-induced follicular rupture.

▶ In this study, clomiphene citrate, not human menopausal gonadotropin (hMG), was used to produce ovarian hyperstimulation. As shown in Abstracts 12–4 and 12–5, this method, which does not require daily ultrasound monitoring, when combined with intrauterine insemination results in increased pregnancy rates in couples with unexplained infertility. Performing insemination after a spontaneous LH surge in women treated with clomiphene without hMG may be more successful than administering hCG when the dominant follicle reaches 18 mm. Daily urinary LH testing is certainly more convenient than daily ultrasonographic monitoring of follicular size. It is of interest that the 9% pregnancy rate per cycle after hCG-induced ovulation in this study is similar to the 9% pregnancy rate obtained by Deaton et al. (Abstract 12–4) with the same technique.—D.R. Mishell, Jr., M.D.

Multiple Follicular Recruitment and Intrauterine Insemination Outcomes Compared by Age and Diagnosis

Horbay GLA, Cowell CA, Casper RF (Univ of Toronto; Toronto Hosp, Ont, Canada)

Hum Reprod 6:947–952, 1991 12–7

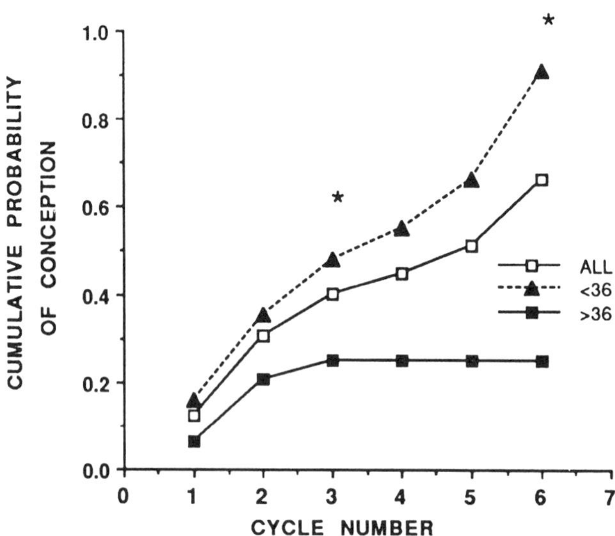

Fig 12–2.—Cumulative probability of conception per MFR-IUI treatment cycle. Derived from life table analysis. (Courtesy of Horbay GLA, Cowell CA, Casper RF: *Hum Reprod* 6:947–952, 1991.)

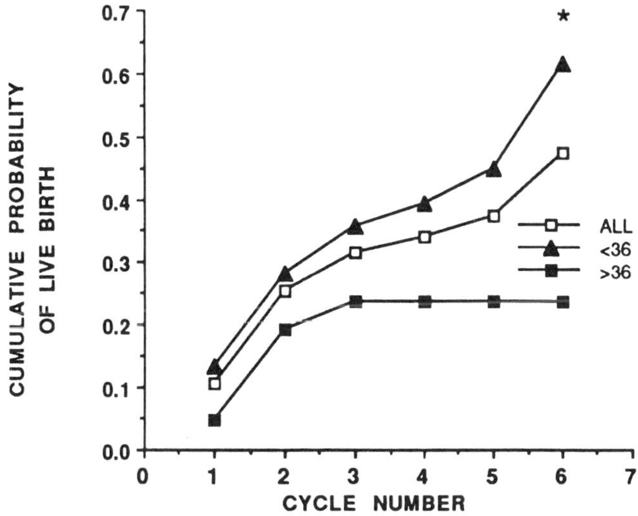

Fig 12–3.—Cumulative probability of live birth per MFR-IUI cycle. Derived from life table analysis. (Courtesy of Horbay GLA, Cowell CA, Casper RF: *Hum Reprod* 6:947–952, 1991.)

Background.—Intrauterine insemination (IUI) of washed semen has been used to treat infertility of various causes with varying results. The outcome of a large IUI plus multiple follicular recruitment (MFR) program in a tertiary care facility was assessed.

Methods.—In all, 190 couples (mean age, 33 years) completed 472 cy-

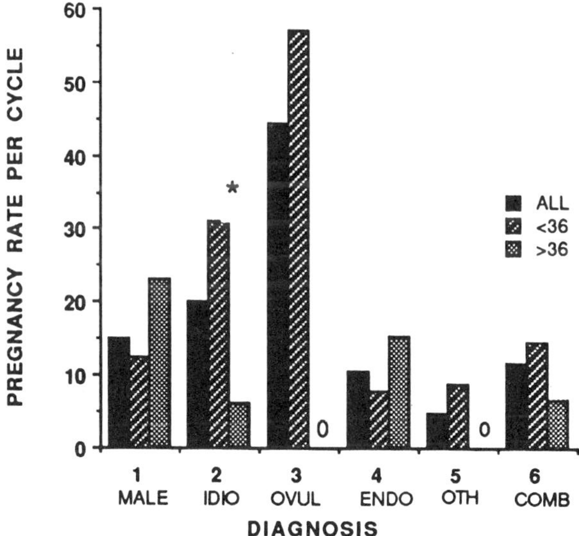

Fig 12–4.—Pregnancy rate per cycle with reference to age (less than age 36 years or age 36 years or older) and diagnosis. *Abbreviations: MALE,* male factor, *IDIO,* idiopathic infertility; *OVUL,* ovulatory disorder; *ENDO,* endometriosis, *OTH,* other; *COMB,* combined factors. (Courtesy of Horbay GLA, Cowell CA, Casper RF: *Hum Reprod* 6:947–952, 1991.)

cles of ovarian MFR and timed IUI in 1988 and 1989. Pure male factor infertility, idiopathic infertility, ovulatory disorder, or other causes of infertility were present. Semen was prepared for IUI by using wash and swim-up methods.

Results.—Pregnancy rates were greater for couples younger than age 36 years. The probability of conceiving after 3 treatment cycles was .402 overall, i.e., .481 for those younger than age 36 years and .252 for those aged 36 years or older. The probability of conceiving for those with male factor was .469, and for those with idiopathic infertility, .411. An age effect was noted only in those with idiopathic infertility (Figs 12–2, 12–3, 12–4).

Conclusions.—Age appears to play a significant role in the ability to conceive after MFR plus IUI. However, pregnancy loss, multiple gestation, and spontaneous pregnancy in nontreatment cycles were unrelated to age. Life-table analyses suggest that patients aged 36 years or older will benefit from a maximum of only 3 MFR plus IUI treatment cycles. Those younger than age 36 years may benefit from up to 4–6 cycles.

▶ Although this study was nonrandomized, it contained a large number of infertile couples and confirmed the effectiveness of ovarian stimulation and washed IUI for the treatment of not only unexplained infertility but also male factor infertility. The interesting but not unexpected conclusions are that pregnancy rates are greater among women younger than age 36 with unexplained infertility than they are in older women, and that there is continued effectiveness in treating these younger women for more than 3 cycles if they do not conceive. If conception fails to occur after 6 cycles of this treatment, in vitro fertilization or gamete intrafallopian transfer can be offered to these couples.—D.R. Mishell, Jr., M.D.

The Value of Menotrophin Treatment for Unexplained Infertility Prior to an In-Vitro Fertilization Attempt

Simon A, Avidan B, Mordel N, Lewin A, Samueloff A, Zajicek G, Schenker JG, Laufer N (Hadassah Univ Hosp, Jerusalem; Hadassah Univ, Jerusalem)

Hum Reprod 6:222–226, 1991 12–8

Purpose and Method.—The efficacy of inducing ovulation with menotropins was compared with that of in vitro fertilization and embryo transfer (IVF-ET) in couples with unexplained infertility for at least 2 years. All women had normal ovulatory cycles. Eighty-seven couples underwent 446 cycles of induction of ovulation with menotropins, and 72 others underwent 108 cycles of IVF-ET. Infertility had lasted longer in those undergoing IVF-ET.

Results.—Comparable pregnancy rates were achieved in the 2 groups on a per patient basis. Similar cumulative pregnancy rates were achieved in 3 cycles of induction of ovulation and 1 cycle of IVF-ET (Fig 12–5). The cumulative live birth rate after 3 cycles of induction of ovulation exceeded that after 1 IVF-ET cycle (Fig 12–6).

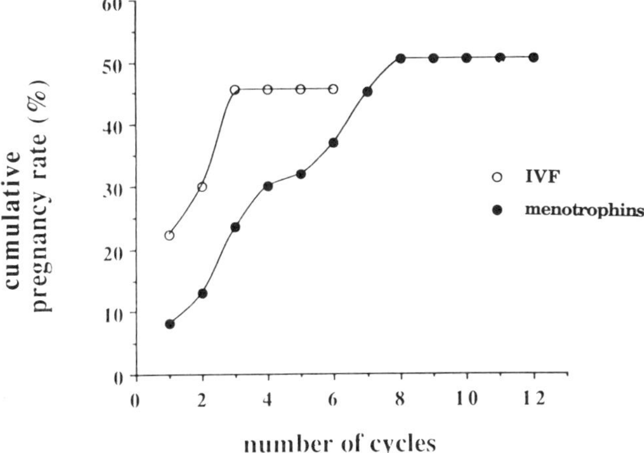

Fig 12–5.—Cumulative pregnancy rates of unexplained infertile patients treated by ovulation induction or in vitro fertilization. (Courtesy of Simon A, Avidan B, Mordel N, et al: *Hum Reprod* 6:222–226, 1991.)

Conclusion.—These results suggest that treatment with menotropin should precede an attempt at IVF in couples with unexplained infertility. In vitro fertilization or a gamete intrafallopian transfer procedure should be attempted if no pregnancy is achieved with 6 or 7 cycles of treatment with menotropin.

▶ It is certainly cost effective and more convenient to administer human menopausal gonadotropin (hMG)-human chorionic gonadotropin (hCG) followed by

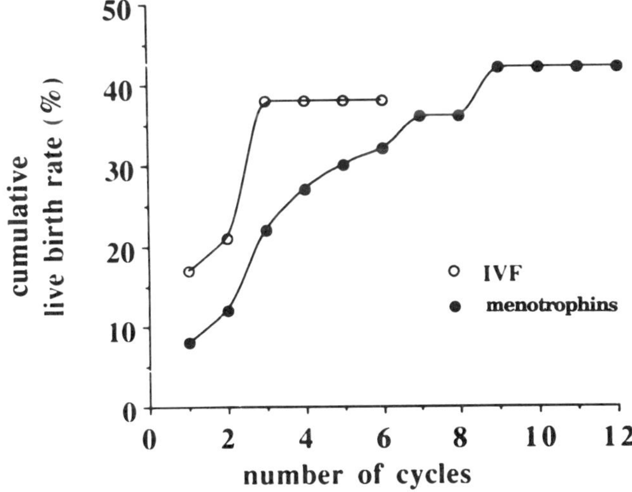

Fig 12–6.—Cumulative live birth rates of unexplained infertile patients treated by ovulation induction or in vitro fertilization. (Courtesy of Simon A, Avidan B, Mordel N, et al: *Hum Reprod* 6:222–226, 1991.)

washed intrauterine insemination (IUI) than to perform IVF or gamete intrafallopian transfer (GIFT). Although this was a retrospective study, the results agree with those reported by others who used similar therapy in couples with unexplained infertility and achieved monthly pregnancy rates of 8% to 20%. Because ovarian ultrasound monitoring is necessary with hMG, and the therapy is expensive for couples with unexplained infertility, we usually try a few cycles of clomiphene, 100 mg a day from cycle days 2–6, followed by washed IUI the day after the spontaneous luteinizing hormone peak. If conception does not occur, a few cycles of hMG-hCG with washed insemination should be tried before proceeding to IVF or GIFT.—D.R. Mishell, Jr., M.D.

A Comparative Analysis of the Cycle Fecundity Rates Associated With Combined Human Menopausal Gonadotropin (hMG) and Intrauterine Insemination (IUI) Versus Either hMG or IUI Alone

Chaffkin LM, Nulsen JC, Luciano AA, Metzger DA (Univ of Connecticut, Farmington)

Fertil Steril 55:252–257, 1991 12–9

Introduction.—Combined treatment with human menopausal gonadotropin (hMG) and intrauterine insemination (IUI) for unexplained infertility is superior to either treatment alone; however, the relative effectiveness of the 2 individual and combined treatments for other causes of infertility is unknown. A retrospective study was done to assess whether cycle fecundity rates were improved with controlled hMG superovulation combined with IUI, and to assess the efficacy of combined therapy in patients in whom previous treatment with either agent alone failed.

Methods.—The records of 322 patients treated with 1 of the 3 regimens over a 3-year period were reviewed. Patients were categorized into 4 infertility subgroups: male factor, with at least 2 semen analyses at least 1 month apart showing less than 20×10^6 sperm per mL, less than 40% motile sperm, and/or less than 40% normal morphology; cervical factor, with poor postcoital test (PCT) and poor cervical mucus, or less than 5 sperm per high-power field; endometriosis, with documented implants; or unexplained infertility of more than 18 months' duration, with documented ovulation, normal semen and normal findings on endometrial biopsy, hysterosalpingography, PCT, and laparoscopy. Timed by the urine luteinizing hormone level, IUI alone was used in 56 patients; hMG superovulation without insemination was used in 131 patients, and combination therapy in 135 patients.

Results.—The IUI-only group included significantly more couples with male factor infertility and fewer couples with endometriosis. No significant differences among the treatment groups were observed for incidence of cervical factor or unexplained infertility. Intrauterine insemination was effective only in couples with cervical or male factor infertility; it was not effective in any couples with both male and cervical factors and pelvic adhesions. AFter 5 cycles of IUI only, the cumulative pregnancy rate was 18% (Fig 12–7). When hMG was given alone, the average cycle fecun-

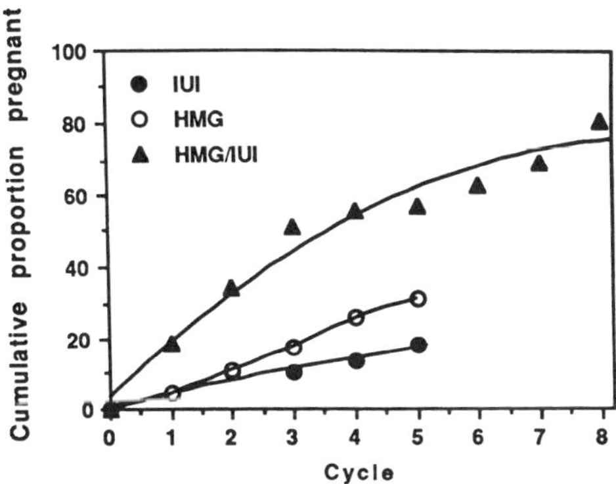

Fig 12–7.—Overall cumulative proportion of pregnant patients comparing hMG, IUI, and combined hMG/IUI therapies. Life table analysis was calculated by the method of Cramer et al., and the curves were fitted by computer analysis of the individual data points. (Courtesy of Chaffkin LM, Nulsen JC, Luciano AA, et al: *Fertil Steril* 55:252–257, 1991.)

dity rate was 6.3%, with a 25.5% pregnancy rate after 4 cycles. Combination therapy resulted in an average cycle fecundity rate of 19.6%, with a 56.8% pregnancy rate after 4 cycles. The cycle fecundity rate was relatively constant for hMG or IUI alone, but it decreased significantly after 3 cycles of combination therapy, explaining the higher pregnancy rate for combination therapy compared to hMG. Among 22 patients who had combination therapy after IUI alone failed there were 7 pregnancies in 40 cycles. Among 29 patients who had combination therapy after hMG alone failed there were 9 pregnancies in 64 cycles. The cumulative pregnancy rate in these groups was similar to that for patients who had combination therapy from the outset.

Conclusion.—Combination therapy with IUI and hMG yields significantly higher cycle fecundity and cumulative pregnancy rates than either method alone. This is true whether the cause of infertility is male factor, cervical factor, or endometriosis, or is unexplained.

▶ Although this study was retrospective and nonrandomized, the high cycle fecundity rate with hMG and IUI, 19.6%, agrees with what other groups have reported previously. A prospective, randomized trial is urgently needed between this approach and the invasive gamete intrafallopian transfer (GIFT) procedure in couples with infertility resulting from causes other than tubal disease. Until that is done, the use of hMG and IUI for at least 4 cycles (cumulative pregnancy rate, 60%) should be offered as an alternative to, or before, GIFT.—D.R. Mishell, Jr., M.D.

Experience With Peritoneal Oocyte and Sperm Transfer as an Outpatient-Based Treatment for Infertility

Sharma V, Campbell S, Pampiglione JS, Riddle A, Mason BA (Hallam Med Centre; King's College School of Medicine and Dentistry, London)

Fertil Steril 55:579–582, 1991 12–10

Introduction.—Several programs now aid in the outpatient treatment of infertility, including intrauterine insemination (IUI), gamete intrafallopian transfer (GIFT), direct intraperitoneal insemination, and peritoneal oocyte and sperm transfer. A large series of peritoneal oocyte and sperm transfer methods using donor [in donor insemination (DI) failure] or partner's semen was evaluated.

Methods.—Patients comprised individuals with unexplained infertility and DI failure who fulfilled specific criteria. The DI failure required at least 6 previous timed inseminations with frozen donor sperm. Each patient had a maximum of 2 stimulated cycles, with ovulation induced by 100 mg of clomiphene citrate from days 2 to 6 of the treatment cycle and human menopausal gonadotropin (hMG). Oocyte retrieval usually was done by the transabdominal route. Up to 4 oocytes and 1 mL of washed sperm solution (4×10^6 motile sperm per mL) were injected into the pouch of Douglas via the aspiration needle.

Findings.—The 59 patients had 81 stimulated cycles for peritoneal oocyte and sperm transfer, with 7 cycles stopped before the surgery because of an inadequate follicular response. Eighteen clinical pregnancies (24%) occurred. Four of 12 patients (33%) became pregnant using their partner's sperm as did 14 of 62 DI-failure patients using donor sperm (23%). The excess oocytes that resulted after 53 peritoneal oocyte and sperm transfers underwent in vitro fertilization, but no differences in pregnancy rates resulted from their use. The 18 pregnancies produced 1 set of triplets, 2 sets of twins, and 13 singleton live births. There were also 1 spontaneous abortion and 1 blighted ovum.

Conclusions.—These results indicate peritoneal oocyte and sperm transfer can work as an outpatient or office-based alternative procedure to the GIFT method. It offers a welcome alternative for patients who do not wish to undergo general anesthesia.

▶ Although the pregnancy rate of 24% per cycle reported with this technique is good, it does not appear to be significantly higher than that occurring with superovulation and intrauterine or intraperitoneal insemination of washed sperm. Whether aspirating the ova and placing them in the peritoneal cavity increases the rate of ovum pickup by the oviduct compared with natural ovulation needs to be established before this unique technique of treating unexplained infertility should be offered to infertile couples.—D.R. Mishell, Jr., M.D.

Transvaginal Intratubal Insemination by Tactile Sensation: A Preliminary Report

Pratt DE, Shangold G, Bieber E, Vignovic E, Barnes R, Schrieber J (Univ of Chicago)

Fertil Steril 56:984–986, 1991 12–11

Background.—Recent studies of ovulation induction with human menopausal gonadotropins (hMG) and intrauterine insemination (IUI) in couples with unexplained infertility have shown pregnancy rates similar to those achieved with laparoscopic gamete intrafallopian transfer

(GIFT). Pregnancies have also resulted from intratubal insemination (ITI) using the laparoscopic approach and a transvaginal approach with ultrasound guidance. The preliminary results of using ITI by transvaginal catheterization of the fallopian tube using fresh and frozen sperm were assessed.

Methods.—Thirty-two women aged 19–24 years underwent transvaginal ITI. Before the procedure patients were stimulated with clomiphene citrate or hMG. Fourteen women were stimulated with clomiphene on days 5–9 of their menstrual cycle. Transvaginal ultrasound and estradiol monitoring was begun on cycle day 13 and continued until at least 1 follicle reached an average diameter of 18 mm and the estradiol level was more than 300 pg/mL. Human chorionic gonadotropin, 10,000 units, was given intramuscularly. Intratubal insemination was done within 34–36 hours after injection of hCG on the dominant follicle side. Eighteen patients were stimulated with hMG beginning on the third day of the cycle. Monitoring began on day 7 and continued until there was at least 1 follicle with a mean diameter of 18 mm, a second with a mean diameter of 16 mm, and a level of estradiol between 750 and 2,000 pg/mL. When these criteria were met, hCG was given and ITI was performed as in the other group.

Results.—Eleven pregnancies occurred after a total of 45 cycles. The pregnancy rate per patient was 34%, and per cycle, 24%. Seven pregnancies resulted during the first ITI cycle and 4 in the second. Six pregnancies occurred with hMG stimulation and 5 during clomiphene-stimulated cycles. Two pregnancies occurred in patients with unexplained infertility, in 3 with ovulatory dysfunction, in 2 with ovulatory dysfunction-male factor, in 2 with male factor only, and in 2 in the frozen donor group; none with unilateral tubal obstruction became pregnant. No ectopic pregnancies or excessive bleeding was associated with the procedure. One patient contracted a severe infection after ITI.

Conclusions.—These preliminary findings show that pregnancies can result from transvaginal ITI. The procedure is easy to perform and requires no analgesia, ultrasound, endoscopic equipment, or fluoroscopy. It may be advantageous compared with IUI because the sperm can be placed in the fallopian tube nearest the ovary with the dominant follicle or with the largest number of mature follicles.

▶ The pregnancy rate of 24% per cycle is identical to that reported in Abstract 12–6 and is similar to the rates achieved by various techniques of sperm transfer after superovulation reported in the European randomized trial (Abstract 12–12). Randomized trials are necessary to determine whether the additional time and effort required to perform direct ITI results in higher pregnancy rates than occur with the simpler technique of IUI.—D.R. Mishell, Jr., M.D.

The ESHRE Multicentre Trial on the Treatment of Unexplained Infertility: A Preliminary Report

Crosignani PG, Walters DE, Soliani A (Univ of Milan, Italy; Cambridge Research Station, Cambridge, England)

Hum Reprod 6:953–958, 1991 12–12

Estimated Mean Pregnancy Rates for 5 Experimental Treatments

Method	Pregnancy rate/cycle First	Second	Combined
IUI	0.271	0.283	0.274
IPI	0.299	0.257	0.270
GIFT	0.284	0.257	0.280
IVF	0.237	0.380	0.257
Superovulation	0.174	0.116	0.152*

Note: Rates derived from statistical analysis.
*Significance probability for comparison superovulation versus remainder was .058.
(Courtesy of Crosignani PG, Walters DE, Soliani A: *Hum Reprod* 6:953–958, 1991.)

Background.—Of an estimated 16% of couples classified as infertile, there is no obvious cause in 10% to 20%. A multicenter study of the treatment of unexplained infertility was done to explore the efficacy of superovulation alone and in combination with intrauterine insemination, intraperitoneal insemination, gamete intrafallopian transfer, or in vitro fertilization.

Methods.—Nineteen European fertility centers in the European Society of Human Reproduction and Embryology participated in this controlled, randomized trial. Each was invited to use 2 of the 5 treatments under study. Individual patients were randomly assigned to a treatment. The patients had more than 36 months of infertility and were younger than age 38 years. They also had normal fallopian tubes and evidence of spontaneous ovulation. Another criterion for study entry was that the male partner have normal fertility.

Results.—By the end of the trial 444 patients had been treated for a total of 649 cycles. Statistical analysis suggested that the pregnancy rate obtained from superovulation alone was inferior to that resulting from superovulation combined with a method of assisted conception. The pregnancy rate associated with each assisted procreation method was much better than various estimates of the spontaneous rates cited in the literature and estimates of the upper limit of the pregnancy rate implied by the pretreatment infertility period (table).

Conclusions.—The use of 1 of the methods of assisted conception enhanced the pregnancy rate beyond that expected from superovulation alone, but there was no evidence that any single individual invasive method was superior. All of the pregnancy rates obtained well exceeded various estimates of spontaneous rates.

▶ The results of these approaches are comparable to those reported in Abstract 12–11. Whether intraperitoneal insemination is better, comparable, or worse than intrauterine insemination after stimulation with human chorionic gonadotropin needs to be studied in a prospective, randomized manner.—D.R. Mishell, Jr., M.D.

A Comparison of Intrauterine Insemination, Intraperitoneal Insemination, and Natural Intercourse in Superovulated Women

Evans J, Wells C, Gregory L, Walker S (Univ Hosp of Wales, Cardiff)

Fertil Steril 56:1183–1187, 1991 12–13

Background.—A simple, safe treatment is needed for couples with unexplained infertility, oligospermia and asthenospermia, cervical mucus hostility, or antisperm antibodies. The results of intrauterine insemination (IUI), intraperitoneal insemination (IPI), and natural intercourse were compared in women receiving comparable ovarian stimulation.

Methods.—Twenty-two couples with unexplained infertility, 22 with oligospermia or asthenospermia, and 12 with antisperm antibodies were recruited. Ovarian stimulation consisted of 100 mg of clomiphene citrate on days 5–9 and 150 IU of human menopausal gonadotropin on days 6, 8, and 10. For continued treatment in that cycle, a maximum of 4 follicles greater than 12 mm was allowed, and at least 1 had to be larger than 16 mm. Those who responded appropriately received 10,000 IU of human chorionic gonadotropin to stimulate maturity of the oocyte and emergence of the corpus luteum. Insemination was done about 42 hours later. Initially, couples were assigned randomly to 1 of the 3 treatments under study. They progressed to the next treatment so that they had 4 cycles of each treatment in rotation.

Results.—Fourteen women became pregnant, for an overall rate of 25%. Seven of them aborted spontaneously. The pregnancy rate per cycle was significantly higher in cycles in which IPI was used, compared with

Overall PR Per Cycle Relating to Type of Treatment in First and Second Part of the Study

Type of treatment	No. of cycles	No. of pregnancies	% Pregnancy/cycle
Natural	63 (90)	2[c] (2)[d]	3.1 (2.2)
IUI	56 (77)	2[c] (2)[e]	3.5 (2.5)
DIPI[f]	84 (130)	10[c] (16)[d,e]	11.9 (12.3)

Notes: Values not in parentheses relate to first part of the study only. Values in parentheses relate to total numbers from the first and second part of the study.

[c]Statistical significance detected when pregnancy occurred after IP insemination compared with pregnancy occurring after natural intercourse and IUI in the first part of the study ($P < .05$).

[d]Statistical significance detected when pregnancies that occur in natural cycles are compared with those that occur after IP insemination in the total numbers from the first and second part of the study ($P < .01$).

[e]Statistical significance detected when pregnancies that occur after IUI are compared with those that occur after IP insemination in the total numbers from the first and second part of the study ($P < .05$).

[f]Intraperitoneal insemination abbreviated DIPI in table.

(Courtesy of Evans J, Wells C, Gregory L, et al: *Fertil Steril* 56:1183–1187, 1991.)

the other 2 methods (table). The pregnancy rate was higher in the group with unexplained infertility, regardless of the method used. The highest pregnancy rate occurred during the cycles in which patients with unexplained infertility underwent IPI, the rate being 17.5%.

Conclusions.—In this series, Pregnancy rates were significantly higher after IPI than after IUI and natural intercourse after superovulation. Pregnancy rates were also higher in patients with unexplained infertility, compared to those with semen factors. Intraperitoneal insemination combined with superovulation appears to be a simple, inexpensive, safe alternative to gamete intrafallopian transfer.

▶ After ovarian hyperstimulation of the woman with unexplained infertility, IPI of washed sperm is being used by several European centers instead of the technique of IUI, which is used widely in the United States. In contrast to the results of the large multicenter study reported in Abstract 12–12, which showed no difference in success rates between the 2 techniques, the results of this randomized trial in one center indicates that IPI results in higher pregnancy rates than IUI or natural intercourse. Obviously, more randomized studies are needed to resolve the different results. Until then, if clinicians do not have good success with IUI of washed sperm, they should consider inseminating the washed sperm into the cul de sac through the vagina wall using a technique similar to culdocentesis.—D.R. Mishell, Jr., M.D.

Pregnancy After Direct Intraperitoneal Insemination

Seracchioli R, Melega C, Maccolini A, Cattoli M, Bulletti C, Bovicelli L, Flamigni C (Univ of Bologna, Bologna, Italy)

Hum Reprod 6:533–536, 1991 12–14

Introduction.—An alternative to gamete intrafallopian transfer (GIFT) is to induce superovulation and then carry out direct intraperitoneal insemination to augment the concentration of motile sperm and bring them closer to the oocytes. This approach was tried in 109 couples whose history of infertility averaged 5.5 years despite multiple attempts at treatment.

Management.—Superovulation was achieved using a combination of purified follicle-stimulating hormone and human menopausal gonadotropin. Semen samples were incubated for 30–45 minutes in Ham's F10 medium before being injected under sterile conditions into the cul de sac via the posterior vaginal fornix. The injection was given about 40 hours after human chorionic gonadotropin. Ultrasonic control was used.

Outcome.—Pregnancy was achieved by 25 of 96 evaluable couples and there were 6 abortions. The pregnancy rate was 20% per cycle and increased with the number of follicles stimulated. It declined with advancing age. Samples that produced pregnancy, were relatively rich in motile spermatozoa.

Discussion.—Direct intraperitoneal insemination and stimulated superovulation provide a cycle fecundity rate comparable to that achieved with GIFT and in vitro fertilization-embryo transfer. Invasive oocyte retrieval is not necessary, and extracorporeal fertilization is avoided. The cost is relatively low.

▶ Several centers in Europe have reported good success with direct intraperitoneal insemination of washed sperm after swim-up separation. Many of the couples in this study had been treated previously with superovulation and intrauterine insemination without conceiving. If prospective, randomized studies confirm the findings reported in this abstract, perhaps the noninvasive technique of intraperitoneal insemination can be used instead of GIFT or in vitro fertilization in infertile women with patent oviducts and no pelvic disease.—D.R. Mishell, Jr., M.D.

Gonadotropin-Releasing Hormone Agonist Improves the Efficiency of Controlled Ovarian Hyperstimulation/Intrauterine Insemination

Gagliardia CL, Emmi AM, Weiss G, Schmidt CL (Univ of Medicine and Dentistry of New Jersey, Newark)

Fertil Steril 55:939–944, 1991 12–15

Introduction.—The addition of a gonadotropin-releasing hormone agonist can improve the quality and quantity of oocytes obtained through controlled ovarian hyperstimulation in in vitro fertilization cycles. It was hypothesized that this improvement may be extended to controlled ovarian hyperstimulation in combination with intrauterine insemination (IUI) cycles.

Study Design.—During an 18-month period, all patients completing a human menopausal gonadotropin (hMG)/IVI cycle (group 1) or a leuprolide acetate (LA)/hMG/IUI cycle (group 2) were assessed for characteristics and outcomes. There were 123 patients in group 1 and 64 in group 2. Patients in group 1 completed 219 cycles and those in group 2, 102 cycles. Twenty-eight patients who did not conceive with hMG/IUI were moved to group 2.

Results.—Patients in group 2 had a significantly greater rate of clinical pregnancies per IUI than did those in group 1 (26.5% and 16%, respectively). Group 1 patients also had a higher live birth per IUI rate, at 21.6% compared with 12.8%. There were no differences in rate of fetal wastage or multiple births.

Conclusion.—The addition of a gonadotropin-releasing hormone agonist to hMG/IUI improved the pregnancy rate in this series of women with recalcitrant infertility.

▶ This study, like most infertility studies, suffers from the problem that it was retrospective and not prospectively randomized. Furthermore, no control group was included; the couples had long-standing infertility, however, and such couples usually resist being part of a control group. Therefore, the conclusions, although worthy of further investigation, cannot be considered definitive. Nevertheless, the 27% pregnancy rate is equivalent to, and the 22% live birth rate higher than, that achieved with 1 or 2 cycles of gamete intrafallopian transfer or in vitro fertilization.—D.R. Mishell, Jr., M.D.

A Novel Superovulation Regimen: Three-Day Gonadotropin-Releasing Hormone Agonist With Overlapping Gonadotropins

Jacobson A, Weckstein L, Galen D, Jacobson J, Milani H (Univ of California, Berkeley)

Fertil Steril 56:1169–1172, 1991 12–16

Background.—Superovulation with gonadotropins, primarily with human menopausal gonadotropin (hMG) especially when combined with intrauterine insemination (IUI), is now an effective alternative to gamete intrafallopian tube transfer and in vitro fertilization for couples with idiopathic or subtle causes of infertility. The results of using leuprolide acetate (LA) for superovulation with gonadotropin in IUI were assessed.

Methods.—Twenty patients with idiopathic or subtle causes of infertility were prospectively randomized to treatment with a regimen of gonadotropin-releasing hormone agonists and gonadotropins. Baseline sonograms were obtained on the second day of the menstrual cycle, and 1 mg of LA was given subcutaneously every day for 3 days if no follicular cysts of more than 15 mm were seen. Human menopausal gonadotropin or follicle-stimulating hormone, 150–225 IU, was given intramuscularly beginning on day 3 for 3–4 days. Doses were adjusted according to patient response to a maximum of 375 IU per day. Levels of estradiol and luteinizing hormone (LH), as well as follicle size, were monitored beginning on day 5 or 6 and every day or every other day thereafter. There were 2 control groups: 1 consisting of 11 patients with similar diagnoses treated at the same time with gonadotropins only, and 1 consisting of 8 patients treated with the new LA and gonadotropin regimen who had immediately previously been given gonadotropins only.

Results.—Among 20 patients in the group given GnRH-a and treated for 24 cycles, 7 conceived. Six had ongoing pregnancies or delivered. In the first control group 11 patients were treated for 13 cycles; 2 became pregnant. In the second control group 8 patients were treated for 9 cycles; 1 conceived, but the pregnancy ended in a spontaneous abortion. The number of premature LH surges and LH surges at good follicular development was significantly less in the LA-treated group than in either of the control groups.

Conclusions.—Three days of LA with overlapping gonadotropin seems to prevent LH surges in superovulation cycles, which may result in good conception rates in a more cost-effective manner. Larger randomized prospective studies are now needed to confirm these findings.

Adjunctive Leuprolide Therapy Does Not Improve Cycle Fecundity in Controlled Ovarian Hyperstimulation and Intrauterine Insemination of Subfertile Women

Dodson WC, Walmer DK, Hughes CL Jr, Yancy SE, Haney AF (Pennsylvania State Univ, Hershey, Pa; Duke Univ, Durham, NC)

Obstet Gynecol 78:187–190, 1991 12–17

Introduction.—Premature luteinization and asynchronous ovarian follicular development occur during controlled ovarian hyperstimulation for intrauterine insemination. These problems are similar to those observed with controlled ovarian hyperstimulation for in vitro fertilization (IVF) and gamete intrafallopian transfer (GIFT). Previous reports have suggested that a higher pregnancy rate per cycle may be associated with the adjunctive use of gonadotropin-releasing hormone agonists (GnRH-a) in IVF and GIFT. Whether adjunctive GnRH-a therapy may have a beneficial effect on cycle quality and fecundity was investigated in subfertile women treated with controlled ovarian hyperstimulation and intrauterine insemination.

Study Design.—In the first cycle of controlled ovarian hyperstimulation and intrauterine insemination, 97 subfertile women were randomly assigned to superovulation treatment with human menopausal gonadotropin (hMG), either with or without leuprolide therapy. A daily dose of 1 mg of leuprolide was given about 4–7 days before the expected onset of the next menstrual period. If pregnancy did not occur during the first cycle, the woman was given the other treatment in the second cycle. No woman received more than 2 cycles of treatment.

Findings.—The leuprolide-treated cycles necessitated a larger amount of hMG and a longer duration of stimulation per cycle, resulting in financial costs that were 40% greater than those in cycles in which no leuprolife therapy was used. The mean estradiol concentration and number of follicles did not differ between the groups, nor did pregnancy rates and cycle fecundity (table).

Clinical Outcome of Superovulation and Intrauterine Insemination

	hMGs	hMGs + leuprolide
Cycles	78	81
Cycles canceled	8 (10%)	9 (11%)
Pregnancies		
Chemical	1	1
Spontaneous abortion	1	1
Ectopic	1	0
Ongoing or delivered	14	7
Cycle fecundity	0.22	0.11
Live births/cycle initiated	0.18	0.09

(Courtesy of Dodson WC, Walmer DK, Hughes CL Jr, et al: *Obstet Gynecol* 78:187–190, 1991.)

Conclusion.—In unselected subfertile women, the adjunctive use of leuprolide for controlled ovarian hyperstimulation and intrauterine insemination does not enhance cycle fecundity.

▶ The results of the small, nonrandomized study by Jacobson et al. (Abstract 12–16) are in agreement with the results reported in Abstract 12–15. However, neither study was prospective nor randomized. In addition, the method of administering the gonadotropin-releasing hormone agonist (GnRH-a) differed in the 2 studies. The prospective, randomized study of the use of hMG with and without a GnRH-a, followed by IUI, performed by Dodson et al., revealed that use of the GnRH-a increased the cost of therapy without increasing cycle fecundability. The data reported in Abstracts 12–15, 12–16, and 12–17 emphasize the absolute necessity to perform prospective, randomized studies for all infertility therapies before concluding that the therapy being advocated is truly effective.—D.R. Mishell, Jr., M.D.

The Gonadotropin-Releasing Hormone Agonist Stimulation Test: A Sensitive Predictor of Performance in the Flare-Up In Vitro Fertilization Cycle

Winslow KL, Oehninger SC, Toner JP, Acosta AA, Brzyski RG, Muasher SJ (Eastern Virginia Med School, Norfolk)

Fertil Steril 56:711–717, 1991 12–18

Objective.—Use of gonadotropin-releasing hormone agonists (GnRH-a) is an established means of initiating ovarian hyperstimulation

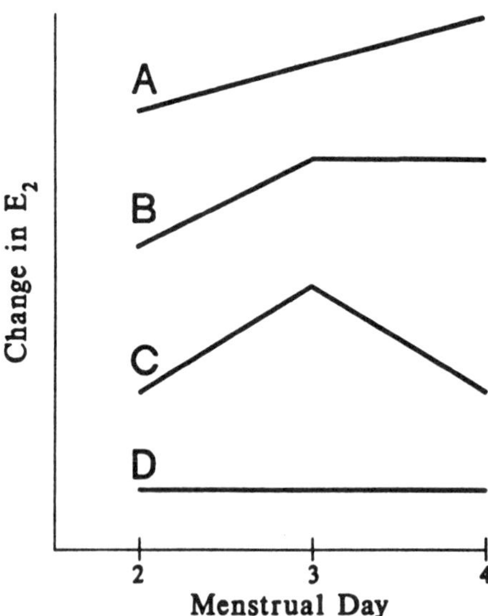

Fig 12–8.—Schematic representation of 4 patterns of E_2 change after administration of 1 mg of LA on days 2, 3, and 4 before initiation of gonadotropin therapy. (Courtesy of Winslow KL, Oehninger SC, Toner JP, et al: *Fertil Steril* 56:711–717, 1991.)

in in vitro fertilization (IVF) cycles. The prognostic value of the early estradiol (E_2) pattern and the initial change in E_2 after administration of a GnRH-a were examined.

Methods.—A prospective group of 228 patients undergoing IVF received stimulation with leuprolide acetate (LA) in a flare-up protocol. In most (72%) of these patients at least 1 attempt at IVF had failed. A dose of 1 mg of LA was given on menstrual days 2, 3, and 4, followed by administration of human menopausal gonadotropin, follicle-stimulating hormone, and human chorionic gonadotropin.

Findings.—Four serum patterns of E_2 were observed on days 2–4 (Fig 12–8). The initial change in E_2, but not in the early E_2 pattern, was predictive of both the number of mature oocytes retrieved and pregnancy. The E_2 pattern was predictive, however, of the amount of gonadotropin needed for stimulation.

Conclusions.—The GnRH-a stimulation test is a simple means of predicting the ovarian response to stimulation in IVF cycles and the chance of pregnancy. Knowledge of the E_2 pattern can help to estimate how many ampules of gonadotropin are required.

▶ I am not sure that we are ready to act on these data yet, although they are of interest. The lack of a good E_2 response after the first few days of GnRH-a therapy, as used in the flare protocol, correlated well with a poor prognosis in terms of ovarian stimulation and, ultimately, embryo transfer. The authors describe 4 patterns of estradiol responses between days 2 and 4 of agonist administration (see Fig 12–8). Seventeen percent of the patients had the A pattern, i.e., increasing levels of E_2 between days 2 and 3 and again on days 3 and 4. Pattern B was the most common, occurring in 43% of the patients; initial doubling was observed between days 2 and 3, then a plateauing of estrogen levels between days 3 and 4. In pattern C, 32% had initial doubling with a falling off of estrogen levels by day 4. Clearly, these first 3 patterns led to reasonable outcomes, the first 2 patterns having the better results. In pattern D, however, which occurred in the minority (only 8%), no E_2 rise whatsoever occurred between days 2 and 4. This obviously resulted in decreased success and a greater gonadotropin requirement.

As stated above, I am not sure that we are ready yet to act on these data, but it is theoretically possible, with our rapid E_2 assays, to be able to acquire this information prospectively. A doubling of E_2 levels between days 2 and 3 would put the patient in a good prognostic category, A pattern of estradiol that does not increase at all might dictate a higher starting dose of gonadotropin on day 4 to compensate for the anticipated lack of response. Again, comparing responses between days 3 and 4, may allow the clinician to determine the possible prognosis.—R.A. Lobo, M.D.

13 Assisted Reproductive Technologies

In Vitro Fertilization-Embryo Transfer (IVF-ET) in the United States: 1989 Results From the IVF-ET Registry

Hartz SC, for the Medical Research International, Society for Assisted Reproductive Technology, American Fertility Society (Med Research Internatl, Burlington, Mass)

Fertil Steril 55:14–23, 1991 13–1

Introduction.—The United States In Vitro Fertilization Registry was established in 1987 to explore the epidemiology of assisted reproductive technology. The growth of this registry is charted in Figure 13–1. Data concerning events reported by member clinics in 1989 were reviewed.

Findings.—A total of 24,183 ovarian stimulation cycles were performed in 17,970 women, resulting in 4,598 clinical pregnancies and 3,472 live births. Twenty heterotopic pregnancies were reported. Embryos were transferred to a host uterus in 198 cycles, 18% of which resulted in pregnancy and 17% in delivery. The clinics performed 18, 211 stimulation cycles for in vitro fertilization (IVF), 85% of which resulted in retrievals and embryo transfers (ET) resulting from 88% of the retrievals. The pregnancy rate after ET was 21% and delivery rate, 16%. A total of 2,876 infants were born. Overall, 24% of pregnancies resulted in multiple delivery. Pregnancy and delivery rates increased with number of embryos transferred, with best results in regimens using gonadotropin-releasing hormone analog; these rates declined with age. Cancellation rates

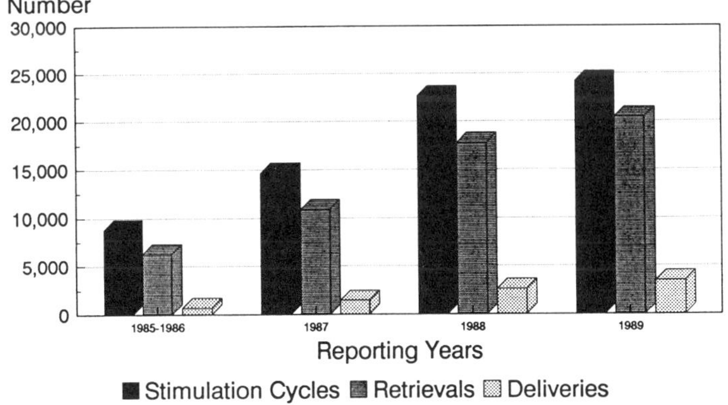

Fig 13–1.—Growth of the United States IVF Registry. (Courtesy of Medical Research International Society for Assisted Reproductive Technology, American Fertility Society: *Fertil Steril* 55:14–23, 1991.)

were between 18% and 20%. Thirty-four chromosomal abnormalities and 28 different congenital malformations were reported. A total of 4,372 stimulation cycles were initiated for gamete intrafallopian transfer (GIFT), with 30% of cycles resulting in pregnancy; the spontaneous abortion rate was 22%. Pregnancy and delivery rates decreased with age. A total of 1,048 stimulation cycles were performed using zygote intrafallopian transfer (ZIFT) or a similar procedure, with 87% resulting in oocyte retrieval and 67% in a transfer cycle. Further, 21% of retrievals resulted in pregnancy and 17% in delivery; 15% of the births were premature. Of 2,124 frozen ET cycles, 11% resulted in pregnancy and 8% in delivery. Of 377 donor transfers in 328 patients, 29% resulted in pregnancy and 21% resulted in delivery.

Discussion.—Reporting clinics increased by 21% during 1988, but the number of stimulation cycles increased by only 7%. The number of assisted reproductive procedures may be leveling off, but the cancellation rate has decreased. Retrieval cycles for IVF, GIFT, and ZIFT increased, and frozen embryo and donor oocyte transfers more than doubled.

▶ These annual surveys provide valuable information for counseling infertile couples who wish to consider the use of assisted reproductive technology. However, those using these surveys must remember that the transmission of data to a national registry is voluntary, not compulsory, and unlike the Internal Revenue Service, reports are not audited for accuracy. Therefore, the final results may be more optimistic than what actually occurs in each IVF clinic. The data provided in the table are particularly important because the etiology of infertility varies. As a result of the low rate of embryo transfer per stimulation cycle in couples with endometrious or male factor infertility, the *delivery* rate per *stimulation* cycle varies from a high of 9% for infertility attributable to tubal disease to a low of 5% for female unexplained infertility, endometriosis, and male factor etiology. In other words, 1 of every 10 women initiating an IVF cycle for tubal blockage will deliver an infant, whereas only 1 in 20 women with the other diagnoses will do so. Patients should be informed of these data at the outset of counseling.—D.R. Mishell, Jr., M.D.

Results of IVF From a Prospective Multicentre Study

Haan G, Bernardus RE, Hollanders JMG, Leerentveld RA, Prak FM, Naaktgeboren N (Univ of Limburg, Maastricht; Free Univ Hosp, Amsterdam; St Radboud Univ Hosp, Nijmegen; Acad Hosp Dijkzigt, Rotterdam; St Elisabeth Hosp, Tilburg; et al, The Netherlands)

Hum Reprod 6:805–810, 1991 13–2

Introduction.—As part of a cost-effectiveness study of in vitro fertilization (IVF) in The Netherlands, the data on clinical results obtained over a predetermined 2-year period were analyzed. Data from all regular IVF treatments performed at 5 major IVF centers were collected prospectively in a uniform way.

Results.—During the 2-year period, 3093 IVF treatments were per-

Estimations for the Logistic Regression Model

	Odds ratio	Reliability interval
Male factor	0.48	0.31 - 0.72
Idiopathic infertility	1.54	1.02 - 2.32
One ovary	0.65	0.50 - 0.85
Woman ≥ 36 years	0.58	0.45 - 0.75
Duration of infertility	0.64	0.52 - 0.79
Treatment episode	0.86	0.77 - 0.95
Constant factor	0.23	0.19 - 0.29

% on-going pregnancy per started cycle: 18.82% (15.61 - 22.50) in the base category

Note: Dependent variable, ongoing pregnancy; explanatory variables, patient characteristics and treatment episode number.

(Courtesy of Haan G, Bernardus RE, Hollanders JMG, et al: *Hum Reprod* 6:805–810, 1991.)

formed at the 5 treatment centers, of which 2466 were continued to follicle aspiration and 2089 to embryo transfer. The clinical pregnancy rate was 20% per embryo transfer and 13.5% per started cycle. Ninety-three clinical pregnancies ended in abortion or ectopic pregnancy. Eighty-four pregnancies were multiple, including 14 triplets and 2 quadruplets. The rate of multiple pregnancy per ongoing pregnancy was significantly related to the number of embryos transferred.

Data Analysis.—Univariate analysis revealed huge differences in results. Those differences were classified and analyzed according to patient characteristics and treatment center. Analysis of the patient characteristics revealed that tubal pathology was present in 90% of all cycles; the tubal factor was the sole indication in almost 75% of patients. Significantly better results were obtained in the group with tubal pathology than in all other categories. When a tubal factor was associated with other factors such as male infertility, older age, or only 1 ovary, however, the favorable prognosis disappeared (table). When the data were analyzed according to treatment center, the average ongoing pregnancy per started IVF treatment was almost 3 times higher in the center with the best results compared with the center having the worst results. But the differences in results at the different treatment centers could not be fully explained. Multivariate analysis confirmed that these differences were attributable primarily to patient characteristics, treatment episode, and treating hospital.

▶ The results of this prospective, multicenter study in which data were accumulated by persons without a vested interest in the individual programs who performed weekly surveys of the centers is probably more valid than the retrospective self-reporting of data to the United States IVF Registry (Abstract 13–1). Thus the article contains much useful data that can be presented to couples contemplating the use of IVF when counseling them regarding pregnancy success. Even though the clinical pregnancy rate for embryo transfer was 20% in this series, the ongoing pregnancy rate per IVF treatment initiated was only half that, 10%. Because couples undergoing IVF wish to have a baby, not just to become pregnant, they should be counseled accordingly.—D.R. Mishell, Jr., M.D.

Age and Pregnancy Rates in In Vitro Fertilization

Dicker D, Goldman JA, Ashkenazi J, Feldberg D, Shelef M, Levy T (Golda Meir Med Ctr, Petah Tikva; Tel-Aviv Univ, Tel-Aviv, Israel)

J In Vitro Fert Embryo Transf 8:141–144, 1991 13–3

Background and Methods.—A woman's age can affect the outcome of in vitro fertilization (IVF). To investigate further, the results of IVF/embryo transfer (ET) were assessed in 1801 women, 301 of whom were aged 40; of this group, 79 were aged at least 43. The ovulation induction protocol consisted of pure follicle-stimulating hormone, human menopausal gonadotropin (hMG), and human chorionic gonadotropin.

Outcome.—Pregnancy rates decreased significantly from an average of 30% per transfer among women younger than age 36 years to about 16% per transfer among women aged 37 years or older. Oocyte production was reduced significantly from 5 at age 30 years or younger to 3 at age 40 years or older; it then decreased to 2 in the 43- to 47-year-old group (table). Women who were 37 years or older required larger amounts of hMG and a longer duration of treatment compared with

In Vitro Fertilization/Embryo Transfer Outcome According to Age

Age (years)	No. patients	No. mean oocytes	Fert. Rate (%)	No. ET	No. clin. preg.	Preg. rate per transfer (%)	No. (%) abortions	No. (%) ect. preg.	No. (%) deliveries
<25	255	5.15	72.2	230	67	29.1	19 (28.4%)	4 (5.9%)	44 (65.7%)
25–26	176	4.98	70.8	145	43	29.6	17 (39.5%)	4 (9.3%)	22 (51.2%)
27–28	154	4.92	71.6	141	44	31.2	18 (40.9%)	4 (9.1%)	22 (50.0%)
29–30	190	4.62	71.3	174	53	30.4	22 (41.5%)	5 (9.4%)	26 (49.1%)
31–32	222	4.65	70.2	203	61	30.0	24 (39.3%)	5 (8.2%)	32 (52.5%)
33–34	186	4.73	70.1	178	54	30.3	21 (38.8%)	5 (9.2%)	28 (52.0%)
35–36	163	4.26	70.6	154	47	30.5	20 (42.5%)	4 (8.5%)	23 (49.0%)
37–38	144	4.02*	72.1	123	21	17.1*	9 (42.8%)	3 (14.3%)	9 (42.9%)
39–40	176	3.73	69.7	167	26	15.6	14** (53.8%)	2 (7.7%)	10** (38.5%)
41–42	89	3.16	69.5	76	12	15.8	8 (66.7%)	1 (8.3%)	3 (25.0%)
43–47	46	2.25	68.1	39	6	15.4	3 (50.0%)	1 (16.6%)	2 (33.4%)
P			NS					NS	
Total	1801			1608	434	26.9%	175 (40.3%)	38 (8.8%)	221 (50.9%)

Abbreviations: fert, fertilization; *ET,* embryo transfer; *clin,* clinical; *preg,* pregnancy; *ect,* ectopic; *NS,* not significant.
$^{*}P < .001$.
$^{**}P < .05$.
(Courtesy of Dicker D, Goldman JA, Ashenkazi J, et al: *J In Vitro Fert Embryo Transf* 8:141–144, 1991.)

younger women. The fertilization rates did not differ among the various age groups, but the reduction in pregnancy rates for a similar number of ETs suggests an alteration in the implantation process. The total pregnancy loss rate increased from between 35% and 50% up to age 36 to between 66% and 75% in the 40 and older age group. Only 2 of the 6 pregnancies in patients older than 43 years proceeded to viability. The pregnancy rates remained stable up to age 38 years and decreased thereafter in those patients with tubal infertility. In the various age groups, pregnancy rates remained stable in those patients with male factor and unexplained infertility; however, the rates decreased in patients 35 or older with endometriosis.

Conclusion.—A woman's age is an important prognostic factor in the success of IVF. The reduction in pregnancy rates is related to a decrease in oocyte production and alteration in implantation.

▶ As women age there is a decrease in conception rates with normal sexual intercourse and, as shown in this report, a similar decrease occurs after superovulation, oocyte retrieval, and IVF/ET. In addition to a decrease in the number of oocytes retrieved per cycle age age 37 (despite an increased amount and duration of hMG therapy), there is also a decreased pregnancy rate per ET. The authors postulate that the latter decrease results from alterations in the process of implantation attributable to aging. However, because of the high pregnancy rates achieved by others after the use of donor oocytes in women in this age group, the decreased pregnancy rate per ET appears to result mainly from problems of embryo quality in older women.—D.R. Mishell, Jr., M.D.

The Predictive Value of Idiopathic Failure to Fertilize on the First In Vitro Fertilization Attempt

Molloy D, Harrison K, Breen T, Hennessey J (Watkins Med Ctr, Brisbane, Queensland, Australia)

Fertil Steril 56:285–289, 1991 13–4

Objective.—Experience in recent years suggests that truly idiopathic failures of fertilization after successful oocyte retrieval are infrequent. The outcome of later treatment cycles was examined in 378 patients in whom oocyte fertilization did not occur in a first treatment cycle. Ninety-four of these patients (25%) had no specific oocyte or sperm defect that could account for the failure.

Observations.—Sixty-four of the 94 study patients sought further treatment, and in 54 of them at least 1 oocyte was fertilized in the next cycle (4 using donor sperm). Fourteen couples had 2 consecutive cycles with failed fertilization using the partner's sperm. Three had successful fertilization with the partner's sperm in a subsequent cycle and another had fertilization with donor sperm. Twenty in vitro fertilization pregnancies occurred with the partner's sperm. The live birth rate per patient with at least 2 treatment cycles was 23%.

Conclusions.—Idiopathic first-cycle fertilization failure is not frequent, but it accounted for a quarter of all couples in whom fertilization did not occur in the primary treatment cycle. Further treatment cycles clearly are warranted; the rate of failure in the second cycle is quite low.

▶ Idiopathic first-cycle in vitro fertilization (IVF) failure is uncommon, occurring in only about 4% of couples initiating an IVF procedure. No sperm or oocyte abnormality or antisperm antibody was found in 25% of these couples whose eggs were not fertilized in the first IVF cycle. The fact that there is a high subsequent pregnancy rate among such couples is useful information when counseling them about proceeding with additional cycles of IVF.—D.R. Mishell, Jr., M.D.

Predictive Value of Pregnancy During Original In Vitro Fertilization Cycle on Implantation and Pregnancy in Subsequent Cryothaw Cycles

Toner JP, Veeck LL, Acosta AA, Muasher SJ (Eastern Virginia Med School, Norfolk)

Fertil Steril 56:505–508, 1991 13–5

Introduction and Method.—The homogeneity of oocyte quality in in vitro fertilization (IVF) is not clear. Therefore, a group of 367 women who had cryopreserved pre-embryos subsequently thawed was studied. The pregnancy and implantation rates of all 367 women were compared in the initial IVF cycle and in subsequent cryothaw cycles.

Results.—Of the 1577 pre-embryos frozen, 1370 (86.7%) were thawed. The pre-embryo survival rate was 64%. Pregnancy in the initial IVF cycle was associated with significantly higher implantation rates and ongoing sac rates in subsequent cryothaw cycles. The differences in sac rates after initial IVF cycles resulted in pregnancy rates that were 50% higher in subsequent cryothaw cycles. Similarly, pregnancy in cryothaw cycles was significantly associated with higher implantation and ongoing sac and clinical pregnancy rates in the initial IVF cycle. These relationships were not affected by certain confounding variables, e.g., patient age, peak estradiol level, number of preovulatry oocytes retrieved or transferred, or pre-embryo survival at thaw.

Conclusion.—Oocytes within a cohort appear to have a similar pregnancy potential.

▶ The fecundability rate (percentage of conception per month in cycles after ovulatory midcycle coitus among fertile couples) in women differs markedly. When fecundability is very low, the couple is designated "infertile" even though, with sufficient time, they may conceive. These couples have a diagnosis of "unexplained infertility." Perhaps one of the reasons for the differences in fecundability rates relates to postfertilization events that occur because of differences in oocyte quality. This paper indicates that if conception occurs after fertilization of one of a cohort of oocytes, this is more likely after fertilization of another of the same cohort than if fertilization did not occur initially.—D.R. Mishell, Jr., M.D.

Selective Drop-Out in Successive In-Vitro Fertilization Attempts: The Pendulum Danger

Haan G, Bernardus RE, Hollanders HMG, Leerentveld BA, Prak FM, Naaktgeboren N (Univ of Limburg, Maastricht; Free Univ Hosp, Amsterdam; St Radboud Univ Hosp, Nijmegen; Academic Hosp Dijkzigt, Rotterdam; St Elizabeth Hosp, Tilburg; et al, The Netherlands)

Hum Reprod 6:939–943, 1991 13–6

Background.—Because in vitro fertilization (IVF) is generally not offered as a single opportunity, information on the success rate of IVF after several treatments seems most useful for patients. The central question is whether success rates decline or increase.

Methods.—Data were collected prospectively concerning all 3092 regular IVF treatments done from 1986 to 1988. In vitro fertilization success rates in the long term were analyzed by calculating a cumulative pregnancy rate after several treatments.

Results.—Outcomes during the IVF treatment phases until embryo transfer were similar, but pregnancy rates declined significantly at higher order attempts. Ongoing rates per started treatment cycle were 12.2% at the first treatment, about 10% at the second and third treatments, and 6.8% at later treatments. Success rates in repeated tries were analyzed in 2 additional ways: by considering couples not treated with IVF before the study period, and by number of attempts made.

Conclusions.—With increasing numbers of treatments, there appears to be a significant decline in the ongoing pregnancy rate per started IVF treatment. After a mean of 2.5 started IVF treatments, 1 in every 4 women achieved an ongoing pregnancy.

► In contrast to most other IVF clinics that report pregnancy rates per follicle aspiration procedure or per embryo transfer, these investigators report ongoing (not clinical) pregnancy rates per started treatment cycle. This method of calculation is a more realistic way to counsel couples embarking on IVF as a method of conceiving. One must remember that success with IVF, as with normal reproduction, declines with age, so this factor needs to be entered into the possibility of conception. It is not surprising that pregnancy rates decline with the number of IVF attempts, as a similar decline occurs in couples attempting to conceive normally. The most fertile conceive earlier, and the least fertile remain attempting to conceive.—D.R. Mishell, Jr., M.D.

The Incidence of Multiple Pregnancy After in Vitro Fertilization and Embryo Transfer, Gamete, or Zygote Intrafallopian Transfer

Bollen N, Tournaye H, Camus M, Devroey P, Staessen C, Van Steirteghem AC (Vrije Universiteit Brussel, Brussels, Belgium)

Fertil Steril 55:314–318, 1991 13–7

Introduction.—Ovarian hyperstimulation has become a standard part of in vitro fertilization and embryo transfer (IVF-ET) procedures, but this method can lead to familial and social problems as well as a poor obstetric outcome. The risk of multiple pregnancies after triple embryo transfers using IVF-ET, gamete intrafallopian transfer (GIFT), or zygote intrafallopian transfer (ZIFT) was assessed retrospectively.

Methods.—In 1987–1988, 2113 oocyte retrievals were performed at a single center. Patients with damage to both fallopian tubes underwent IVF-ET only, whereas those with only 1 healthy tube had either IVF-ET, GIFT, or ZIFT. Ovarian hyperstimulation was induced by human menopausal gonadotropin (hMG) and either clomiphene citrate or gonadotropin-releasing hormone analogs. In the planned IVF-ET treatments, the 3 best embryos were transferred to the uterus. In the GIFT technique, a maximum of 3 mature oocytes were transferred; in the ZIFT procedure, 3 zygotes were transferred.

Results.—For IVF-ET, 1592 pick-ups were performed and 213 pregnancies occurred, of which 33% were multiple pregnancies. There were 6 ectopic pregnancies in this group. The implantation rate after the 3-embryo transfer was 13.7%. Of the 203 GIFT procedures, 37 achieved a clinical pregnancy, 7 of which were multiple. The implantation rate was 8.4% per transferred embryo. Of the 317 pick-ups for the ZIFT procedure, 161 used 3 zygotes that resulted in 62 pregnancies, of which 21 were multiple. The implantation rate was 18.2%.

Conclusion.—The ZIFT procedure led to the highest pregnancy rates without significantly increasing the risk of multiple pregnancy. These results need to be confirmed in a controlled, prospective, clinical trial before the ZIFT technique can be recommended for general use. Physicians should focus on improving embryo quality and uterine receptivity.

▶ Although this study was retrospective, the pregnancy rate was higher with ZIFT than with GIFT or IVF-ET. In contrast to the findings reported by these authors, most other clinics report higher pregnancy rates with GIFT than with IVF-ET. Because GIFT is easier to carry out than ZIFT, the former technique is more commonly performed in the United States. If a prospective study confirms the finding of this retrospective study, (i.e., that ZIFT is more effective than GIFT), there should be greater use of that technique.—D.R. Mishell, Jr., M.D.

Heterotopic Pregnancies After In Vitro Fertilization and Embryo Transfer

Rizk B, Tan SL, Morcos S, Riddle A, Brinsden P, Mason BA, Edwards RG (Bourn Hallam Med Ctr, London)

Am J Obstet Gynecol 164:161–164, 1991 13–8

Background.—The management of combined intrauterine and extrauterine pregnancy is difficult. Measurement of β-human chorionic gonadotropin (β-hCG) levels, which are usually low in ectopic pregnancy, is not helpful in combined pregnancy. Laparotomy during the first trimester may threaten the intrauterine pregnancy. Previous studies have shown that the incidence of combined intrauterine and extrauterine pregnancy is higher after in vitro fertilization and embryo transfer (IVF-ET) than in spontaneous pregnancies.

Findings.—Between 1985 and 1989, a total of 1648 clinical pregnancies resulted from IVF, 17 of which were combined intrauterine and extrauterine. These 17 patients were aged 20–37 years. Nine patients had abdominal pain and vaginal bleeding, 3 had acute surgical abdominal emergencies, and 5 had no symptoms. Ten patients underwent transabdominal ultrasonography, and 5 patients had both transabdominal and transvaginal ultrasound before treatment of the ectopic pregnancy. The ectopic pregnancy ruptured before ultrasound could be done in the other 2 patients.

Outcome.—All 5 patients who had both transabdominal and transvaginal ultrasonography had a correct diagnosis, whereas only 5 of the 10 patients who had transabdominal ultrasonography only had a correct diagnosis. Fourteen of the 17 patients were treated by surgical excision, 2 were treated with local potassium chloride injection into the fetal heart and aspiration of the gestation sac under transvaginal ultrasound guidance, and 1 had spontaneous resolution of the extrauterine gestation sac. Eight patients had spontaneous rupture of the extrauterine gestation sac. Only 1 of the 9 patients with viable intrauterine pregnancies miscarried. The other intrauterine pregnancies progressed uneventfully.

Discussion.—A high index of suspicion of heterotopic pregnancy after IVF-ET is warranted. Transvaginal ultrasonography is superior to transabdominal ultrasonography in the diagnosis of extrauterine pregnancy. Early diagnosis of an ectopic pregnancy after IVF-ET avoids mortality and morbidity and provides an opportunity for more conservative treatment of the ectopic pregnancy in patients with viable intrauterine pregnancies.

▶ The 1% incidence of heterotopic pregnancy after IVF in this study is similar to the rate reported in other centers. The incidence of heterotopic pregnancy after normal conception is between 1/4,000 to 1/7,000 pregnancies. Thus the incidence after IVF with multiple ETs is 30–60 times higher than occurs with unassisted conception. For these reasons, women conceiving after IVF should be monitored carefully with transvaginal ultrasound to determine whether a heterotopic pregnancy is present so that the tubal gestation can be easily removed before enlargement and/or rupture and allow the intrauterine gestation to continue normally.—D.R. Mishell, Jr., M.D.

A Report on 100 Cycles of Oocyte Donations; Factors Affecting the Outcome

Abdalla HI, Baber R, Kirkland A, Leonard T, Power M, Studd JWW (Lister Hosp, London)

Hum Reprod 5:1018–1022, 1990 13–9

Background.—Assisted conception now routinely uses oocyte donation for patients with premature ovarian failure. Results of the first 100 attempted cycles of occyte donation were reviewed and the factors defined that affect the overall pregnancy and patient outcome of these procedures.

Methods.—Eighty-two patients (mean age, 37 years) underwent 100 cycles of ovum donation. Primary ovarian failure in 16 and secondary ovarian failure in 50 patients was the indication for participation in this program. Patients with genetic factors and repeated failure previously with in vitro fertilization-embryo transfer comprised the remainder. All patients received a hormone replacement regimen of estradiol valerate, 2 mg/day for 11 days, and then the addition of norgestrel, .5 mg/day for 10 more days. The gamete intrafallopian transfer (GIFT) or the zygote intrafallopian transfer (ZIFT) techniques were used if the tubes were patent. Otherwise, intrauterine embryo transfer was performed. In asynchronous cycles the embryos were frozen and then transferred at a later cycle. Forty-two of 68 donors, included unpaid volunteers recruited by the patients or through the media.

Results.—A total of 27 pregnancies occurred among the 82 patients, for a 33% success rate per patient and a 27% success rate per cycle. Six patients had a miscarriage between 7 and 14 weeks' gestation, 2 experienced ectopic pregnancies, 12 delivered, and 7 pregnancies were ongoing at the time of this study. The fresh ZIFT pregnancy rate was about 42%; the fresh GIFT rate, 40%; and the frozen ZIFT rate, 30%. The frozen embryo transfer pregnancy rate was 9.7%, whereas the fresh embryo transfer rate was 30%. Intrafallopian transfer produced a significantly higher pregnancy rate than did intrauterine transfer (36% vs. 15%, respectively). Patients with primary ovarian failure had a significantly higher pregnancy rate (50%) than did patients with secondary ovarian failure (18%).

Implications.—These findings indicate that oocyte donation can successfully result in pregnancy and live births while protecting the anonymity of donors. From these data, intrafallopian transfer appears to produce significantly better outcomes than intrauterine transfer of oocytes. Young patients with primary ovarian failure had the best overall results with this method.

▶ This study reports a high success rate of pregnancy after transferring either fresh or frozen embryos fertilized from anonymous oocyte donors in women with ovarian failure as well as those who did not become pregnant after numerous in vitro fertilization or GIFT procedures previously. These authors used both tubal and uterine embryo transfer and noted a higher pregnancy rate with the tubal transfer procedure. The techniques were not randomized, however, and the women with blocked tubes who received uterine embryo transfers were different from the women with patent tubes who received tubal transfer, as reported in Abstract 13–10. In that study, intrauterine transfer of donor embryos in women with ovarian failure was very successful and avoided the necessity of general anesthesia and laparoscopy.—D.R. Mishell, Jr., M.D.

Oocyte and Pre-embryo Donation to Women With Ovarian Failure: An Extended Clinical Trial

Sauer MV, Francis MM, Paulson RJ, Lobo RA, Macaso TM (Univ of Southern California, Los Angeles)

Fertil Steril 55:39–43, 1991 13–10

Introduction.—Oocyte transfer has become an accepted technique, with many methods of oocyte retrieval and pre-embryo donation under development. The authors previously reported their initial study of pre-embryo donation from fertile female oocyte donors to women with ovarian failure. The results of this technique were assessed in 31 consecutive patients.

Methods.—Oocyte donors were younger than 40 years, had proven fertility, and no history of medical or psychiatric disorders. All underwent psychological analysis and testing for syphilis. hepatitis, and HIV. A hormonal regimen was used to synchronize donors and recipients, with the latter group synchronized for embryo transfer (ET) on day 18 of the simulated cycle. All recipients had verified ovarian failure for at least 2 years. All spouses of the recipients underwent HIV testing and semen analysis. Oocyte recovery, fertilization, and ET were performed using standard in vitro fertilization (IVF) methods.

Findings.—Twenty-six women underwent 45 cycles of controlled ovarian hyperstimulation to donate oocytes to 31 infertile couples. The table presents the results of the 45 cycles. A total of 20 clinical pregnancies occurred, with 12 women delivering, 2 having a spontaneous abortion, and 6 pregnancies continuing. The ongoing pregnancy rate per ET

Cumulative Statistics for Cycles Performed Between April 1, 1988 and August 1, 1990

	Statistics
No. of oocytes/recipient	13.7 ± 1.1 (3 to 42)*
Fertilization rate (%)	60 (395 of 657 oocytes)
Transfer cycles/initiated recipient cycles	47 of 49 (96)†
Pre-embryos transferred/ET	4.5 ± .2/couple (1 to 6)†
Implantation rate (%)	21/pre-embryo transferred
Pregnancies/ET (%)	53 (25 of 47)
No. of preclinical	5
No. of clinical	20
No. of ongoing or delivered/ET	18 (38)†; 18 of 31 participants (58)†

*Values are mean ±SEM with ranges in parentheses.
†Numbers in parentheses are percents.
(Courtesy of Sauer MV, Francis MM, Paulson RJ, et al: *Fertil Steril* 55:39–43, 1991.)

procedure was 38%. Fourteen patients (70%) had bleeding in the first trimester. One patient had twins at 27 weeks and 1 had a 1000-g infant that died after 12 hours. One patient had intrauterine fetal demise after 41 weeks' gestation. Ten of the 12 delivered patients had a cesarean section and all breast-fed their infants easily.

Conclusions.—These findings indicate that oocyte and pre-embryo donation is a safe and effective method of managing patients with ovarian failure who wish to become pregnant. The outcome of these patients demonstrated the ease of transfer and goodwill between donors and patients in a nonanonymous setting.

▶ Many centers are now providing oocyte donations for women with ovarian failure who wish to become pregnant. Some use anonymous donors, whereas others, such as this one, use nonanonymous women as donors, especially younger family members who are ovulatory. The high rate of pregnancy success per cycle of ET and low rate of spontaneous abortion indicates that aging of the oocyte is the most common cause of declining fertility rates in women older than age 35.—D.R. Mishell, Jr., M.D.

Consecutive Pregnancies in a Menopausal Woman Following Oocyte Donation

Sauer MV, Paulson RJ (Univ of Southern California, Los Angeles)

Gynecol Obstet Invest 32:118–120, 1991 13–11

Background.—Previously, the successful implementation of a nonanonymous donor oocyte program was announced. Pregnancies occurred in functionally agonadal women aged 24–47 years and were achieved in about 40% of embryo transfer cycles. One oocyte donation recipient older than age 40 years, however, gave birth at term to a stillborn infant. A second ongoing pregnancy was established in this patient.

Case Report.—Woman, gravida 1, para 1, was first seen at age 41 years. She had hypergonadotropic hypogonadism with amenorrhea and a serum level of follicle-stimulating hormone (FSH) exceeding 100 mIU/mL. The patient was synchronized to the menstrual cycle of a gravida 2, para 2, oocyte donor aged 31 years who had controlled ovarian hyperstimulation and transvaginal ultrasound-directed follicle aspiration. The oocytes were fertilized in vitro with the sperm of the patient's husband and 5 embryos were transferred transcervically to the patient. Rising serum β-human chorionic gonadotropin (β-hCG) titers were observed. She had a normal ultrasound examination at 40 weeks' gestation; a nonstress test done at that time was reactive. When she was in early labor, she was told to return once active labor began. About 48 hours later she returned in active labor and was found to have intrauterine fetal demise. About 6 months after this stillbirth the patient returned and requested a second attempt at pregnancy. She was matched to the same donor, and another oocyte donation cycle was done in the identical manner. A preclinical pregnancy occurred, but ended shortly thereafter. About 3 months later the patient wished to try again. The same donor and procedure were used. Five embryos were transferred and serum β-hCG titers rose normally within 9 days and 14 days after transfer. A singleton pregnancy with cardiac activity and embryonic development was noted on ultrasonography at 7 weeks' gestation. The pregnancy continued to progress normally into the third trimester.

Conclusions.—This is believed to be the first published report of consecutive pregnancies in the same woman after oocyte donation. This menopausal patient successfully became pregnant on multiple occasions. Older recipients are likely to be at higher obstetric risk than younger women, however.

▶ Older women who become pregnant as a result of oocyte donation from young women experience the same obstetric problems as do older women who conceive spontaneously, except for a lower incidence of early spontaneous abortion and a lower incidence of chromosomal anomalies in the fetus. Considering the time, effort, and expense necessary to achieve a viable pregnancy after oocyte donation, it would appear prudent not to allow such pregnancies to continue past 40 weeks' gestation. Standard obstetric texts state that a high rate of fetal death occurs in women of advanced reproductive age; therefore, it is reasonable to avoid postterm gestation.—D.R. Mishell, Jr., M.D.

Ureaplasma in Semen and IVF

Montagut JM, Leprêtre S, Degoy J, Rousseau M (Laboratoire de Biologie de la Reproduction; Clinique Saint-Jean Languedoc, Toulouse, France)

Hum Reprod 6:727–729, 1991 13–12

Introduction.—Screening for *Ureaplasma urealyticum* was carried out before in vitro fertilization (IVF) cycles in 306 couples. Males provided first urinary stream and split ejaculate specimens, and urethral and cervical samples were studied. In addition, 70 endometrial biopsy specimens obtained after unsuccessful IVF were examined.

Findings.—In 42% of couples at least 1 partner was *Ureaplasma* positive. About half of the semen infections were associated with male or female urethral infection, and 70% were associated with endocervical infection. After treatment with 200 mg of doxycycline daily for 3 weeks, reinfection or new infection was found chiefly in previously infected couples. Only 1 pregnancy occurred when reinfection by *U. urealyticum* was present on the day of IVF. The rate of pregnancy per embryo transfer was 16% when the semen was infected and 32% in uninfected cases.

Implications.—The presence of *U. urealyticum* appears to affect nidation negatively without influencing fertilization or embryo cleavage rates. Preliminary studies of endometrial biopsy samples may confirm that *U. urealyticum* in semen reflects the severity of sexually transmitted *U. urealyticum* related disease.

▶ One of the vexing problems of IVF procedures is failure of pregnancy to occur after normal fertilization and embryo cleavage. It has been hypothesized that these conception failures result from some factor that interferes with the process of implantation of the normally cleaving embryos into the endometrium. This study supports the possibility that the presence of *U. urealyticum* in the semen reduces the occurrence of implantation of normally cleaving embryos. If confirmed, treatment of the infected male partner may increase the rate of success of IVF procedures.—D.R. Mishell, Jr., M.D.

Positive Chlamydial Serology and Its Effect on Factors Influencing Outcome of IVF Treatment

Driscoll GL, Dodd J, Tyler JPP, Howard B, Lamont B, Coles R (Integrated Fertility Services, Westmead, NSW, Australia)

Aust NZ J Obstet Gynaecol 31:145–147, 1991 13–13

Objective.—The relationship between *Chlamydia trachomatis* and the outcome of in vitro fertilization (IVF) was examined in 49 couples having 98 IVF treatment cycles. The female partner in all couples was seropositive for *C. trachomatis*. In another 176 couples, both partners were seronegative for *C. trachomatis*.

Findings.—Sperm from all 5 men having positive chlamydial titers were able to fertilize their partners' oocytes with a normal cleavage rate. Seropositivity did not influence the overall fertilization rate or the ability of fertilized oocytes to cleave and form 2- or 4-cell embryos. Seven couples with a seropositive female partner (15%) achieved pregnancy. Three aborted spontaneously, and 1 pregnancy was ectopic. In the seronegative group, 16% of the women conceived, 43% of those who conceived aborted, and 1 pregnancy was ectopic.

Conclusions.—The success of IVF was not influenced by exposure to *C. trachomatis* in this study. No only was the IVF pregnancy rate the same as in uninfected couples, but there were no significant differences in fertilization or embryo cleavage rates.

▶ This report indicates that a history of infection by *Chlamydia* in either partner does not influence the results of IVF therapy for infertility. Even though this organism can persist in the tissues of the genital tract for a long time, its possible asymptomatic presence does not influence IVF results.—D.R. Mishell, Jr., M.D.

Relationship Between Sperm Motility Assessed With the Hamilton-Thorn Motility Analyzer and Fertilization Rates In Vitro

Liu DY, Clarke GN, Baker HWG (Univ of Melbourne; Royal Women's Hosp, Melbourne, Vic, Australia)

J Androl 12:231–239, 1991 13–14

Introduction.—Sperm motility is thought to be an important characteristic in assessment of the fertility potential of ejaculated spermatozoa. However, sperm motility examined microscopically does not correlate well with in vivo or in vitro fertilization, except when the spermatozoa are absolutely immotile.

Methods.—To determine which sperm movement characteristics are related to in vitro fertilization rates, semen and swim-up preparations used for in vitro fertilization in 108 patients were analyzed using the Hamilton-Thorn HTM-2030 Motility Analyzer (HTMA) and other sperm tests.

Results.—The correlation between manual and HTMA results for sperm concentration and percentage of motile spermatozoa was highly significant. Compared with semen, the insemination medium after selection of motile spermatozoa by the swim-up method had significantly higher prcentages of motile spermatozoa with average path velocities greater than 10 μm/sec and 20 μm/sec, straight line and curvilinear velocity, linearity, amplitude of lateral head displacement, and beat-cross frequency. According to a nonparametric test, linearity, the percentage of morphologically normal spermatozoa and straight line velocity in semen, and the percentage of motile spermatozoa with average path velocities of greater than 10 μm/sec in both semen and insemination medium were correlated significantly with the in vitro fertilization rate. According to logistic regression analysis, the diagnoses of male infertility and tubal disease, linearity in semen, and the percentage of motile spermatozoa with average path velocities of 10–20 μm/sec in insemination medium correlated significantly with in vitro fertilization rates. None of the other variables was significant. In patients with poor sperm morphology, linearity in semen and the proportion of spermatozoa with normal intact acrosomes in the insemination medium were the only factors significantly associated with in vitro fertilization rates.

Conclusion.—The HTMA measures of linearity in semen and the percentage of motile spermatozoa with average path velocities of 10–20 μm/sec in insemination medium are most significantly related to the fertilization rate in vitro, along with the diagnoses of male infertility and tubal disease. Thus movement characteristics may be important for fertilization in vitro.

▶ Reasonably good correlation between manual and the HTMA results. Probably cost effective when patient volume is high.—C.A. Paulsen, M.D.

Sperm Morphological Assessment Based on Strict Criteria and In-Vitro Fertilization Outcome

Kobayashi T, Jinno M, Sugimura K, Nozawa S, Sugiyama T, Iida E (Keio Univ; Ogikubo Hosp, Tokyo)

Hum Reprod 6:983–986, 1991 13–15

Background.—Sperm morphology assessed by new, strict criteria reportedly is a good predictor of in vitro fertilization (IVF) outcome. The results of an IVF program were analyzed to clarify the relationship between sperm morphology evaluated by modified strict criteria and outcome measured by rates of embryo cleavage, embryo transfer, pregnancy, and miscarriage.

Methods.—Analysis was made of 123 IVF cycles in 115 patients. Samples in which the sperm concentration was less than 15×10^6 or in which motility was less than 30% were not included. The 123 cycles were divided into 3 groups: in 13 the percentage of strictly normal morphology (%SNM) was less than 12%; in 68, %SNM was between 12% and 40%; and in 42, it was equal to or greater than 40%.

Results.—Differences in semen volume and sperm concentrations among the 3 groups were not significant. Motility was significantly higher in the third group, and the cleavage rates per oocyte were significantly higher in the second and third groups. The embryo transfer rate per cycle rose with rising %SNM, although the differences were nonsignificant. The overall pregnancy rate per cycle also increased, as %SNM did; it was significant higher in the group with %SNM of 40% or above. The ongoing pregnancy rate also rose with increasing %SNM, with a significantly higher rate in group 3. The miscarriage rate was lower in the third group than in the second group, but the difference was nonsignificant.

Conclusions.—The rates of embryo transfer, overall pregnancy, and ongoing pregnancy per cycle increase with increasing %SNM when 12% and 40% are the cutoff points. The miscarriage rate also appears to be lower in the highest %SNM group. The cleavage rate per oocyte is higher in the group with %SNM of at least 12% than in the group with %SNM of less than 12%.

▶ One of the variables in this study is the definition of "strictly normal sperm morphology." These investigators used the strict criteria for normality described by Kruger et al. (1), with some modifications of their own. Using these strict definitions they found that the pregnancy rate per IVF treatment cycle correlated directly with the percentage of sperm with normal morphology. A prospective study needs to be undertaken to determine the predictive value of sperm morphology as it relates to the success of IVF.—D.R. Mishell, Jr., M.D.

Reference

1. Kruger TF, et al: *Fertil Steril* 49:112, 1988.

Total Acrosin Activity Correlates With Fertility Potential After Fertilization In Vitro

Tummon IS, Yuzpe AA, Daniel SAJ, Deutsch A (Univ of Western Ontario, London, Ont, Canada; Bioscreen Inc, New York)

Fertil Steril 56:933–938, 1991 13–16

Background.—Acrosin is an acrosomal enzyme that probably is responsible at least in part for sperm binding to the zone and subsequent transit to the oolemma. Sperm that lack acrosin are infertile, and infertile men have lower levels of acrosin than those who are fertile.

Objective.—Acrosin activity in spermatozoa was related to fertility potential after in vitro fertilization (IVF) in 99 women who had a total of 101 retrievals. Mature oocytes were obtained in 89 cycles. A miniature assay was used to estimate total acrosin activity in the semen sample used for IVF.

Findings.—Total acrosin activity in spermatozoa correlated with both the proportion of mature oocytes fertilized and the proportion that were transferred as cleaving embryos. Total acrosin activity was higher in cycles in which at least 1 mature oocyte was fertilized than in cycles where all mature oocytes failed to fertilize.

Conclusions.—Total acrosin activity in spermatozoa correlates with indices of fertility potential after IVF. The determination therefore is a reasonable test of the fertilizing capacity of sperm.

▶ Acrosin determinations may be useful in comparing populations of men, but there is too much overlap for this assay to be useful in the clinic.—C.A. Paulsen, M.D.

Gamete Intrafallopian Transfer: Assessment of the Optimal Number of Oocytes to Transfer

Penzias AS, Berger MJ, Alper MM, Thompson IE, Oskowitz SP (Boston IVF, Brookline, Mass; Beth Israel Hosp, Boston)

Fertil Steril 55:311–313, 1991 13–17

Introduction.—In gamete intrafallopian transfer (GIFT), the optimum number of oocytes that should be transferred is extremely valuable information considering that recent advances in cryopreservation allow excess

Pregnancy Rates for GIFT Cycles as a Function of the Number of Oocytes Transferred

No. of oocytes transferred	No. of GIFT procedures	No. of clinical pregnancies	No. of multiple pregnancies
1	8	1 (12.5)	0 (0.0)
2	36	4 (11.1)	1 (2.8)
3	47	5 (10.6)	1 (2.1)
4	132	29 (22.0)	9 (6.8)
5	51	19 (37.3)	5 (9.8)
6	95	28 (29.5)	6 (6.3)
7	22	8 (36.4)	3 (13.6)
8	8	2 (25.0)	1 (12.5)
Totals	399	96 (24.1)	26 (6.5)

Notes: Values in parentheses are percents.

(Courtesy of Penzias AS, Berger MJ, Alper MM, et al: *Fertil Steril* 55:311–313, 1991.)

oocytes retrived in a given cycle to be fertilized and frozen as embryos for later transfer. In a preliminary study, the results of 399 consecutive GIFT procedures were evaluated retrospectively as a function of the number of oocytes transferred.

Methods.—In nearly all patients, controlled ovarian hyperstimulation with clomiphene citrate or human menopausal gonadotropin followed by intrauterine insemination was performed. One to 8 oocytes with approximately 2×10^5 spermatozoa were placed into either one or both fallopian tubes.

Results.—Clinical pregnancy was achieved in 24% of GIFT procedures. It was 3 times more likely in women who received 4 or more oocytes, compared to those who received 3 or fewer (table). The transfer of 5 oocytes (37%) was marginally better than the transfer of 4 oocytes (22%), but there appeared to be no advantage to the transfer of 6 or more oocytes.

Conclusion.—The optimum number of oocytes that should be transfered with GIFT appears to be 4 or 5. Oocytes in excess of 5 may be used more effectively if they are fertilized and frozen as embryos for later transfer.

▶ This study confirms the findings of the larger study by Craft et al. (1) that for optimal pregnancy rates with the GIFT procedure, it is necessary to transfer at least 4 oocytes. In both studies, pregnancy rates were significantly increased when 4 or more oocytes were transferred, compared with 3 or less. However, the rate of multiple gestation also tripled when 4 or more oocytes were transferred. Patients wishing to have GIFT should be appropriately counseled about this risk.—D.R. Mishell, Jr., M.D.

Reference

1. Craft I, et al: *Lancet* 1:1094, 1988.

Comparison of Unilateral and Bilateral Tubal Transfer in Gamete Intrafallopian Transfer (GIFT)

Penzias AS, Alper MM, Oskowitz SP, Berger MJ, Thompson IE (Beth Israel Hosp, Boston; Boston IVF, Brookline, Mass)

J In Vitro Fert Embryo Transf 8:276–278, 1991 13–18

Background.—Usually, gamete intrafallopian transfer (GIFT) is done by transferring gametes into the ampulla of 1 or both fallopian tubes. This decision is made by the surgeon at laparoscopy and is based on the anatomical findings, number of available oocytes, and the surgeon's judgment. A large series of GIFT procedures was reviewed to evaluate the effects of fallopian tubes on outcome.

Methods.—In an 18-month period, 399 transfers were performed in 335 patients. In each procedure, 1–8 oocytes and about 2×10^5 spermatozoa were placed into 1 or both fallopian tubes by laparoscopic oocyte

Pregnancy Rates in GIFT Cycles as a Function of Unilateral or Bilateral Tubal Transfer

	Transfers	Clinical pregnancies	Multiple pregnancies
Unilateral	113	34 (25.6%)†, *	10 (29.4%)†
Bilateral	266	62 (23.3%)††	16 (25.8%)††
Total	399	96 (24.1%)	26 (27.1%)

*No significant difference ($P > .05$) between superscript† and superscript‡.
(Courtesy of Penzias AS, Alper MM, Oskowitz SP, et al: *J In Vitro Fert Embryo Transf* 8:276–278, 1991.)

retrieval and tubal cannulation. There were 133 unilateral transfers and 266 bilateral transfers.

Results.—Of 586 GIFT cycles, 187 were cancelled. The pregnancy rate was 25.6% after unilateral transfer and 23.3% after bilateral transfer, not a significant difference (table). Unilateral transfer of 4 oocytes appeared to have a significant advantage, but the biological significance of that finding was questionable. There were 5 ectopic pregnancies, but they were evenly distributed.

Conclusions.—In GIFT, unilateral vs. bilateral fallopian tube transfer makes no difference in outcome. Thus, although the outcome is no better with the use of 1 tube rather than 2, it is easier to use 1. The clinician should always use the more "normal" tube, avoiding those with peritubular adhesions. Either tube may be used when both are normal.

▶ It is technically easier to transfer gametes into 1 oviduct than into both, and this report indicates that there is no difference in pregnancy rates whether gametes were transferred into 1 or both oviducts. Some clinicians suggest using both oviducts when 4 or more oocytes are available to transfer, and 1 oviduct with 3 or less oocytes. Whether differences in pregnancy rates actually occur when 1 or more oviducts are used can be determined only in a randomized, prospective manner. Such a technique was not used in this retrospective analysis.—D.R. Mishell, Jr., M.D.

Gamete Intrafallopian Transfer By Hysteroscopy as an Alternative Treatment for Infertility

Possati G, Pareschi A, Seracchioli R, Maccolini A, Melega C, Flamigni C (Univ of Bologna, Bologna, Italy)

Fertil Steril 56:496–499, 1991 13–19

Objective.—The efficacy and safety of hysteroscopic cannulation of the fallopian tubes for gamete intrafallopian transfer (GIFT) were studied.

Procedure.—A group of 26 women aged 21–41 years was treated during a 6-month period. The causes of infertility included terminal tubal damage, male factors, unexplained factors, and endometriosis. Those patients with uterine tubal ostia unsuitable for gamete transfer or cervical incontinence were excluded. All of the procedures were performed without hospitalization and general anesthesia. Ovulation was induced, and oocyte retrieval was performed by transvaginal ultrasonically guided puncture. Gamete transfer was performed with CO_2 hysteroscopic visualization using a flexible endoscopic catheter put through the operating channel. The swim-up method was used to retrieve motile sperm.

Outcome.—The mean number of oocytes retrieved per cycle was 4.8, and the mean number of mature oocytes transferred per hysteroscopic GIFT was 3.7. Only 1 tube was used for hysteroscopic GIFT. There were 7 clinical pregnancies, for a pregnancy rate of 25.9% per cycle. Two of the patients aborted during the first weeks of pregnancy, but none of the patients had an ectopic pregnancy. The procedure was well accepted and patients reported only low distress.

Conclusion.—Hysteroscopic GIFT is a safe and effective noninvasive alternative for the treatment of infertility.

▶ The major disadvantage of GIFT, as now performed, is the necessity for general anesthesia and laparoscopy. The technique of aspirating oocytes by transvaginally placed needles under ultrasonic guidance is well established. The technique of cannulating the oviduct with a flexible catheter placed through the endometrial cavity under hysteroscopic visualization is being performed in only a few centers. However, if the results of this study can be repeated elsewhere, the technique will markedly reduce the cost and increase the safety of performing GIFT, because laparoscopy and general anesthesia can be avoided.—D.R. Mishell, Jr., M.D.

Ultrasound-Guided Embryo Transfer: A Controlled Trial

Hurley VA, Osborn JC, Leoni, MA, Leeton J (Epworth Hosp, Melbourne, Vic, Australia)

Fertil Steril 55:559–562, 1991 13–20

Background.—Most failures in human in vitro fertilization (IVF) procedures appear after normal embryo transfer (ET) to the uterus at an established time in the early luteal phase of the menstrual cycle. Ultrasound represents the major means of coordinating IVF-ET programs. The results of a controlled trial of transvaginal ultrasound guidance for ET were reviewed to evaluate the accuracy of clinical judgment for this procedure and whether ultrasound guidance can improve pregnancy rates.

Methods.—Ninety-four patients participated in the IVF-ET program between October 1988 and March 1989. Controls included a group of 246 matched patients from this same time period. Patients underwent ultrasound guidance unanesthetized and without premedication.

Technique.—The inner transfer catheter is inserted up to the uterine fundus by feel, followed by reinsertion of the ultrasound probe. After the transfer catheter is identified in the uterine cavity, it is moved to within 1 cm of the fundal limit of the uterine cavity. At this point, the embryo(s) are introduced via injection of 30 μL of culture medium containing the embryo(s). The catheter is removed and the patient monitored by ultrasound to insure that the transferred embryos remained at the location.

Results.—In 8 of the 94 patients, the transfer catheter and embryos could not be seen after insertion. Therefore, these embryos were considered not correctly placed. The catheter insertion was then repeated. No pregnancies occurred in these 8 patients. In 12 patients the tip of the catheter was placed in the lower part of the uterus when it was thought to be in the fundus. The pregnancy rate in the patients having ultrasound-guided transfer was 20.2%, whereas controls had a 17.5% pregnancy rate. The difference was not significant overall. For a single ET, however, those having ultrasound-guided transfer had a significantly greater increase in pregnancy rate than did controls.

Implications.—The patients and their partners reacted positively to visualization of the ultrasound-guided transfer process. The patients experienced less anxiety, allowing an easier transfer procedure. Clinical operators also demonstrated a high acceptance of ultrasound guidance of ET.

▶ It is interesting that several times when the operator thought the tip of the transfer catheter was in the fundus, ultrasonographic visualization found it to be in the lower uterine segment. Ultrasonographic visualization is certainly a simple technique to master and should not increase the expense of IVF because ultrasound equipment is available in all IVF labs. Whether consistent high fundal placement of embryos increases pregnancy rates after ET remains to be determined.—D.R. Mishell, Jr., M.D.

A Controlled Study of Gonadotropin-Releasing Hormone Agonist (Buserelin Acetate) for Folliculogenesis in Routine In Vitro Fertilization Patients

Polson DW, Wood C, MacLachlan V, Healy DL, Krapez JA (Infertility Med Ctr, Epworth Hosp, Richmond, Vic, Australia)

Fertil Steril 56:509–514, 1991 13–21

Objective.—A prospective, randomized study was undertaken to determine whether gonadotropin-releasing hormone agonist (GnRH-a) and gonadotropin therapy can improve folliculogenesis and pregnancy rates in women with previously satisfactory responses to clomiphene citrate and human menopausal gonadotropin (hMG).

Treatment.—A group of 157 women with tubal or idiopathic infertility was assigned to receive treatment with either hMG alone or with 600 μg or 1,200 μg of the GnRH-a buserelin acetate plus hMG per day. Buserelin acetate treatment was begun on day 3 of the menstrual cycle.

Outcome.—Pretreatment with buserelin acetate significantly increased the pregnancy rate per treatment cycle, compared with hMG alone. There was no difference in the pregnancy rates between the 2 doses of buserelin acetate. Of the hMG cycles, 27% were abandoned, usually because of a premature luteinizing hormone (LH) surge; however, only 6% of the buserelin acetate cycles were abandoned and none because of an

LH surge. Pretreatment with buserelin acetate significantly increased the duration and dosage of hMG, compared with hMG alone. The number of oocytes retrieved and the fertilization rates were similar between groups, despite significantly lower serum estradiol concentrations in buserelin acetate cycles.

Conclusion.—Pretreatment with the GnRH-a buserelin acetate increases the pregnancy rate per treatment cycle because of a significant reduction in the number of abandoned cycles rather than any improvement in folliculogenesis. The higher pregnancy rate is achieved at the expense of a longer duration of stimulation and a higher dosage of hMG. In view of these findings, the routine use of GnRH-a in in vitro fertilization programs must be questioned.

Comparison of Ovarian Stimulation Regimens for In Vitro Fertilization (IVF) With and Without a Gonadotropin-Releasing Hormone (GnRH) Agonist: Results of a Randomized Study

van de Berg-Helder A, Helmerhorst FM, Blankhart A, Brand R, Waegemaekers C, Naaktgeborne N (Univ Hosp Leiden, Leiden, The Netherlands)

J In Vitro Fertil Embryo Transf 7:358–362, 1990 13–22

Introduction.—Gonadotropin-releasing hormone agonists (GnRH-a) are sometimes used to diminish cancellation rates caused by a premature endogenous luteinizing hormone (LH) surge or poor ovarian response. Three regimens for stimulation of follicular growth for in vitro fertilization were compared, 2 of which included buserelin treatment.

Methods.—Women with tubal infertility were randomized into 3 groups: group I received conventional treatment with human menopausal gonadotropin (hMG) alone; group II was given hMG shortly after the LH surge caused by a GnRH-a; and group III was given hMG when they achieved a hypogonadotropic state after long-term treatment with buserelin. The latter drug was given in a dose of 200 μg intranasally 3 times daily. The average numbers of embryos per transfer were 2.5 in group I, 2.9 in group II, and 2.6 in group III.

Results.—Group I included 52 cycles, of which 9 were cancelled; group II, 51 cycles, of which 3 were cancelled; and group III, 50 cycles, of which 11 were cancelled. The average length of hMG treatment was 8 days in groups I and II and 10 days in group III. The average number of hMG ampules used was 10 in group I, 17 in group II, and 26 in group III. There were no differences in number of oocytes retrieved or fertilization rates. Pregnancy rates were 7.7% in group I, 19.6% in group II and 12% in group III.

Conclusions.—Patients treated with buserelin from the first day of hMG stimulation to the day of human chorionic gonadotropin administration have a higher pregnancy rate per cycle than those stimulated with hMG without buserelin. There is no difference in the take-home infant rate per cycle in these groups. Buserelin treatment is effective in preventing the premature onset of the LH surge.

▶ The results of the randomized studies of IVF, reviewed in Abstracts 13–21 and 13–22, in patients with either blocked oviducts or a previous satisfactory response to clomiphene citrate and hMG indicate that the use of a GnRH-a does not significantly increase the number of oocytes retrieved or fertilization rates. Use of the agonists increases the pregnancy rate per initiated treatment cycle because these drugs decrease the number of cancelled cycles as the result of a premature LH surge. However, use of the agonist increases the expense of IVF because of the need for a higher dosage and duration of treatment with hMG. Routine use of agonist therapy in women who respond satisfactory to hMG alone is probably unnecessary.—D.R. Mishell, Jr., M.D.

The Use of the GnRH Analogue Buserelin for IVF: Does It Improve Fertility?

Shelton K, Fishel S, Jackson P, Webster J, Faratian B, Johnson J (AMI Park Hosp; Queen's Med Ctr, Nottingham, England)

Br J Obstet Gynaecol 98:544–549, 1991 13–23

Background.—Gonadotropin-releasng hormone in the form of its analogue buserelin is increasingly used in conjunction with human menopausal gonadotropin (hMG) for in vitro fertilization. The agonist is able to recruit large numbers of follicles while eliminating adversely high luteinizing hormone (LH) levels and the spontaneous LH surge.

Objective.—The effects of a brief course of buserelin and hMG were examined in a prospective series of 373 infertile couples. The women were younger than 46 years of age and had normal ovulatory cycles. Clomiphene was given on cycle days 2–6 with hMG from days 5 onward in 151 instances. In the other 222 couples, buserelin was given from day 1 to day 3 of the menstrual cycle, and hMG from day 2 onward. The dose of buserelin was 500 μg.

Observations.—More women given buserelin/hMG treatment were discharged because they failed to respond and fewer because of a poor or inappropriate response. Oocyte recovery and embryo transfer were possible in similar proportions of the 2 groups. Women given clomiphene had higher plasma levels of estradiol-17 and progesterone than the others, as well as higher plasma LH levels. Pregnancy occurred in 38% of the group given buserelin/hMG and in 35% of the group given clomiphene/hMG. Miscarriages, multiple pregnancies, and live deliveries were comparably frequent in the 2 groups.

Conclusion.—Given adequate follicular-phase management, the chance of pregnancy is not improved by short-term buserelin/hMG treatment. The risk of hyperstimulation has prompted the return to milder stimulation using clomiphene and hMG in women with normal cycles.

▶ This study shows that a short course of a GnRH agonist was ineffective in producing higher rates of fertilization, as well as pregnancy, among a group of ovulatory women.—D.R. Mishell, Jr., M.D.

Early Pituitary Densensitization and Ovarian Suppression With Leuprolide Acetate Is Associated With In Vitro Fertilization-Embryo Transfer Success

Seifer DB, Thornton KL, DeCherney AH, Lavy G (Yale Univ)
Fertil Steril 56:500–504, 1991 13–24

Introduction.—The use of gonadotropin-releasing hormone agonists enhances the efficiency of in vitro fertilization-embryo transfer (IVF-ET). A retrospective study was conducted to determine whether the timing of the onset of pituitary desensitization and ovarian suppression using follicular-phase leuprolide acetate (LA) was associated with IVF-ET success for pregnancy.

Treatment.—In preparation for 80 cycles of IVF-ET, 78 patients received LA on day 1 of their menstrual cycle. Controlled ovarian hyperstimulation was started after satisfactory ovarian suppression was achieved after 10 days of LA, with serum estradiol (E_2) levels <40 pg/mL (group 1), whereas LA was continued for 1–3 weeks in those without ovarian suppression at 10 days (group 2). The mean estradiol (E_2) response, ampules of human menopausal gonadotropin (hCG), cancellation rates, number of oocytes retrieved, fertilization rates, and pregnancy rates per cycle were compared between groups.

Results.—After 11 days of LA, 47 cycles (59%) were suppressed (group 1); 33(41%) cycles were not adequately suppressed, requiring a mean of 9 additional days to achieve suppression (group 2). The number of ampules of hCG and the number of oocytes retrieved did not differ between the 2 groups. Compared with group 2 patients, group 1 patients had a higher E_2 response on the day of hCG administration, greater fertilization rates, higher pregnancy rates per cycle (34% vs. 12%), and a trend toward fewer cancellations before transfer.

Conclusion.—Women in whom pituitary desensitization and ovarian suppression are achieved within 11 days of initiating LA appear to have a more favorable outcome for IVF-ET than those in whom desensitization and suppression do not occur within this time.

▶ When a gonadotropin-releasing hormone agonist is given in conjunction with human menopausal gonadotropin for ovarian hyperstimulation before IVF, this study shows that a lesser amount of agonist is better than a greater amount. Studies should be performed to help clarify the mechanism responsible for this finding.—D.R. Mishell, Jr., M.D.

Serum Progesterone Levels Predict Success of In Vitro Fertilization/Embryo Transfer in Patients Stimulated With Leuprolide Acetate and Human Menopausal Gonadotropins

Silverberg KM, Burns WN, Olive DL, Riehl RM, Schenken RS (Univ of Texas, San Antonio)
J Clin Endocrinol Metab 73:797–803, 1991 13–25

Purpose.—Reportedly, serum progesterone (P_4) levels of more than 2.86 nmol/L on the day of human chorionic gonadotropin (hCG) administration are associated with decreased pregnancy rates in women undergoing in vitro fertilization/embryo transfer (IVF-ET). The relationship between elevated P_4 levels and IVF-ET cycle outcomes was further examined in 115 patients.

Methods.—The patients underwent ovarian stimulation for IVF-ET with midluteal leuprolide acetate and human menopausal gonadotropins (hMG). All were given leuprolide acetate beginning 10 days after spontaneous ovulation. Cycle outcome was correlated retrospectively with P_4 levels on the day of hCG administration.

Results.—Two patients had their stimulations canceled. Uterine transfer of pronuclear stage embryos was performed in 109 of the remaining 113 patients (96.5%) 1 day after oocyte retrieval, and 26 of them (23.9%) subsequently had positive serum pregnancy tests. The clinical pregnancy rate was 18.3%, and the delivered pregnancy rate was 15.6%. During the same period, 42 patients underwent frozen ET with an ongoing/delivered pregnancy rate of 9.5%. Two critical breakpoints in serum P_4 levels on the day of hCG administration were identified, 1.27 nmol/L and 2.86 nmol/L. When patients were divided into 3 groups according to their P_4 levels, clinical pregnancy was found to occur in 9 of 18 patients with P_4 levels of less than 1.27 nmol/L, 11 of 18 patients with P_4 levels of 1.27–2.86 nmol/L, and in none of 14 patients with P_4 levels of more than 2.86 nmol/L (table). However, 2 patients with P_4 levels of more than 2.86 nmol/L subsequently conceived viable pregnancies with oocytes obtained from an elevated P_4 cycle, indicating that the adverse effect of P_4 is not exclusively on the oocyte. The number of oocytes retrieved per patient was significantly correlated with serum P_4 levels. There was no difference in either the number or the quality of oocytes retrieved from patients with increased P_4 levels, but both the number of oocytes retrieved and the number of mature oocytes recovered from patients with P_4 levels of less than 1.27 nmol/L were significantly lower than in those with increased P_4 levels.

Conclusion.—Even modest increases in serum P_4 levels are associated

Pregnancy Rate and Outcome by Serum P_4 Level on the Day of hCG Administration

	Group I, $P_4 \leq 1.27$ nmol/L (0.4 ng/mL)	Group II, $1.27 < P_4 < 2.86$ nmol/L	Group III, $P_4 \geq 2.86$ nmol/L (0.9 ng/mL)
No. of patients	18	81	14
No. of patients receiving ET	17	76	14
No. with positive hCG/ET (%)	9 (52.9)^{a,b}	17 (22.4)^{a,c}	$0^{b,c}$
No. of clinical pregnancies/ET (%)	9 (52.9)^{d,e}	11 (14.5)^{d,f}	$0^{e,f}$
Ongoing/delivered pregnancies/ET (%)	7 (41.2)^{g,h}	10 (13.2)^{g,i}	$0^{h,i}$

$^{a,g,h}P \leq .01$.
$^{b,d,e}P = .001$.
$^{c,f,i}P$ = NS.

(Courtesy of Silverberg KM, Burns WN, Olive DL, et al: *J Clin Endocrinol Metab* 73:797–803, 1991.)

with reduced pregnancy rates in IVF-ET cycles. However, the mechanism may not involve poor oocyte quality exclusively.

▶ This is now the second paper to indicate that elevated circulating progesterone levels on the day of hCG administration are associated with a poor pregnancy rate after IVF-ET, despite the fact that more oocytes are retrieved per patient and more are fertilized among women with the highest progesterone levels. The association of elevated progesterone levels and a reduced pregnancy rate may be linked to poor embryo quality or diminished receptiveness of the endometrium.—D.R. Mishell, Jr., M.D.

Co-treatment With Growth Hormone, After Pituitary Suppression, for Ovarian Stimulation in In Vitro Fertilization: A Randomized, Double-Blind, Placebo-Control Trial

Owen EJ, Ostergaard H, Shoham Z, Jacobs HS, Mason BA (Univ College and Middlesex Hosp, London; Hallam Med Ctr, London; Novo Nordisk A/S, Denmark)

Fertil Steril 56:1104–1110, 1991 13–26

Background.—Co-treatment with growth hormone (GH) can improve the ovarian response to gonadotropins in patients with hypogonadotropic hypogonadism and in those with polycystic ovaries. Whether co-treatment with GH in in vitro fertilization cycles after gonadotropin-releasng hormone analog (GnRH-a) treatment would yield better results than co-treatment with placebo, as found previously in patients with hypogonadotropic hypogonadism was determined.

Methods.—The study subjects were 25 patients who had in vitro fertilization and had responded suboptimally to GnRH-a in a previous treatment cycle. Eighteen patients had ultrasound findings of polycystic ovaries. The main outcome measures were the amount of gonadotropin used, development of follicles of 14 mm or greater, and number of oocytes collected, fertilized, cleaved, and replaced, as well as insulin-like growth factor I (IGF-I) levels in the serum and follicular fluid.

Results.—Co-treatment with GH produced a significant decrease in the amount of gonadotropins required. More follicles developed and more oocytes were collected, fertilized, and cleaved in patients with polycystic ovaries. Significantly greater follicular fluid IGF-I levels were found in patients receiving GH co-treatment compared with those given placebo.

Conclusions.—There may be a place for biosynthetic GH treatment in selected in vitro fertilization cycles after pituitary suppression.

Co-Treatment With Growth Hormone of Suboptimal Responders in IVF-ET

Owen EJ, WEst C, Mason BA, Jacobs HS (Middlesex Hosp, London; Hallam Med Ctr, London)

Hum Reprod 6:524–528, 1991 13–27

Introduction.—Several growth factors influence the ovarian response to gonadotropin. The interaction of growth hormone (GH) in the ovarian response to clomiphene and gonadotropins used for in vitro fertilization and embryo transfer (IVF-ET), was examined.

Patients.—Twenty women who had failed to respond optimally to clomiphene and gonadotropin stimulation received intramuscular injections of 24 IU of GH or placebo on alternate days, along with the same daily dose of gonadotropin. The most common indication for IVF-ET was tubal damage, but 6 women had unexplained infertility. Infertility had been present for a median of 5.5 years.

Outcome.—There was no overall improvement in ovarian responses to stimulation with GH treatment, although more follicles tended to develop. In women with polycystic ovaries, however, more oocytes were collected and urinary estrogen production was higher after GH treatment. Treatment with GH caused no adverse effects. Serum estradiol and follicle-stimulating hormone levels were similar in GH-augmented and placebo cycles.

Conclusions.—The use of GH in conjunction with conventional ovarian stimulation may be worthwhile in women with ultrasound-confirmed polycystic ovaries who fail to respond optimally to standard treatment. Co-treatment with GH appears to be safe.

▶ The studies reviewed in Abstracts 13–26 and 13–27 indicate that patients with polycystic ovaries who do not respond optimally to stimulation with clomiphene and gonadotropins alone, or human menopausal gonadotropin (hMG) plus a GnRH-a may have better results if GH is added to the ovarian stimulation treatment regimen. The findings of this center need to be confirmed elsewhere before advising the addition of GH to hMG in women with polycystic ovaries who enter an in vitro fertilization program and in whom ovarian hyperstimulation fails to produce a satisfactory number of oocytes.—D.R. Mishell, Jr., M.D.

Controlled Preparation of the Endometrium With Exogenous Estradiol and Progesterone in Women Having Functioning Ovaries

de Ziegler D, Hazout A, Cornel C, Bouchard P, Bergeron C, Frydman R (Hôpital A Béclère, Clamart; Hôpital de Bicêtre; Institut de Pathologie et Cytologie Appliquée, Paris)

Fertil Steril 56:851–855, 1991 13–28

Background.—Timing embryo transfers in women with irregular menstrual cycles or with luteal phase defect can be problematic. Although temporary suppression of ovarian function with a long-acting agonist of gonadotropin-releasing hormone (GnRH-a) with exogenous estradiol (E_2) and progesterone allows reliable synchronization of endometrial receptivity, this approach is rather complex and associated with the cumbersome side effects of GnRH. A simplified hormone regimen was developed for preparation of endometrium receptivity in women with functioning ovaries.

Treatment.—Six female volunteers with problems of timing embryo transfers in their menstrual cycles received transdermal E_2 starting on day 1 of spontaneous or induced menstrual cycles and vaginal progesterone on days 15–28 without previous ovarian suppression with GnRH-a. The hormone regimen was designed to duplicate the plasma E_2 and progesterone levels seen in the menstrual cycle. Hormonal changes in the blood were monitored. Endometrial biopsy was performed on day 20.

Results.—Plasma luteinizing hormone (LH) reached surge levels on day 11 in 1 woman, on day 12 in 2, and on day 14 in 3. Pelvic ultrasound on days 9 and 14 showed no follicular growth in all patients, and the plasma progesterone level did not increase before the progesterone administration. Endometrial specimens on day 20 showed typical early secretory changes, similar to those previously observed in women treated with Gn-Rh-a, E_2, and progesterone.

Conclusions.—Controlled preparation of the endometrium in women with functioning ovaries can be achieved with exogenous E_2 and progesterone without previous ovarian suppression with a GnRH-a. This approach is a simpler and less costly alternative to combined GnRH-a and E_2 plus progesterone regimen.

▶ I welcome the trend to simplify and streamline various strategies of assisted reproductive technologies. In women who have irregular cycles, the replacement of cryopreserved embryos has necessitated the use of down-regulation followed by E_2 and progesterone supplementation, or the induction of ovulation with clomiphene. The authors propose here that a similar synchronized approach using transdermal E_2 and vaginal progesterone may be all that is required. Indeed, in this preliminary pilot study the authors have demonstrated the feasibility of this.

Their approach is to use Estraderm, .1 mg/day on days 1 through 7, starting on day 1 of the menstrual cycle, and then .2 mg on days 8 through 11, .4 mg on days 12 through 14, .3 mg on days 15 to 18, .2 mg on days 18 to 25, and .1 mg on days 25 to 28. Micronized progesterone is added on days 15 through 28. These high doses of estrogen are thought to suppress ovulation, which would otherwise interfere with this menstrual plan. The authors emphasize, however, that it is important to measure serum progesterone levels before starting progesterone vaginally; because the patients do not have a functioning corpus luteum, continued luteal support is necessary until pregnancy is documented. Transdermal estrogen used in this way sometimes causes skin reactions; the same approach might be used with E_2 in oral form. A study of oral E_2 is underway.—R.A. Lobo, M.D.

Does Ovarian Stimulation for In-Vitro Fertilization Induce a Hypercoagulable State?

Aune B, Høie KE, Øian P, Holst N, Østerud B (Univ of Tromsø, Norway)

Hum Reprod 6:925–927, 1991 13–29

Background.—Estrogens have a role in thrombosis and overall cardiovascular disease, but it is not known whether the role is protective or deleterious. Studies using different types of estrogens, endogenous or exogenous, natural or synthetic, have produced conflicting results. The effects of a brief increase of endogenous estrogens on blood coagulation and fibrinolysis were evaluated in 12 healthy women aged 25–37 years who were accepted for in vitro fertilization (IVF) because of tubal infertility.

Methods.—Blood samples were taken before the women received follicle-stimulating hormone (FSH) on days 3 and 4 of the menstrual cycle and after ovulation induction with human chorionic gonadotropin (hCG) on days 10–12. The day after ovulation induction was the day of maximum serum estradiol levels. Whole blood clotting time, whole blood clot lysis time, plasma fibrinogen, factor VII, and antithrombin III (AT-III) were measured.

Findings.—Ovarian stimulation for IVF produced significant changes in the coagulation and fibrinolytic system. During ovarian stimulation, the mean serum levels of estradiol increased and the whole blood clotting time was slightly but not significantly reduced. The plasma fibrinogen level was significantly increased, the AT-III level was reduced, and there was no change in factor VII.

Conclusion.—During IVF treatment a significant reduction in fibrinolytic activity has been observed. A slight but not significant shortening of the whole blood clotting time and a significant increase occurred in the procoagulant factor fibrinogen concomitant with a decrease in the most important physiologic inhibitor of blood coagulation, AT-III. There was no compensatory increase in the fibrinolytic system and, in fact, there was a decrease in fibrinolytic activity as measured by the whole blood clot lysis time. The implication is that ovarian stimulation for IVF treatment is associated with a hypercoagulable state.

▶ Although this paper specifically suggests the effect of IVF on coagulation factors, similar data have been described for induction of ovulation. Systemic increases in estrogen can result in stimulation of hepatic procoagulant factors, but the estrogen levels must be significantly elevated. This occurs to a greater extent with high oral doses of estrogen. A higher level of estrogen is required for a longer time to affect hepatic factors when delivered nonorally. This study showed that when estrogen levels at midcycle reach threshold levels averaging 1800 pg/mL, certain changes favoring coagulant activity can occur. This is not a new finding, but it is important to note that in susceptible individuals this may be a risk factor for thrombosis. The changes, although significant, were not out of the normal range, and even reductions in AT III may not be of any clinical significance, unless an individual is at risk (e.g., the patient who has a personal or family history of recurrent thrombotic episodes).

Another significant factor is the known complication of coagulopathy associated with the hyperstimulation syndrome. Whereas this is in part the result of intervascular contraction in these patients, the increase in procoagulant factors, and potentially the decrease in fibrinolytic activity associated with high levels of estrogen, poses an additional risk.—R.A. Lobo, M.D.

14 Early Pregnancy

The Obstetric and Neonatal Outcome of Pregnancy in Women With a Previous History of Infertility: A Prospective Study

Li TC, MacLeod I, Singhal V, Duncan SLB (Univ of Sheffield; Jessop Hosp for Women, Sheffield, England)

Br J Obstet Gynaecol 98:1087–1092, 1991 14–1

Background.—Many physicians have studied the outcomes of pregnancy in women with a history of infertility. This issue was further explored in a prospective cohort study to establish the frequency of common antepartum complications, the amount of antepartum surveillance, and the obstetric and neonatal outcome.

Methods.—The cohort consisted of 114 women with a history of infertility who reached 16 weeks' gestation with live singletons. Outcomes in this group were compared with those in an age- and parity-matched group of 114 control women.

Results.—Women with a history of infertility did not have an increased number of common antenatal complications compared with the control group. The relative risk of needing an emergency cesarean section in the group with a history of infertility was 2.43 when compared with women in the control group. Birth weights and neonatal outcomes in the groups did not differ significantly.

Conclusions.—Once singleton pregnancy is established beyond 16 weeks, women with a history of infertility had obstetric and neonatal outcomes not significantly different from those of women without a history of infertility, although those with such a history have an increased likelihood of undergoing emergency cesarean section. The idea that successful treatment of infertility produces pregnancies in women who have adverse biological characteristics is not justified.

▶ Many women who conceive after treatment for infertility are concerned that the incidence of obstetric complications in later pregnancy may be increased. Although such women do have a higher rate of ectopic pregnancies than women without a history of infertility, the results of this prospective age- and parity-matched study indicate that when pregnancy has progressed beyond 16 weeks, the incidence of pregnancy-associated problems, except for emergency cesarean delivery, as well as birth weight and neonatal outcome is not significantly different compared with women who became pregnant without a history of infertility. These data should relieve some of the anxiety of infertile women who conceive.—D.R. Mishell, Jr., M.D.

Subfertility and the Risk of Low Birth Weight

Williams MA, Goldman MB, Mittendorf R, Monson RR (Harvard School of Public Health; St Margaret's Hosp for Women, Boston; Tufts Univ)
Fertil Steril 56:668–671, 1991 14–2

Objective.—The evidence has suggested that women with previous infertility are at increased risk of delivering low-birth-weight (LBW) infants. The relationship between subfertility and delivery of LBW infants was further examined, as was the role of excessive coffee consumption during pregnancy.

Study Design.—During a 3-year period obstetric and delivery information was obtained on 12,718 women from medical record review and by personal interview. This analysis was restricted to nondiabetic married women who planned their pregnancies, who reported the date they last used contraception, and who subsequently delivered singletons of 20 or more gestational weeks. A total of 3,622 women met the study criteria. Subfertility was defined as the failure to achieve a clinically recognized pregnancy within 1 year of unprotected intercourse. Low birth weight was defined as a birth weight of less than 2,500 g.

Results.—There were 644 subfertile women and 2,978 fertile women. Thus, among the 3,622 nondiabetic, married women who planned their pregnancies and subsequently delivered a viable singleton, nearly 18% required more than 12 months to conceive. Sixty-two subfertile women (9.6%) and 146 fertile women (4.9%) delivered a LBW infant. The relative risk (RR) of delivering a LBW infant for subfertile women compared with fertile women was 1.9. This increased RR persisted after adjustment for maternal age, race, educational attainment, parity, history of cervical incompetence, in utero exposure to diethylstilbestrol, spontaneous abortion, cigarette smoking, low ponderal index, suboptimal pregnancy weight gain, gestational bleeding, and history of assisted conception. The adjusted RR estimate for LBW was elevated for every category of LBW (table). After adjusting for potential confounding factors, the RR of intrauterine growth retardation was 2.3 for subfertile women relative to fertile women. Subfertility was associated with a mean birth weight re-

Distribution of Subfertile and Fertile Subjects

Category of low birth weight	Subfertile*		Fertile*		RR †	95% CI
g						
<1,500	15	(2.3)	32	(1.1)	2.0	0.8, 4.8
1,500 to 2,499 (<37 weeks)	29	(4.5)	63	(2.1)	1.7	1.0, 3.1
1,500 to 2,499 (≥37 weeks)	18	(2.8)	51	(1.7)	2.3	1.2, 4.4
Total (<2,500)	62	(9.6)	146	(4.9)	1.9	1.3, 2.8

Abbreviation: CI, confidence interval; *RR,* relative risk.
*Values are numbers with pecents in parentheses. Subfertile number = 644; fertile number = 2,978.
†Relative risk adjusted for maternal age, race, educational attainment, parity, history of cervical incompetence, in utero exposure to DES, spontaneous abortion, cigarette smoking, low ponderal index, subuptimal pregnancy weight gain, gestational bleeding, and history of assisted conception.
(Courtesy of Williams MA, Goldman MB, Mittendorf R, et al: *Fertil Steril* 56:668–671, 1991.)

duction of 93 g among all delivered infants and with a mean birth weight reduction of 58 g among term-only deliveries. There was no statistical interaction between subfertility and excessive coffee consumption during pregnancy. Thus the subfertility-LBW relationship was not modified by excessive coffee consumption.

Conclusion.—Subfertility is associated with suboptimal intrauterine growth in the subsequent pregnancy, which may increase a woman's risk of delivering a LBW infant.

▶ The results of this study disagree with those reported in Abstract 14–1, providing further evidence that epidemiology is not an exact science. Factors such as differences in study design (prospective, matched vs. cross-sectional, adjusted), methodology, and populations may each have contributed to the different results.— D.R. Mishell, Jr., M.D.

Perinatal Outcome and Congenital Malformations in In-Vitro Fertilization Babies From the Bourn-Hallam Group

Rizk B, Doyle P, Tan SL, Rainsbury P, Betts J, Brinsden P, Edwards R (Bourn Hallam Med Ctr, London and Cambridge, England; London School of Hygiene and Tropical Medicine; King's College, London)

Hum Reprod 6:1259–1264, 1991 14–3

Background.—It is unclear whether the perinatal outcome of infants conceived as a result of in vitro fertilization (IVF) differs from that after natural conception. The perinatal outcomes of infants born between 1978 and 1987 after IVF-embryo transfer (IVF-ET) at 2 centers in England were analyzed.

Methods.—During the study period 1,360 infants were born after IVF-ET at these 2 centers. Congenital abnormalities were compared with those from 3 sources of control data.

Findings.—In all, 961 infants were born to 763 residents of England. Of these, 62% were singletons, 30% were twins, and 9% were triplets. There were no quadruplets or quintuplets. The multiple birth rate was therefore 23%. Twins accounted for 19% of all deliveries and triplets for 4%. The rate of premature deliveries was high at 25%. The incidence of prematurity was closely related to birth multiplicity, rising from 14% among singletons to 38% for twins. Overall, 32% of the infants had a low birth weight, and 6% had a very low birth weight. Also, 14% of singletons had a low birth weight, compared with 7% of all births in England and Wales. The overall rates of stillbirth and perinatal and infant mortlaity in infants born after IVF were double to triple those of infants born after natural conception, but when maternal age and multiplicity were controlled for, perinatal mortality among IVF infants was not significantly higher. Fetal and infant mortality rose significantly with multiplicity, with stillbirth rates of 20.8 and 24.7 per thousand for twin and triplet infants, respectively, compared with 5.07 per thousand for singletons. Perinatal mortality was 13.5, 38.2, and 37 per thousand births for singletons, twins, and triplets. The overall prevalence of major congenital malformations was 3%. At least 1 major malformation was diagnosed in the first week of life in 2.5% of the infants, which was within the range of expected values in the United Kingdom. There was no significant increase in any specific malformations, but a higher than expected number of CVS, chromosomal, and urogenital and extremity malformations was observed.

Conclusions.—The infants in this series were born after IVF treatment in 2 closely linked centers having similar scientific programs and are therefore of special interest. Most studies of perinatal outcome after IVF have involved a small number of pregnancies from single centers or large numbers from many centers with different protocols.

▶ Several findings from this large study are helpful when counseling women regarding the outcome of pregnancies occurring after IVF. First, the rate of major congenital malformations is not significantly increased. Second, when the factors of age and multiple births are controlled, there is no significant increase in perinatal morbidity. Third, multiple gestations are associated with a much higher rate of prematurity, stillbirths, and perinatal mortality. The latter finding provides support for the concept of avoiding hyperstimulation and performing IVF in normal ovulatory cycles. The goal of IVF is to deliver a healthy viable baby, not to have multiple fetuses that do not survive.—D.R. Mishell, Jr., M.D.

Thromboxane Dominance and Prostacyclin Deficiency in Habitual Abortion

Tulppala M, Viinikka L, Ylikorkala O (Univ Central Hosp, Helsinki)

Lancet 337:879–881, 1991 14–4

Background.—In recurrent spontaneous abortion (RSA), usually no cause can be found. Microthrombosis, vasospastic changes, and necrosis are common, suggesting that changes in the production of vasoactive and/or platelet-active compounds play a role. The relationship was examined between pregnancy outcome and prostacyclin and thromboxane A_2 (TxA_2) production in early pregnancy in women with RSA.

Methods.—The urinary excretion of prostacyclin metabolites and TxA_2 metabolites was examined during 25 pregnancies in 22 women with RSA. Sixteen pregnant women with no history of spontaneous abortion were studied for comparison.

Findings.—A living fetus was identified by ultrasound examination in 23 pregnancies in women with RSA. Nine ended in abortion and 14 continued to term. All pregnancies in the control group continued to term. Compared with women in the control group, women with RSA had a lower ratio of prostacyclin to thromboxane between the fourth and seventh weeks of gestation and a lower output of prostacyclin metabolite 2,3-dinor-6-keto-$PGF_{1\alpha}$ between 8 and 11 weeks. Women who aborted had a higher output of TxA_2 metabolite 2,3-dinor-TxB_2 between weeks 4 and 7 and lower excretion of 2,3-dinor-6-keto-$PGF_{1\alpha}$ between weeks 8 and 11 when compared with women whose pregnancies proceeded to term.

Conclusions.—In women with RSA, changes in the output of prostacyclin and TxA_2 metabolites occur in early pregnancy. Up to 11 weeks' gestation, pregnancy in women with RSA was associated with a lower ratio of prostacyclin to TxA_2. The changes seen in this series were greater in women whose pregnancy ended in abortion.

▶ Recurrent spontaneous abortion is a difficult and heterogenous problem. There are multiple causes for recurrent loss, and most cases do not have a specific diagnosis to explain them. Among the new theories advocated as possibilities are problems with an elevated level of luteinizing hormone in the follicular phase, and abnormalities in the ratio of prostacyclin to thromboxane, which is the focus of this paper. The vasodilatory prostacyclin, and specifically the 2,3-dinor metabolite of the stable marker (6-keto-$PGF_{1\alpha}$), which reflects more the systemic circulation, is counterbalanced by the thrombotic tendency of thromboxane and its 2,3-dinor metabolite. In this study, although the patients with recurrent miscarriage clearly had lower levels of 6-keto-$F_{1\alpha}$, and abnormalities of thromboxane resulting in an abnormal ratio of prostacyclin to thromboxane metabolites, the data are not very precise. Although they had histories of recurrent loss, patients whose pregnancies went to term, as well as those ending in abortion, had similar ratios and levels of these metabolites. Therefore, there is more than meets the eye in terms of implicating a direct link in abnormal prostacyclin/thromboxane metabolism. Perhaps these findings reflect not the cause but, rather, the result of some other immunologic deficiency that has yet to be uncovered.—R.A. Lobo, M.D.

15 Basic Investigations

Influence of Porcine Follicular Fluid on the Fertilizing Capacity of Human Spermatozoa

Siegel MS, Graczykowski JW (Univ of Southern California, Los Angeles)

Fertil Steril 55:1204 1206, 1991 15–1

Introduction.—Follicular fluid (FF) from human preovulatory follicles enhances hamster egg penetration test scores. Human FF can also stimulate the acrosome reaction in mice and rats; thus FF factors that stimulate sperm may not be species specific. The effect of porcine FF on the fertilizing ability of human spermatozoa was studied.

Methods.—Ejaculates were obtained from 10 healthy men. Capacitated sperm solution was mixed with an equal volume of 1 of 5 fluids: S25, 25% porcine FF solution from follicles less than 3 mm; S50, 50% porcine FF solution from follicles less than 3 mm; L25, 25% porcine FF solution from follicles of more than 8 mm; L50, 50% porcine FF solution from follicles greater than 8 mm; and, as the control fluid, Ham's medium. Sperm were incubated with porcine FF for 20 minutes at 37° C, then washed, centrifuged, resuspended in medium, and used for hamster egg penetration tests.

Results.—Although the attachment score did not differ significantly among the porcine FF treatments, there seemed to be a tendency for the L25 and L50 treatments to be higher than control values. In the S25 and S50 treatment groups there was a significant reduction in percent of eggs penetrated compared with controls. The penetration scores in sperm treatments with L25 and L50, however, were more than 3 times those of controls. The 25% and 50% FF solutions from either small or large follicle treatment groups did not differ significantly. The attachment index was decreased for S50 and increased for L25 and L50, with that for L50 being greater than for L25 and about twice that of the control value. Penetration indices for S25 and S50 were comparable to those in the control condition. However, this index was increased for the L25 and L50 conditions compared with controls, with that of L50 being greater than that of L25. All of the treatments had comparable percentages of sperm motility and straight-line velocity after incubation.

Conclusion.—Factors that affect human sperm fertilizing potential appear to be present in porcine FF. Fluid from developmentally mature follicles seem to stimulate sperm, whereas fluid from immature follicles can inhibit sperm.

► This is another in the series of studies showing the beneficial effect of follicular fluid of various in vitro tests of sperm function. How does this relate to in vivo fertilization?—C.A. Paulsen, M.D.

DNA Hybridization Study Using Y-Specific Probes in an XX-Male

Fuse H, Satomi S, Kazama T, Katayama T, Nagabuchi S, Tamura T, Nakahori Y, Nakagome Y (Toyama Med and Pharmaceutical Univ, Toyama; Natl Children's Med Research Ctr, Tokyo)
Andrologia 23:237–239, 1991 15–2

Background.—When a crossing-over event between the X and Y chromosomes occurs proximal to the short arms of these chromosomes, the result is an XX-male. A male with an XX karyotype was studied using the Southern blot technique to evaluate the presence or absence of 23 loci on the Y chromosome.

Case Report.—Man, 30, complained of infertility. At his birth, his mother and father were ages 35 and 38 years, respectively. He had no history of any diseases. The patient had bilateral small testes, and his semen contained no sperm. Hormonal studies indicated hypergonadotropic hypogonadism. Cytogenic studies revealed a 46,XX karyotype. High-resolution banding showed no abnormalities in either X chromosome. Histologic examination of the testes revealed germinal aplasia and the proliferation of Leydig cells. These findings suggested a diagnosis of an XX-male. A DNA hybridization study using 17 Y-specific probes detected the presence of a major part of the short arm of the Y chromosome that apparently had been translocated to the X chromosome. The translocated Y short arm contained a small deletion.

Conclusions.—In this patient, 3 crossing-over events in paternal meiosis between loci 50f2D and 87-4, 87-17B and 52dC, and between 52dB and 52dC may have been involved in the development of the abnormalities. Or it may be that a single crossing-over event between 50f2D and 87-4 was associated with an interstitial deletion involving 52dC.

▶ Careful study of the sex chromosomal composition in an XX male. The testicular determining factor present on the portion of the short arm Y translocated to the X chromosome.—C.A. Paulsen, M.D.

Sperm Surface Fibronectin: Expression Following Capacitation

Fusi FM, Bronson RA (State Univ of New York, Stony Brook)
J Androl 13:28–35, 1992 15–3

Background.—The Arg-Gly-Asp (RGD) amino acid sequence is important in many recognition systems involved in cell-to-cell and cell-to-matrix adhesion. Several fibronectin-derived RGD-containing oligopeptides competitively inhibit the adhesion of human spermatozoa to hamster eggs and their penetration, implicating integrin receptors in gamete interactions. The major cell-binding domain of fibronectin possesses an RGD sequence, but it is not clear whether fibronectin itself has a role in gamete interactions.

Objective.—An attempt was made to learn whether fibronectin is present on the surface of living human spermatozoa, and whether its expression varies with the functional status of the spermatozoa. Motile sperm were selected by swim-up separation in specimens from 10 healthy donors.

Findings.—Most fresh spermatozoa lacked fibronectin on their plasma membranes, but up to 16% were positive. In contrast, 18% to 100% of spermatozoa incubated overnight under capacitating conditions reacted with antifibronectin antibody. Induction of an acrosome reaction with progesterone did not alter the number of sperm with surface fibronectin. Antifibronectin significantly reduced both sperm-oolemmal adhesion and the ability of human spermatozoa to penetrate hamster eggs.

Conclusions.—Human spermatozoa bear fibronectin on their surfaces, and fibronectin may well participate in sperm-oolemmal adhesion. Defective expression of fibronectin might contribute to sperm dysfunction and infertility.

▶ Another significant piece of the fertilization puzzle. What we need is a clear picture of specific "rate-limiting" biochemical events in the cascading process.—C.A. Paulsen, M.D.

The Form and Function of the Leydig Cells in Hypophysectomized Rams Treated With Pituitary Extract When Spermatogenesis Is Disrupted by Heating the Testes

Setchell BP, Locatelli A, Perreau C, Pisselet C, Fontaine I, Kuntz C, Saumande J, Fontaine J, Hochereau-de Reviers M-T (INRA Station de Physiologie de la Reproduction, Nouzilly, France)

J Endocrinol 131:101–112, 1991 15–4

Background.—It was once thought that Leydig cells are unaffected by brief, moderate heating of the testes sufficient to disrupt spermatogenesis. More recently, however, evidence that heat-induced aspermatogenesis is associated with reduced in vivo Leydig cell function was obtained in rats.

Study Design.—Leydig cell function was monitored in 16 rams after spermatogenesis was disrupted by a single testicular exposure to 42° C for 45 minutes. Some of the animals were surgically hypophysectomized at the time of testicular heating and received pituitary extract.

Observations.—The heated testes decreased in size by about 50% in the next 20 days, whether or not the hypophysis was removed. Secretion of testosterone was markedly reduced. The heat-exposed testes contained fewer but larger Leydig cells than those of intact rams. Leydig cells were most numerous in unheated, hormone-treated animals.

Implications.—Leydig cells hypertrophy when spermatogenesis is disrupted by heating the testes if gonadotropic stimulation is maintained. The reduction in secretion of testosterone is related more to decreased blood plasma flow through the testes than to the number or size of the Leydig cells.

▶ Another example showing that Leydig cells are not as resistant to heat as previously thought.—C.A. Paulsen, M.D.

Expression of Messenger Ribonucleic Acids That Encode for 3β-Hydroxysteroid Dehydrogenase and Cholesterol Side-Chain Cleavage Enzyme Throughout the Luteal Phase of the Macaque Menstrual Cycle

Bassett SG, Little-Ihrig LL, Mason JI, Zelenik AJ (Univ of Pittsburgh; Univ of Texas, Dallas)

J Clin Endocrinol Metab 72:362–366, 1991 15–5

Background.—In macaque monkeys, secretion of progesterone by the corpus luteum is absolutely dependent on luteinizing hormone (LH) during the luteal phase of the menstrual cycle. There appears to be no direct correlation, however, between changes in the pattern of LH secretion and luteal function. Luteal regression may be caused by intrinsic changes in luteal cells rather than changes in the pattern of LH secretion per se.

Methods.—Corpora lutea were obtained from cynomolgus macaques at defined stages of the luteal phase to examine steady-state levels of mRNAs that encode for the 2 major enzymes involved in progesterone biosynthesis—cytochrome P450 cholesterol side chain cleavage ($P450_{scc}$) and 3β-hydroxysteroid dehydrogenase (3βHSD).

Findings.—The steady-state levels of mRNAs for both $P450_{scc}$ and 3βHSD were maximal or near maximal shortly after ovulation and luteinization (days 3–5 of the luteal phase). The relative intensity of the $P450_{scc}$ mRNA declined slightly, but not significantly, throughout the remainder of the luteal phase, and the values fell to undetectable levels upon luteal regression. The steady-state levels of 3βHSD mRNA were significantly lower in corpora lutea removed during the midluteal phase than in newly formed corpora lutea, and they declined to 10% of the early luteal phase values by days 13–15 of the luteal phase. The 3βHSD mRNA values fell to nondetectable levels after menses. In contrast, serum progesterone concentrations were very low after ovulation and increased during the midluteal phase.

Discussion.—A paradoxical relationship was found between the steroidogenic activity of the primate corpus luteum in vivo and the steady-state levels of mRNAs that encode for the 2 major enzymes in progesterone biosynthesis. Expression of these enzymes declines independently of the overall pattern of progesterone and, by inference, LH secretion during the luteal phase. This suggests that the lifespan of the corpus luteum is set at the time of ovulation, and the decline in luteal cell function may be caused, in part, by decay of specialized luteal cell mRNAs with finite half-lives.

▶ This is an interesting paper concerning key enzymes in the corpus luteum of the macaque. Of note in this paper was the finding that these enzymes, which encode key enzymes in steroidogenesis in the corpus luteum, peaked at the time of ovulation and declined gradually thereafter. This is different from the pattern of luteal progesterone as measured in blood, which peaks some days after the onset of ovulation. This dissociation, if you will, suggests that the inherent capacity of the corpus luteum to produce messages for these enzymes is programmed at the time the dominant follicle becomes the corpus luteum and then gradually ages. On the other hand, the functional capacity of the corpus luteum with these enzymes to produce progesterone is affected by other factors such as stimulation of the LH surge, which occurs progressively throughout the luteal phase. The authors used classic Northern analysis to determine production of these enzymes by the corpus luteum. Of interest in the future, perhaps the use of such techniques as in situ harvesting may be useful in determining the various types of luteal cells responsible for these shifts of steroidogenesis.—R.A. Lobo, M.D.

Titrating Luteinizing Hormone Surge Requirements for Ovulatory Changes in Primate Follicles: I. Oocyte Maturation and Corpus Luteum Function

Zelinski-Wooten MB, Lanzendorf SE, Wolf DP, Chandrasekher YA, Stouffer RL (Oregon Regional Primate Research Ctr, Beaverton; Oregon Health Sciences Univ, Portland)

J Clin Endocrinol Metab 73:577–683, 1991 15–6

Background.—The surge of luteinizing hormone (LH) seen during the normal menstrual cycle typically is attenuated or absent during ovarian stimulation to promote follicle development. There is evidence from animal studies that the threshold of gonadotropin exposure varies for different events during the ovulatory process.

Objective and Methods.—Periovulatory requirements of LH were titrated by administering follicle-stimulating hormone (FSH) with and without LH to female rhesus monkeys for 9 days, starting at the menses. Groups of animals subsequently received 1000 IU of human chorionic gonadotropin (hCG) intramuscularly, 1 or 3 subcutaneous injections of 100 μg of gonadotropin-releasing hormone (GnRH), or 2 subcutaneous injections of 50 μg of a GnRH agonist at an 8-hour interval.

Observations.—Levels of estradiol rose to similar peaks on day 10 in all groups. Treatment with hCG markedly increased circulating LH-like bioactivity for up to 3 days. Both 3 injections of GnRH and agonist treatment extended the time of increased LH bioactivity, compared with a single injection of GnRH. Levels of progesterone were consistently increased only in hCG-treated animals, and these animals had by far the highest proportions of oocytes in metaphase I or II of meiosis.

Conclusions.—Exposure to LH alone is not sufficient to routinely reinitiate meiotic maturation of oocytes or support early function of the corpus luteum in primates. Further studies are needed to learn why the primate follicle requires prolonged exposure to LH for ovulatory events to take place.

▶ I thought this was an interesting paper because it dissects the requirements of LH at midcycle, which is important in terms of induction of ovulation as well as cycling for in vitro fertilization. The focus here is on the requirements for oocyte maturation and subsequent corpus luteum development rather than just the release of oocytes and the process of ovulation. On a practical note, it has been suggested that stimulation regimens using gonadotropins result in attenuation or elimination of the spontaneous LH surge. This clearly happens now that we are using the GnRH agonist.

Questions have arisen that perhaps we do not need to use hCG in midcycle to trigger ovulation because hCG is responsible for hyperstimulation under most circumstances. It has been suggested that recombinant pure LH can be used effectively to trigger ovulation, and in the monkey this has been shown by Hodgen and colleagues. There has also been interest recently in the use of the GnRH agonist to trigger ovulation. Well, this paper does study the use of GnRH to induce a normal LH surge: native GnRH in 1 or 3 doses as well as 2 doses of the GnRH agonist in lieu of hCG.

Of some surprise in this paper, but of potential importance, is that although the bioactivity of LH was similar or was similarly increased by these regimens, normal oocytes in metaphase 2 occurred after hCG administration. Whereas 86% of the monkeys studied had this response to hCG, even 3 injections of GnRH to raise Lh levels produced only 43% of mature oocytes. These data suggest that 15 or more hours of LH exposure are required, out of the normal 48-hour LH surge. One must remember this concept in determining newer strategies for triggering ovulation. Although hCG was found to be beneficial under these conditions, the actual amount of hCG required has not been determined.—R.A. Lobo, M.D.

Sustained Hyperglycemia Results in Testicular Dysfunction and Reduced Fertility Potential in BBWOR Diabetic Rats

Cameron DF, Rountree J, Schultz RE, Repetta D, Murray FT (Univ of South Florida, Tampa; Univ of Florida, Gainesville)

Am J Physiol 259:E881–E889, 1990 15–7

Introduction.—Previous studies in hyperglycemia male rats with short-term diabetes demonstrated reduced fertility and diminished serum testosterone levels. The effects of long-term diabetes with sustained hyperglycemia on testicular function and fertility potential were investigated in male rats. Because the pharmaceuticals used to induce experimental diabetes also can induce definite toxicity, the study was performed in spontaneousy diabetic BB rats.

Methods.—Testicular morphology, testicular function, and fertility potential were examined in spontaneously diabetic hyperglycemic BB rats, age-matched normoglycemia BB rats, and normal control Wistar rats. All rats with diabetes had been hyperglycemic for more than 180 days, with serum glucose levels ranging from 300 mg to 350 mg.

Results.—Chronic hyperglycemia of more than 180 days' duration was associated with reduced testis weights, daily sperm production, and total trunk testosterone levels. Morphological examination of the testes showed seminiferous epithelial dissolution and depletion of germ cells. The number of Leydig cells per testis in diabetic rats was not reduced and the blood-testis barrier appeared intact. There was a significant reduction

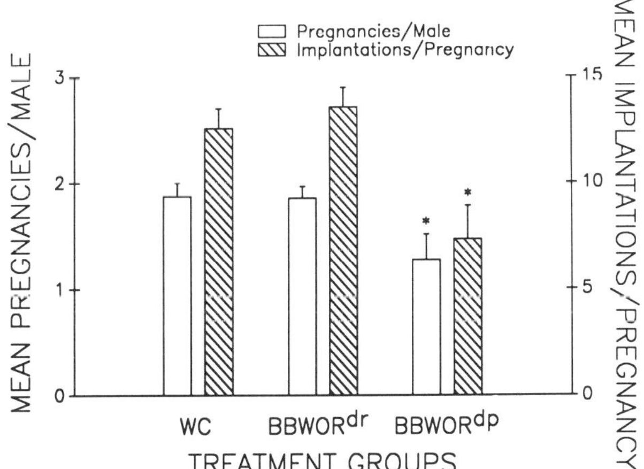

Fig 15–1.—Graph illustrating measurements of fertility parameters for nondiabetic WC and BBWOR^{dr} rats and diabetic BBWOR^{dp} rats. *Significantly ($P < .05$) less than all other treatment groups. (Courtesy of Cameron DF, Rountree J, Schultz RE, et al: *Am J Physiol* 259:E881–E889, 1990.)

in the number of pregnancies per rat and in the number of implantations per pregnancy (Fig 15–1).

Conclusion.—Long-term diabetes with sustained hyperglycemia in spontaneously diabetic male rats is associated with significant testicular disruption and reduced fertility potential.

▶ To my way of thinking, there has not been adequate studies in diabetic men and women to carefully document the impact of hyperglycemia on their reproductive systems. There has not been sufficient attention to this problem. Recent publications by some investigators, however, have provided important data derived from studies in diabetic women (1–3).—C.A. Paulsen, M.D.

References

1. Mills JL, et al: *N Engl J Med* 318:671, 1988.
2. Mills JL, et al: *N Engl J Med* 319:1617, 1988.
3. Fuhrmann K, et al: *Exp Clin Endocrinol* 83:173, 1984.

Subject Index

A

D

E

G

H

K

L

M

W

X

Y

Z

Author Index

A

B

C

D

K

L

M

N

A Simple, Once-a-Year Dose!

Review the partial list of titles below. And then request your own FREE 30-day preview. When you subscribe to a Year Book, we'll also send you an automatic notice of future volumes about two months before they publish.

This system was designed for your convenience and to take up as little of your time as possible. If you do not want the Year Book, the advance notice makes it easy for you to let us know. And if you elect to receive the new Year Book, you need do nothing. We will send it on publication.

No worry. No wasted motion. And, of course, every Year Book is yours to examine FREE of charge for thirty days.

Year Book of **Anesthesia**® (22141)
Year Book of **Cardiology**® (22640)
Year Book of **Critical Care Medicine**® (22639)
Year Book of **Dermatology**® (22645)
Year Book of **Dermatologic Surgery**® (21171)
Year Book of **Diagnostic Radiology**® (22613)
Year Book of **Digestive Diseases**® (22625)
Year Book of **Drug Therapy**® (22630)
Year Book of **Emergency Medicine**® (22080)
Year Book of **Endocrinology**® (21174)
Year Book of **Family Practice**® (22124)
Year Book of **Geriatrics and Gerontology** (22611)
Year Book of **Hand Surgery**® (22618)
Year Book of **Hematology**® (22646)
Year Book of **Health Care Management**® (21177)
Year Book of **Infectious Diseases**® (22650)
Year Book of **Infertility** (22637)
Year Book of **Medicine**® (22638)
Year Book of **Neonatal-Perinatal Medicine** (22629)
Year Book of **Nephrology** (21175)
Year Book of **Neurology and Neurosurgery**® (22616)
Year Book of **Neuroradiology**® (21849)
Year Book of **Nuclear Medicine**® (22627)
Year Book of **Obstetrics and Gynecology**® (22636)
Year Book of **Occupational and Environmental Medicine** (22619)
Year Book of **Oncology** (22651)
Year Book of **Ophthalmology**® (22133)
Year Book of **Orthopedics**® (22644)
Year Book of **Otolaryngology – Head and Neck Surgery**® (22609)
Year Book of **Pathology and Clinical Pathology**® (21176)
Year Book of **Pediatrics**® (22130)
Year Book of **Plastic and Reconstructive Surgery**® (22635)
Year Book of **Psychiatry and Applied Mental Health**® (22649)
Year Book of **Pulmonary Disease**® (22624)
Year Book of **Sports Medicine**® (22111)
Year Book of **Surgery**® (22641)
Year Book of **Transplantation**® (21854)
Year Book of **Ultrasound** (21169)
Year Book of **Urology**® (22621)
Year Book of **Vascular Surgery**® (22612)

Mosby-Year Book, Inc. • 11830 Westline Industrial Drive • St. Louis, MO 63146